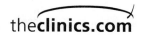

ANESTHESIOLOGY CLINICS

Pain Management

GUEST EDITOR
Howard S. Smith, MD, FACP

CONSULTING EDITOR
Lee A. Fleisher, MD

December 2007 • Volume 25 • Number 4

SAUNDERS

An Imprint of Elsevier, Inc.
PHILADELPHIA   LONDON   TORONTO   MONTREAL   SYDNEY   TOKYO

W.B. SAUNDERS COMPANY
A Division of Elsevier Inc.

1600 John F. Kennedy Boulevard, Suite 1800 • Philadelphia, Pennsylvania 19103-2899

http://www.theclinics.com

ANESTHESIOLOGY CLINICS	Volume 25, Number 4
December 2007	ISSN 1932-2275
Editor: Rachel Glover	ISBN-13: 978-1-4160-5671-3
	ISBN-10: 1-4160-5671-8

The ideas and opinions expressed in *Anesthesiology Clinics* do not necessarily reflect those of the Publisher. The Publisher does not assume any responsibility for any injury and/or damage to persons or property arising out of or related to any use of the material contained in this periodical. The reader is advised to check the appropriate medical literature and the product information currently provided by the manufacturer of each drug to be administered to verify the dosage, the method and duration of administration, or contraindications. It is the responsibility of the treating physician or other health care professional, relying on independent experience and knowledge of the patient, to determine drug dosages and the best treatment for the patient. Mention of any product in this issue should not be construed as endorsement by the contributors, editors, or the Publisher of the product or manufacturers' claims.

Anesthesiology Clinics (ISSN 1932-2275) is published quarterly by Elsevier Inc., 360 Park Avenue South, New York, NY 10010-1710. Months of issue are March, June, September, and December. Business and Editorial Offices: 1600 John F. Kennedy Blvd., Suite 1800, Philadelphia, PA 19103-2899. Customer Service Office: 6277 Sea Harbor Drive, Orlando, FL 32887-4800. Periodicals postage paid at New York, NY and additional mailing offices. Subscription prices are $111.00 per year (US student/resident), $222.00 per year (US individuals), $271.00 per year (Canadian individuals), $332.00 per year (US institutions), $403.00 per year (Canadian institutions), $147.00 per year (Canadian and foreign student/resident), $289.00 per year (foreign individuals), and $403.00 per year (foreign institutions). To receive student and resident rate, orders must be accompanied by name of affiliated institution, date of term, and the *signature* of program/residency coordinator on institutions letterhead. Orders will be billed at individual rate until proof of status is received. Foreign air speed delivery is included in all *Clinics'* subscription prices. All prices are subject to change without notice. POSTMASTER: Send address changes to *Anesthesiology Clinics*, Elsevier Periodicals Customer Service, 6277 Sea Harbor Drive, Orlando, FL 32887-4800. **Customer Service: 1-800-654-2452** (US). From outside of the US, call **1-407-345-4000**. E-mail: hhspcs@wbsaunders.com.

Anesthesiology Clinics, is also published in Spanish by McGraw-Hill Inter-americana Editores S. A., P.O. Box 5-237, 06500 Mexico D. F., Mexico.

Anesthesiology Clinics, is covered in *Index Medicus, Current Contents/Clinical Medicine, Excerpta Medica, ISI/BIOMED*, and *Chemical Abstracts*.

Printed in the United States of America.

CONSULTING EDITOR

LEE A. FLEISHER, MD, Robert D. Dripps Professor of Medicine; Chair, Anesthesiology and Critical Care, University of Pennsylvania School of Medicine, Philadelphia, Pennsylvania

GUEST EDITOR

HOWARD S. SMITH, MD, FACP, Associate Professor and Director of Pain Management, Albany Medical College, Department of Anesthesiology, Albany, New York

CONTRIBUTORS

STACY ACKERLIND, PhD, Director of Assessment, Evaluation, and Research in Student Affairs, University of Utah, Salt Lake City, Utah

ALLEN CARL, MD, Professor, Department of Orthopaedic Surgery, Albany Medical Center, Albany, New York

STEVEN P. COHEN, MD, Associate Professor, Pain Management Division, Department of Anesthesiology, Johns Hopkins School of Medicine, Baltimore, Maryland; Department of Surgery, Walter Reed Army Medical Center, Washington, DC

ANTHONY DRAGOVICH, MD, Fellow in Pain Management, Department of Surgery, Walter Reed Army Medical Center, Washington, DC

NASR ENANY, MD, Assistant Professor, Department of Anesthesiology, University of Cincinnati College of Medicine, Cincinnati, Ohio

STEVEN H. HOROWITZ, MD, Clinical Professor of Neurology, University of Vermont College of Medicine, Burlington, Vermont; Assistant in Neurology, Department of Neurology, Massachusetts General Hospital, Boston, Massachusetts

MOHAMMED A. KHALEEL, MS, Department of Orthopaedic Surgery, Albany Medical Center, Albany, New York

KENNETH L. KIRSH, PhD, Assistant Professor, Pharmacy Practice and Science, University of Kentucky, Lexington, Kentucky

HELENA KNOTKOVA, PhD, Research Scientist, Department of Pain Medicine and Palliative Care, Beth Israel Medical Center, New York, New York

ELIZABETH DEMERS LAVELLE, MD, Clinical Instructor, Department of Anesthesiology, Albany Medical Center, Albany, New York

LORI LAVELLE, DO, Medical Clinician, Department of Rheumatology, Altoona Arthritis and Osteoporosis Center, Altoona, Duncansville, Pennsylvania

WILLIAM LAVELLE, MD, Chief Resident, Department of Orthopaedic Surgery, Albany Medical Center, Albany, New York

JOHN D. MARKMAN, MD, Assistant Professor of Anesthesiology, Neurology, and Neurosurgery, University of Rochester School of Medicine and Dentistry; Director, The Pain Management Center at University of Rochester Medical Center, Rochester, New York

GARY McCLEANE, MD, FFARCSI, Consultant in Pain Management, Rampark Pain Centre, Lurgan, Northern Ireland, United Kingdom

JAMES McLEAN, MD, Pain Fellow, Department of Physical Medicine and Rehabilitation, Northwestern University, Feinberg School of Medicine; Sports and Spine Rehabilitation Center, Rehabilitation Institute of Chicago, Chicago, Illinois

MUHAMMAD A. MUNIR, MD, Assistant Professor and Program Director of Pain Medicine, Department of Anesthesiology, University of Cincinnati College of Medicine, Cincinnati, Ohio

AKIKO OKIFUJI, PhD, Associate Professor of Anesthesiology, Pain Research and Management Center, University of Utah, Salt Lake City, Utah

MARCO PAPPAGALLO, MD, Director for Research, Department of Anesthesiology, Mount-Sinai Hospital, New York, New York

ANNIE PHILIP, MD, Senior Instructor of Anesthesiology, University of Rochester School of Medicine and Dentistry, Rochester, New York

LYNN RADER, MD, Clinical Instructor, Department of Physical Medicine and Rehabilitation, Northwestern University, Feinberg School of Medicine; Attending Physician, Chronic Pain Care Center, Rehabilitation Institute of Chicago, Chicago, Illinois

HOWARD S. SMITH, MD, FACP, Associate Professor and Director of Pain Management, Albany Medical College, Department of Anesthesiology, Albany, New York

STEVEN P. STANOS, DO, Clinical Instructor, Department of Physical Medicine and Rehabilitation, Northwestern University, Feinberg School of Medicine; Medical Director, Chronic Pain Care Center, Rehabilitation Institute of Chicago, Chicago, Illinois

JUN-MING ZHANG, MSc, MD, Associate Professor and Director of Research, Department of Anesthesiology, University of Cincinnati College of Medicine, Cincinnati, Ohio

CONTENTS

> Neuropathic pain is initiated or caused by damage or dysfunction of the peripheral or central nervous systems in various disorders, each having pain-related symptoms and signs thought secondary to common pain mechanisms. Ancillary testing may demonstrate associated nervous system abnormalities, however its specificity is inadequate at present, as it makes inferential conclusions from indirect data. Symptom assessment and physical findings remain paramount in the diagnosis of neuropathic pain.

> Pain is a complex, idiosyncratic experience. When pain is the primary complaint for seeking medical attention, understanding of multiple factors is essential in guiding successful treatment. Behavioral medicine, a branch of psychology, has been an integral part of interdisciplinary/multidisciplinay care of pain patients. In this article, we provide an overview of behavioral medicine approaches to pain, including assessment and commonly used therapeutic methods. Particular attention is given to cognitive-behavioral therapy and motivational enhancement therapy.

> A physical medicine and rehabilitation approach to acute and chronic pain syndromes includes a wide spectrum of treatment

focus. Management includes an assessment and treatment model based on a biopsychosocial approach. Assessment includes a focus on pain behaviors, posture, muscle imbalances, and gait impairments. Effective treatment programs rely on appropriate and realistic goal setting. Treatment options may include physical therapy, polypharmacy, cognitive behavioral therapy, and passive modalities. Treatment goals emphasize achieving analgesia, improving psychosocial functioning, and reintegration of recreational or leisure pursuits. More complicated multidimensional chronic pain conditions may require a more collaborative continuum of multidisciplinary and interdisciplinary treatment approaches. Progress in all therapies necessitates close monitoring by the health care provider and ongoing communication between members of the treatment team.

Nonopioid analgesics represent a varied collection of analgesic agents, many of which also possess antipyretic or anti-inflammatory actions. As a group, nonopioid analgesics represent reasonable first-line analgesics for a variety of mild to moderate painful conditions and also often may be useful in conjunction with other analgesics (eg, opioids) for a myriad of severe painful conditions. Clinicians treating pain should be familiar with the actions, adverse effects, and individual agents in the group of nonopioid analgesics.

Adjuvant analgesics represent a diverse group of drugs that were originally developed for a primary indication other than pain. Many of these medications are currently used to enhance analgesia under specific circumstances. The proper use of adjuvant drugs is one of the keys to success in effective pain management. Since adjuvant analgesics are typically administered to patients who take multiple medications, decisions regarding administration and dosage must be made with a clear understanding of the stage of the disease and the goals of care. The article discusses major classes of adjuvant analgesics, with the focus on the mechanism of action, clinical application, and risks and benefits associated with each particular class of adjuvants.

This article concentrates on recent evidence about opioid analgesics for persistent noncancer pain. Evidence confirms that opioids are drugs with a definite risk of adverse events. Therefore, before prescribing opioids, careful consideration must be given to be certain that the intended benefit of a particular opioid merits its use despite the potential side effects and to determine if the co-prescription of other pharmacologic agents could reduce the risk of adverse events. Strong opioids should be reserved for patients who fail to respond to other lower-risk options and only after proper consideration is given to the long-term consequences of strong opioid use. Problems associated with opioids dictate that more efficacious and safer drugs need to be found.

phenomena. Trigger points may be relieved through noninvasive measures, such as spray and stretch, transcutaneous electrical stimulation, physical therapy, and massage. Invasive treatments for myofascial trigger points include injections with local anesthetics, corticosteroids, or botulism toxin or dry needling. The etiology, pathophysiology, and treatment of myofascial trigger points are addressed in this article.

FORTHCOMING ISSUES

RECENT ISSUES

THE CLINICS ARE NOW AVAILABLE ONLINE!

For more information about Clinics:
http://www.theclinics.com

ELSEVIER
SAUNDERS

Anesthesiology Clin
25 (2007) xi–xii

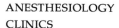

ANESTHESIOLOGY
CLINICS

Foreword

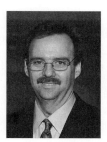

Lee A. Fleisher, MD
Consulting Editor

Chronic pain management has taken on increasing importance for the general public. A large percentage of our health care expenditures are focused on treatment of chronic pain syndromes. It has become increasingly recognized that the treatment of chronic pain conditions extends beyond the traditional silos within departments or subspecialties and, in fact, a more interdisciplinary approach is often required to provide the patient with optimal care. For these reasons, *Medical Clinics of North America* has recently published a two-volume series on chronic pain edited by an anesthesiologist, Howard S. Smith, MD. Given the outstanding quality of this series and the importance of chronic pain treatment to anesthesiologists, I and the publishers of the *Clinics* series felt that selected articles from this series published in the *Anesthesiology Clinics* would be of tremendous value to our readership.

Howard S. Smith, MD is uniquely qualified to bring together an interdisciplinary issue on pain management that would be of value to the anesthesiologist. Smith is a graduate of the Chicago Medical School and completed both his anesthesiology residency and fellowship in pain management at Albany Medical College, where he is currently the Academic Director of Pain Management in the Department of Anesthesiology and Associate Professor of Anesthesiology. He is board-certified in internal medicine and anesthesiology and has certification in pain management and hospice and palliative medicine. He is Chair of the Training and Education Committee of the American Pain Society and a member of numerous other subspecialty

doi:10.1016/j.anclin.2007.08.004   *anesthesiology.theclinics.com*

groups. He has enlisted an excellent group of authors, whose writings will help educate us on this important topic.

Lee A. Fleisher, MD
Anesthesiology and Critical Care
University of Pennsylvania
6 Dulles, 3400 Spruce Street
Philadelphia, PA 19104, USA

E-mail address: fleishel@uphs.upenn.edu

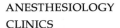

ANESTHESIOLOGY
CLINICS

Anesthesiology Clin
25 (2007) xiii–xiv

Preface

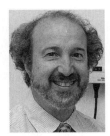

Howard S. Smith, MD, FACP
Guest Editor

Pain and suffering continue to be a challenging clinical dilemma. Providing comfort and alleviation of pain and suffering remains a primary and crucial goal of patient care. The management of pain has been and will continue to be a significant part of what anesthesiologists are involved in, both in the perioperative period and beyond (including patients with pain who have never had surgery).

Furthermore, the degree to which the anesthesiologist is able to achieve optimal analgesia with minimal adverse effects may potentially: abort certain persistent pain states, improve and expedite healing, decrease length of stay, improve and expedite optimal patient physical and/or emotional functioning, diminish morbidity, and improve quality of life. Additionally, the manner in which this is accomplished, as well as how well these goals are reached, may be reflected in how individual anesthesiologists, anesthesiology departments, and institutions are viewed by regulatory agencies, the media, other medical and nonmedical disciplines, referring physicians, other health care providers, and most importantly patients and their families.

Although initial pilot data have not been promising for back pain [1], strategies to combat proinflammatory cytokines may still be worthwhile pursuing for certain painful states. It may someday be possible to utilize gene therapy in attempts to manipulate the supraspinal endogenous pain modulatory system in efforts to restore balance between the pronociceptive dorsal reticular nucleus and the antinociceptive caudial ventrolateral medulla [2].

At higher levels of the central nervous system, it appears that at nociceptive levels of stimulation, pain intensity ratings positively correlate with

1932-2275/07/$ - see front matter © 2007 Elsevier Inc. All rights reserved.
doi:10.1016/j.anclin.2007.08.001

baseline fluctuations in the anterior cingulate cortex (an area involved in the affective dimension of pain), suggesting that baseline brain activity fluctuations may profoundly modify our conscious perception of the external world [3].

Pain is an integral part of the specialty of anesthesiology, its publications, and its missions of clinical care, education, and research. Despite the explosion of basic science research related to nociception, human pain continues to be a significant and suboptimally addressed clinical dilemma. Although clinicians have also made significant strides and have helped millions of patients achieve analgesia, there still remains much room for improvement. This issue of the *Anesthesiology Clinics* reflects a number of analgesic therapeutic options that anesthesiologists/pain specialists may find themselves involved with in some capacity. Thus, exposure to these various treatments may be helpful.

It is our hope that this volume will help anesthesiologists become more familiar with the evaluation and management of patients with persistent pain.

Howard S. Smith, MD, FACP
Albany Medical College
Department of Anesthesiology
47 New Scotland Avenue, MC-131
Albany, NY 12208, USA

E-mail address: smith@mail.amc.edu

References

[1] Cohen SP, Wenzell D, Hurley RW, et al. A double-blind, placebo-controlled, dose-response pilot study evaluating intradiscal etanercept in patients with chronic discogenic low back pain or lumbosacral radiculopathy. Anesthesiology 2007;107:99–105.

[2] Tavares I, Lima D. From meuroanatomy to gene therapy: searching for new ways to manipulate the supraspinal endogenous pain modulatory system. J Anat, in press.

[3] Boly M, Balteau E, Schnakers C, et al. Baseline brain activity fluctuations predict somatosensory perception in humans. Proc Natl Acad Sci USA, in press.

ANESTHESIOLOGY
CLINICS

ELSEVIER
SAUNDERS

Anesthesiology Clin
25 (2007) 699–708

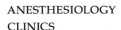

The Diagnostic Workup of Patients with Neuropathic Pain

Steven H. Horowitz, MD[a,b,*]

[a]*University of Vermont College of Medicine, Burlington, VT 05405, USA*
[b]*Department of Neurology, Massachusetts General Hospital,*
55 Fruit Street, Boston, MA 02114, USA

Current concepts of acute and chronic pain disorders distinguish "nociceptive," "inflammatory," "functional," and "neuropathic" pains [1]. Nociceptive pain is the common pain experienced from trauma, cancer, and so forth in which pain receptors (nociceptors) are activated. Transduction, conduction, and transmission of nociceptor activity to a conscious level involves peripheral and central nervous system pain pathways, which, when intact, function in a protective and adaptive manner [1]. However, damage to, or dysfunction of, these pain pathways, peripherally or centrally, can result in a different, much less frequent, but nevertheless important pain picture—that of neuropathic pain.

Neuropathic pain is not a disease in and of itself, but rather a manifestation of multiple and varied disorders affecting the nervous system, particularly its somatosensory components. They include polyneuropathies such as those secondary to diabetes mellitus, alcoholism, and amyloidosis; idiopathic small-fiber neuropathy; hereditary neuropathies; mononeuropathies such as trigeminal, glossopharyngeal, and post-herpetic neuralgias; entrapment neuropathies; and traumatic nerve injuries producing complex regional pain syndrome (CRPS) type II. CRPS type I is also considered a neuropathic pain disorder, although evidence for nerve damage as the underlying mechanism is more controversial. Neuropathic pain can occur in central nervous system disorders, especially spinal cord injury, multiple sclerosis, and cerebrovascular lesions of the brainstem and thalamus. Neuropathic pain in these conditions confers no functional benefit and may be considered a "maladaptive" response of the nervous system to the primary pathology [1].

A version of this article originally appeared in the 91:1 issue of Medical Clinics of North America.

* Department of Neurology, Massachusetts General Hospital, 55 Fruit Street, Boston, MA 02114, USA.

E-mail address: shhorowitz@partners.org

Unfortunately, the diagnosis of neuropathic pain is often problematic. Clinically, a distinction between nociceptive and neuropathic types of pain is not precise and conditions such as diabetes mellitus, cancer, and neurologic diseases with dystonia or spasticity can produce mixed pain pictures [2]. As with other pains, the perception of neuropathic pain is purely subjective, not easily described, nor directly measured. Also, pain pathway responses to damage are not static, but dynamic; signs and symptoms change with pathway activation and responsiveness, and with chronicity. Further, the multiplicity of disorders that have neuropathic pain as a component of their clinical presentations makes a single underlying pathophysiologic mechanism unlikely; more than one type of pain, and therefore probably more than one pain mechanism, can occur in a single patient, and some symptoms can be attributed to multiple mechanisms [2,3]. For these and other reasons the current management of neuropathic pain should be mechanistic in approach rather than disease-based [1]. Existing disease-based symptom palliation strategies should be supplemented with "targeted" mechanism-specific pharmacologic management [4].

History

Despite these complexities, there are several unique features to the clinical presentation of neuropathic pain that can be used to support its diagnosis and should be sought during history taking. In the case of mononeuropathies secondary to trauma, the severity of the pain often exceeds the severity of the inciting injury. CRPS can follow minor skin or joint trauma, bone fractures, or injections. The pain is stimulus-independent and described as "burning," "lancinating," "electric shock–like," "jabbing," or "cramping"; it is often accompanied by pins-and-needles sensations and sometimes by intractable itching (these are considered positive symptoms). These symptoms don't adhere to specific peripheral nerve distributions and often begin and remain most pronounced distally. The pain may be worse at night or during cold, damp weather, and is exacerbated by movement of the affected limb. Multiple types of pain (constant pain with paroxysms and stimulus-evoked pains) can be experienced simultaneously. It is useful to separate stimulus-independent and stimulus-evoked pains to differentiate ongoing from provoked activities [3]. Spread of symptoms outside the initial site of injury is common; in the case of unilateral pain there may be spread to homologous sites in the opposite limb (mirror pain). Positive and negative (numbness, loss of sensation) symptoms can occur concurrently and can be accompanied by autonomic symptoms. Spontaneous pain, often without complaints of sensory loss, is a feature of the cranial mononeuralgias—trigeminal, glossopharyngeal, and post-herpetic. Of course, location, intensity, and duration of pain are extremely important.

In generalized polyneuropathies, rapid progression solely affecting sensory fibers is more likely to be painful, especially if inflammation and ischemia are prominent pathological features, as occurs in the vasculitides [2]. In painful polyneuropathies, eg, idiopathic small-fiber neuropathy, diabetic polyneuropathy with predominant small-fiber (Aδ- and C-fibers) damage, the "burning," "lancinating," "jabbing" pains with pins-and-needles sensations are nerve-length dependent and bilaterally symmetric, beginning distally in the feet. With worsening, symptoms ascend to involve more proximal portions of the lower extremities and may eventually affect the hands. This centripetal progression can also occur in intercostal nerve distributions, beginning anteriorly over the midline of the torso with later symmetric lateral extension to the flanks. Autonomic complaints, eg, abnormal sweating, impotence, orthostatic hypotension, and gastrointestinal symptoms, are frequent.

Clinical examination

Among the more common and important clinical signs in neuropathic pain disorders are positive sensations: stimulus-evoked hypersensitivities such as allodynia to innocuous stimulation, eg, light touch and cold, and hyperalgesia to noxious stimulation, eg, pinprick. They occur focally in mononeuropathies and distally and symmetrically in polyneuropathies. Various forms of hyperalgesia have been described, including touch-evoked (or static) mechanical hyperalgesia to gentle pressure, pinprick hyperalgesia, blunt pressure hyperalgesia, and punctate hyperalgesia that increases with repetitive stimulation (windup-like pain) [2,3]. Paradoxically, these hypersensitivities can occur in areas in which the patient also complains of and demonstrates loss of sensation. There can be persistence of stimulus-evoked pain after the stimulus has been withdrawn (aftersensation) in the same anatomic distributions. As with symptoms, spread of allodynia and hyperalgesia outside the original site of injury is common and may extend to homologous sites in the opposite limb. Focal autonomic abnormalities after nerve injury, especially of sweating, skin temperature, and skin color, in conjunction with the aforementioned pain, fulfill the diagnostic criteria of CRPS (vide infra). With chronicity, trophic changes of the skin and nails develop, as do motor symptoms such as weakness, tremor, and dystonia. Nerve percussion at points of compression, entrapment, or irritation can elicit pins-and-needles or "electrical" sensations (Tinel's sign).

In small-fiber neuropathies, deficits are found in thermal and pain perceptions and sometimes touch, whereas large-fiber functions, eg, muscle strength, reflexes, and perception of vibratory and proprioceptive stimuli, are normal. In combined large- and small-fiber polyneuropathies, all these functions are compromised. Symmetrical distal autonomic dysfunction is often present but rarely severe.

While it is common for there to be relatively modest demonstrable clinical neurological deficits in patients with significant neuropathic pain, in some conditions there may be completely normal clinical examinations. This is the rule in trigeminal and glossopharyngeal neuralgias and it occurs more than occasionally in post-herpetic neuralgia. But some patients, particularly with what appear to be small-fiber neuropathies or specific nerve injuries, who describe their pains with the aforementioned typical neuropathic pain adjectives, also have normal examinations. There is the temptation to attribute their pain complaints to functional etiologies; however, at least from a logical perspective, that cannot always be the case, and if they are known to have a particular disease such as diabetes, or suffered an injury in which nerve damage is likely, pain may be their only manifestation of neural dysfunction. In such situations and, of course, in most cases in which further diagnostic information would be helpful, ancillary testing can be used.

Ancillary tests

Any consideration of the utility of ancillary tests to support the diagnosis of specific neuropathic pain mechanisms must take into account several factors: (1) Currently, available tests only evaluate nervous system structures and functions presumed to be relevant to pain perception and transmission; from their results the presence, extent, and mechanisms of neuropathic pain are, at best, inferred. This situation is somewhat similar to testing for diabetes mellitus with peripheral nerve, ophthalmologic, and renal studies without the availability of plasma glucose levels. (2) There is a spectrum of clinical and physiological manifestations of neural injury within each disorder, with chronic pain occurring in only a small percentage of affected patients. For example, neuropathic pain occurs in ~16% of patients with diabetes mellitus and a third of those with diabetic neuropathy [5]; post-herpetic neuralgia, defined as chronic pain present 4 or more months after resolution of the acute herpes zoster (shingles) rash, occurs in 13% to 20% of patients [6]; and following direct nerve injury, as occurs during venipuncture, persistent pain is rare, perhaps occurring in 1:1,500,000 procedures [7]. (3) The causes of this clinical variability are less than certain, but the presence of pain is presumed to reflect damage to the small myelinated (Aδ-) and unmyelinated (C-) fibers within peripheral nerves [2]. As these fiber types also mediate other clinical functions that are measurable, eg, appreciation of painful stimuli, temperature perception, and autonomic activity, many tests have focused on demonstrating defects in these modalities to verify Aδ- or C-fiber damage.

Clinical neurophysiology

Neurophysiologic testing, principally nerve conduction studies and electromyography, are frequently used in suspected disorders of the peripheral nervous system. The usual techniques, with surface electrodes for nerve stimulation and evoked potential recording, measure activity of the largest and fastest conducting sensory and motor myelinated nerve fibers (Aαβ-).

The most significant measured parameters are maximum conduction velocity (NCV) for the segment of nerve between the stimulating and recording electrodes, and amplitude and configuration of the resulting signals—the compound motor action potential (CMAP) evoked from motor fibers and the sensory nerve action potential (SNAP) evoked from sensory fibers. For central nervous system or proximal peripheral nerve disorders, somatosensory and magnetic evoked potential studies can be helpful. Electromyography (EMG) is the needle evaluation of muscles and evaluates muscle and motor nerve fiber activities.

Unfortunately, Aδ- and C-fiber activities cannot be tested with these techniques. Slowing in maximum NCVs or loss of CMAP or SNAP amplitudes, indicative of peripheral nerve disease either focally or generally, occur as a consequence of large fiber dysfunction. Abnormal EMG features such as acute and chronic denervation indicate involvement of large motor nerve fibers, also focally or generally, from the anterior horn cell distally. If present in a patient with neuropathic pain, these abnormalities can be used to corroborate the clinical impression of damage to a specific peripheral nerve or to peripheral nerves in general as in a polyneuropathy, eg, diabetic or alcoholic neuropathy. However, polyneuropathies or focal nerve lesions with only small-fiber involvement can have normal NCVs and EMG despite significant nerve damage and neuropathic pain.

Quantitative sensory testing

Quantitative sensory testing (QST) is used with increasing frequency, especially in clinical therapeutic trials, and measures sensory thresholds for pain, touch, vibration, and hot and cold temperature sensations. A number of devices are commercially available and range from handheld tools to sophisticated computerized equipment with complicated testing algorithms, standardization of stimulation and recording procedures, and comparisons to age- and gender-matched control values. With this technology, specific fiber functions can be assessed: Aδ-fibers with cold and cold-pain detection thresholds, C-fibers with heat and heat-pain detection thresholds, and large fiber (Aαβ-) functions with vibration detection thresholds. Elevated sensory thresholds correlate with sensory loss and lowered thresholds occur in allodynia and hyperalgesia [8]. In a generalized polyneuropathy when all quantitative sensory thresholds are elevated, it is inferred that all fiber types are affected, whereas if a dissociation exists wherein vibration thresholds are normal, but the other thresholds are elevated, the presence of a small-fiber neuropathy is suspected. In asymptomatic patients, abnormal QST thresholds suggest subclinical nerve damage.

The advantages of quantitation of sensory perception are that by enumerating an individual patient's findings and comparing them with normative values a clearer distinction between normal and abnormal responses occurs, thereby allowing analyses across patient and disease groups and for baseline standards in longitudinal studies. However, it must be appreciated that QST is a psychophysical test and therefore is dependent upon patient motivation, alertness, and concentration. Patients can willingly perform poorly, and even when not doing so there are large intra- and interindividual variations. Further, abnormal findings are not specific for peripheral nerve dysfunction; central nervous system disorders will also affect sensory thresholds.

Autonomic function testing

The evaluation of autonomic functions in patients suspected of having neuropathic pain can be important because of anatomic similarities between pain and autonomic fibers outside the central nervous system (CNS), and because disorders productive of neuropathic pain frequently have signs and symptoms of autonomic dysfunction (dry eyes or mouth, skin temperature and color changes, sweating abnormalities, orthostatic hypotension, heart rate responses to deep breathing, edema, and so forth). The majority of autonomic tests study skin temperature, and sudomotor, baroreceptor, vasomotor, and cardiovagal functions; they have been extensively reviewed [9,10]. A semiquantitative composite autonomic symptoms score (CASS), composed of the results of sudomotor, cardiovagal, and adrenergic testing, has been devised [11]. Less frequently, pupillary, gastrointestinal, and sexual function tests are helpful.

The value of autonomic testing in patients with a general neuropathic pain disorder, painful small-fiber neuropathy with burning feet, has been illustrated in several studies [12,13] in which many patients had normal or only mildly abnormal electrophysiologic (NCVs/EMG) findings. Autonomic abnormalities were seen in more than 90% of patients, the most useful tests being the quantitative sudomotor axon reflex test (QSART), thermoregulatory sweat test, heart rate responses to deep breathing, Valsalva ratio, and surface skin temperature [12,13]. However, in a recent study of patients with diabetic polyneuropathy, discordance was noted between efferent C-fiber responses in sudomotor tests (QSART and sweat imprint), and primary afferent (nociceptor) C-fiber axon-reflex flare responses. These findings indicate that these two C-fiber subclasses can be differentially affected in diabetic small fiber polyneuropathy. There may be involvement of one subclass and not the other or there may be different patterns of regeneration and reinnervation [14]. Autonomic functions can also be abnormal in peripheral neuropathies not associated with pain.

The relationship between autonomic dysfunction and pain is more complicated in CRPS in which focal sudomotor and vasomotor abnormalities are thought to be essential for the diagnosis [15] and sympathetic blockade has been a mainstay of diagnosis and therapy for decades. As would be expected, the vast majority of patients with CRPS were found to have autonomic abnormalities, particularly involving sweating and skin temperature [16]. However, there are patients with identical focal pain, but no clinical evidence of autonomic dysfunction. These patients do not meet the current definition of CRPS and have been termed "post-traumatic neuralgia" [17]; their autonomic functions have not been well studied.

Skin biopsy

For the past decade the histological study of unmyelinated nerve fibers in the skin has grown in importance in the diagnosis of peripheral nerve disorders, both generalized and focal, including those associated with neuropathic pain. When a skin punch biopsy is fixed with certain antibodies, most frequently protein gene product (PGP) 9.5, epidermal fibers can be stained and visualized [18,19]. Epidermal nerve fiber density and morphology, eg, tortuosity, complex ramifications, clustering, and axon swellings, can be quantified [18,19] and compared with control values [20]. A reduced density of epidermal nerve fibers is seen in small-fiber neuropathies [21], diabetic neuropathy, and impaired glucose tolerance neuropathy [22], each of which is associated with neuropathic pain. In a subgroup analysis of one such study, the skin biopsy findings were found to be a more sensitive measure than QSART or QST in diagnosing neuropathy in patients with burning feet and normal NCVs [23]. Conversely, disorders with severe loss of pain sensation such as congenital insensitivity to pain with anhidrosis (hereditary sensory and autonomic neuropathy IV; HSAN IV) and familial dysautonomia with sensory loss (Riley-Day; HSAN III) also have severe loss of epidermal fibers, as does a predominantly large fiber neuropathy, Friedreich's ataxia, in which pain is unusual [18,19]. Thus, the loss of epidermal small fibers is not specific for the presence of neuropathic pain.

Additional tests that may be of value in patients with neuropathic pain, particularly in focal pain syndromes such as CRPS, are bone scintigraphy, bone densitometry, and nerve or sympathetic ganglion blockade. Serum immunoelectrophoresis can be helpful in painful polyneuropathies associated with monoclonal gammopathies and acquired amyloid polyneuropathy. Specific serum antibody tests are valuable in painful neuropathies associated with neoplasia, celiac disease, and human immunodeficiency virus [24].

Summary

Determining the causes of neuropathic pain is more than an epistemological exercise. At its essence, it is a quest to delineate mechanisms of dysfunction through which treatment strategies can be created that are effective in reducing, ameliorating, or eliminating symptomatology. To date, predictors of which patients will develop neuropathic pain or who will respond to specific therapies are lacking, and present therapies have been developed mainly through trial and error [25]. Our current inability to make therapeutically meaningful decisions based on ancillary test data is illustrated by the following:

In a study specifically designed to assess the response of patients with painful distal sensory neuropathies to the 5% lidocaine patch, no relationship between treatment response and distal leg skin biopsy, QST, or sensory nerve conduction study results could be established [25]. From a mechanistic perspective, the hypothesis that the lidocaine patch would be most effective in patients with relatively intact epidermal innervation, whose neuropathic pain is presumed attributable to "irritable nociceptors," and least effective in patients with few surviving epidermal nociceptors, presumably with "deafferentation pain," was unproven [25]. The possible explanations are multiple and outside the scope of this review. However, these findings, coupled with the disparity in C-fiber subtype involvement in diabetic small-fiber neuropathy [14], and the recently reported inability of enzyme replacement therapy in Fabry disease to influence intraepidermal innervation density, while having mixed effects on cold and warm QST thresholds, and beneficial effects on sudomotor findings [26,27], when therapeutic benefit was demonstrated [27], lead one to conclude that the specificity of ancillary testing in neuropathic pain is inadequate at present, and reinforce the aforementioned caveats about inferential conclusions from indirect data. The diagnosis of neuropathic pain mechanisms is in its nascent stages and ancillary testing remains "subordinate," "subsidiary," and "auxiliary" as defined in Webster's Third New International Dictionary.

As a consequence of these difficulties, the recent approach by Bennett and his colleagues [28] may have merit. They have hypothesized (and provide data in support) that chronic pain can be more or less neuropathic on a spectrum between "likely," "possible," and "unlikely," based on patient responses on validated neuropathic pain symptom scales, when compared with specialist pain physician certainty of the presence of neuropathic pain on a 100-mm visual analog scale. The symptoms most associated with neuropathic pain were dysesthesias, evoked pain, paroxysmal pain, thermal pain, autonomic complaints, and descriptions of the pain as being sharp, hot, or cold, with high sensitivity. Higher scores for these symptoms correlated with greater clinician certainty of the presence of neuropathic pain mechanisms. Considering each individual patient's chronic pain as being somewhere on a continuum between "purely nociceptive" and "purely neuropathic" may have diagnostic and therapeutic relevance by enhancing specificity, but this requires clinical confirmation. Thus, symptom assessment remains indispensable in the evaluation of neuropathic pain, ancillary testing notwithstanding [28].

References

[1] Woolf CJ. Pain: moving from symptom control toward mechanism-specific pharmacologic
     management. Ann Intern Med 2004;140:441–51.

[2] Scadding JW, Koltzenburg M. Painful peripheral neuropathies. In: McMahon SB, Koltzenburg M, editors. Wall and Melzack's textbook of pain. 5th edition. Philadelphia (PA): Elsevier Churchill Livingstone; 2006. p. 973–99.

[3] Jensen TS, Baron R. Translation of symptoms and signs into mechanisms of neuropathic pain. Pain 2003;102:1–8.

[4] Smith HS, Sang CN. The evolving nature of neuropathic pain: individualizing treatment. Eur J Pain 2002;6(Suppl B):13–8.

[5] Daousi C, MacFarlane IA, Woodward A, et al. Chronic painful peripheral neuropathy in an urban community: a controlled comparison of people with and without diabetes. Diab Med 2004;21:976–82.

[6] Jung BF, Johnson RW, Griffin DRJ, et al. Risk factors for postherpetic neuralgia in patients with herpes zoster. Neurology 2004;62:1545–51.

[7] Newman BH. Venipuncture nerve injuries after whole-blood donation. Transfusion 2001;41: 571.

[8] Suarez GA, Dyck PJ. Quantitative sensory assessment. In: Dyck PJ, Thomas PK, editors. Diabetic neuropathy. 2nd edition. Philadelphia (PA): Saunders; 1999. p. 151–69.

[9] Low PA, Mathias CJ. Quantitation of autonomic impairment. In: Dyck PJ, Thomas PK, editors. Peripheral neuropathy. 4th edition. Philadelphia (PA): Elsevier Saunders; 2005. p. 1103–33.

[10] Hilz MJ, Dutsch M. Quantitative studies of autonomic dysfunction. Muscle Nerve 2006;34: 6–20.

[11] Low PA. Composite autonomic scoring scale for laboratory quantification of generalized autonomic failure. Mayo Clin Proc 1993;68:748–52.

[12] Novak V, Freimer ML, Kissel JT, et al. Autonomic impairment in painful neuropathy. Neurol 2001;56:861–8.

[13] Low VA, Sandroni P, Fealey RD, et al. Detection of small-fiber neuropathy by sudomotor testing. Muscle Nerve 2006;34:57–61.

[14] Berghoff M, Kilo S, Hilz MJ, et al. Differential impairment of the sudomotor and nociceptor axon-reflex in diabetic peripheral neuropathy. Muscle Nerve 2006;33: 494–9.

[15] Merskey H, Bogduk N. Classification of chronic pain: descriptions of chronic pain syndromes and definitions of pain terms. In: Merskey H, Bogduk N, editors. Task force on taxonomy of the International Association for the study of pain. Seattle (WA): IASP Press; 1994. p. 39–43.

[16] Chelimsky TC, Low PA, Naessens JM, et al. Value of autonomic testing in reflex sympathetic dystrophy. Mayo Clin Proc 1995;70:1029–40.

[17] Wasner G, Schattschneider J, Binder A, et al. Complex regional pain syndrome—diagnostic, mechanisms, CNS involvement and therapy. Spinal Cord 2003;41:61–75.

[18] Kennedy WR. Opportunities afforded by the study of unmyelinated nerves in skin and other organs. Muscle Nerve 2004;29:756–67.

[19] Kennedy WR, Wendelschafer-Crabb G, Polydefkis M, et al. Pathology and quantitation of cutaneous innervation. In: Dyck PJ, Thomas PK, editors. Peripheral neuropathy. 4th edition. Philadelphia (PA): Elsevier Saunders; 2005. p. 869–95.

[20] Umapathi T, Tan WL, Tan NCK, et al. Determinants of epidermal nerve fiber density in normal individuals. Muscle Nerve 2006;33:742–6.

[21] Holland NR, Stocks A, Hauer P, et al. Intraepidermal nerve fiber density in patients with painful sensory neuropathy. Neurol 1997;48:708–11.

[22] Polydefkis M, Griffin JW, McArthur J. New insights into diabetic polyneuropathy. JAMA 2003;290:1371–6.

[23] Periquet MI, Novak V, Callino MP, et al. Painful sensory neuropathy: prospective evaluation using skin biopsy. Neurol 1999;53:1641–7.

[24] Mendell JR, Sahenk Z. Painful sensory neuropathy. N Engl J Med 2003;348: 1243–55.

[25] Herrmann DN, Pannoni V, Barbano RL, et al. Skin biopsy and quantitative sensory testing do not predict response to lidocaine patch in painful neuropathies. Muscle Nerve 2006;33: 42–8.

[26] Schiffmann R, Hauer P, Freeman B, et al. Enzyme replacement therapy and intraepidermal innervation density in Fabry disease. Muscle Nerve 2006;34:53–6.

[27] Schiffmann R, Floeter MK, Dambrosia JM, et al. Enzyme replacement therapy improves peripheral nerve and sweat function in Fabry disease. Muscle Nerve 2003;28:703–10.

[28] Bennett MI, Smith BH, Torrance N, et al. Can pain be more or less neuropathic? Comparison of symptom assessment tools with ratings of certainty by clinicians. Pain 2006;122: 289–94.

ELSEVIER
SAUNDERS

Anesthesiology Clin
25 (2007) 709–719

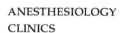
ANESTHESIOLOGY
CLINICS

Behavioral Medicine Approaches to Pain

Akiko Okifuji, PhD[a],*, Stacy Ackerlind, PhD[b]

[a]Pain Research and Management Center, Department of Anesthesiology, University of Utah,
615 Arapeen Drive, Suite 200, Salt Lake City, UT 84108, USA
[b]Student Affairs, University of Utah, A Ray Olpin Union Building,
200 S. Central Campus Drive, Room 270, Salt Lake City, UT 84132, USA

In the early 1970s, the term "behavioral medicine" began appearing in the literature as a branch of behavioral science that applies scientific knowledge and techniques to prevention, diagnosis, treatment, and rehabilitation of physical illness and maintenance of physical health [1]. A fundamental aspect of behavioral medicine is the recognition that psychological and behavioral factors reciprocally and dynamically interact with physical health/illness. Linear causality does not exist in this reciprocal relationship. Instead, behavioral medicine interventions assume that by addressing psychosocial and behavioral factors relevant to the illness in question, the overall clinical picture of the condition will improve.

In the early days of pain medicine, treatments for pain patients were primarily biomedical in nature, targeting specific anatomy, physiology, and neurochemistry to alter nociceptive input. However, the proliferation of behavioral research indicates that a number of behavioral and psychological factors contribute to the experience of pain, particularly chronic cases, which has prompted the application of behavioral medicine approaches to pain treatment.

Complex pain cases, particularly noncancer chronic pain, often require multidimensional conceptualization and treatment. Accordingly, multimodal approaches aimed at reduction of pain and resumption of a productive life are considered critical. Behavioral medicine is generally imbedded in a comprehensive multimodal pain treatment program. One of the most commonly used behavioral medicine approaches for pain is cognitive-behavioral therapy, specifically addressing pain-related cognitions and behaviors.

A version of this article originally appeared in the 91:1 issue of Medical Clinics of North America.

This work was supported by Grant No. AR48888 from the National Institutes of Arthritis, Musculoskeletal, and Skin Diseases to the first author.

* Corresponding author.

E-mail address: akiko.okifuji@hsc.utah.edu (A. Okifuji).

doi:10.1016/j.anclin.2007.07.009
anesthesiology.theclinics.com

Accumulated research in the past 3 decades strongly suggests that multimodal interventions that include cognitive-behavioral therapy modalities is beneficial and cost-effective [2,3].

Underlying the cognitive-behavioral perspective is the integration of cognitive, affective, and behavioral factors into an overall clinical picture and treatment of pain patients. In the model, each patient is considered as an active processor of external cues that modulates his/her internal state. Psychological variables such as anticipation, avoidance, contingencies of reinforcement, and mood factors are of particular interest. Clearly, the cognitive-behavioral model is not just patients' responses to actual events, but also learned responses to predict and summon appropriate reactions to actual or anticipated events. The cognitive-behavioral framework assumes that how patients perceive their situation and what they expect from their conditions are significant contributors to their health status and disability.

There are five central assumptions that characterize the cognitive-behavioral perspective on pain management (see Box 1). The first assumption is that all people are active processors of information rather than passive entities reacting to events or physical cues. Information is processed through use of well-developed cognitive schemes that people have developed as a result of their learning histories. The process is generally overlearned and automated, and thus people are often not aware that they are operating from a set of assumptions that guide their behavior. Nevertheless, people are constantly engaged in this process in their attempt to make sense of the world around them. People can and do adjust their cognitive schemes to adapt to changing environmental demands.

A second assumption of the cognitive-behavioral perspective is that one's cognitive attributions, beliefs, and expectancies can elicit or modulate affect

---

Box 1. Basic assumptions of cognitive-behavioral treatment

1. People are active processors of information rather than passive reactors to environmental contingencies.
2. Thoughts (for example, appraisals, attributions, expectancies) can elicit or modulate physiological and affective responses, both of which may serve as impetuses for behavior. Conversely, affect, physiology, and behavior can instigate or influence one's thinking processes.
3. Behavior is reciprocally determined by both the environment and the individual.
4. In the same way as people are instrumental in the development and maintenance of maladaptive thoughts, feelings, and behaviors, they can, are, and should be considered active agents of change of their maladaptive modes of responding.

and physiological arousal, both of which may serve as impetuses for behavior. Conversely, affect, physiology, and behavior can instigate or influence one's thinking processes. This cycle is dynamic and continuous, and a causal direction is less of a concern than awareness that this interactive process extends over time with the interaction of thoughts, feelings, physiological activity, and behavior.

The third assumption of the cognitive-behavioral perspective is that behaviors occur as a function of reciprocal interaction between the environment and the individual. Given an event, people respond to the environment, which may in turn alter the environment and elicit others to behave in certain ways. In a very real sense, people are the most prominent contributors to their environments. The chain of such interactions over time makes each person's behavioral pattern unique and idiosyncratic. Ironically, most people are not aware of this process and make external attributions for their failures and successes. For pain patients, it is important to help them recognize how they influence their environment to increase support and decrease hindrances to treatment success.

The final assumption of the cognitive-behavioral perspective is that people create their own reality. Just as they are instrumental in the development and maintenance of maladaptive thoughts, feelings, and behaviors, they can, are, and should be considered active agents of change. Pain patients can replace maladaptive modes of responding with more adaptive ones. Pain patients, no matter how severe their pain and despite their common beliefs to the contrary, are not helpless pawns of fate. They can and should become instrumental in learning and carrying out more effective modes of responding to their environment and their situation.

Behavioral medicine assessment of pain patients

The main vehicle of behavioral medicine assessment is a clinical interview with a patient and, if available and feasible, his or her family members. As supplemental informational sources, standardized self-report inventories may be used. The main goals of assessment are to (1) evaluate psychosocial and behavioral factors relevant to the patient's pain and (2) organize and evaluate the relevant information to direct treatment plans. Attention is also given to identification of any factors that might be impediments to rehabilitation as well as factors that may facilitate the rehabilitative processes.

Typically, the assessment protocol consists of three parts. The first part focuses on understanding a clinical picture of the patient's experience of pain. Specifically, a brief history of pain, learning current pain parameters (eg, quality of pain, time parameters, aggravating/relieving factors), other relevant medical history, and assessing current functional levels, including sleep quality and functional impairment due to pain. It is also important to assess how the patient conceptualizes his or her own pain, the patient's understanding of the potential etiological factors, whether he or she believes adequate diagnostic work has been done, and his or her expectations as to what types of treatments may affect adherence to the treatment regimen and ultimately the success of treatment.

The second part of assessment focuses on gaining a broader understanding of the patient. This includes psychosocial history, including family and personal history of pain, functional abilities and limitations, psychological disorders, and problems with substances (including prescription drugs). This information should help the assessor gain a better understanding of how the patient has historically coped with illness and stress, current life circumstances that may aid/impede treatment efforts, and the level of coping resources available to the patient.

The third part of the assessment is a psychological examination to assess the patient's current mental status, mood functions, and any maladaptive behavioral patterns that may influence the course of pain rehabilitation. Because of the high rate of depression and anxiety among pain patients, it is important to address these issues. All of this information is integrated with biomedical information and is used in treatment planning. There should be a close relationship between the data acquired during the assessment phase and the nature, focus, and goals of the therapeutic regimen.

Cognitive-behavioral therapy: self-management of pain

As noted previously, cognitive-behavioral therapy (CBT) is the most commonly used approach in behavioral medicine for pain patients. There are three main components of CBT for pain: patient education, behavioral skill training, and cognitive-skill training.

Patient education

Since the patient's active participation is critical for successful CBT, it is often essential that patients attain some understanding of the basic psychophysiological processes related to pain, sleep, function, and mood. The difference between acute pain and chronic pain, hurt versus harm concept, and what to expect from rehabilitation processes versus acute pain therapy can set the stage for skill training. Knowledge related to the behavioral principles, such as conditioning, reinforcement, pain/illness behaviors, and how those principles interact with pain and disability can also help patients prepare for the behavioral skills training phase.

Behavioral skills training

Relaxation and controlled breathing exercises are especially useful in the skills-acquisition phase because they can be readily learned by almost all patients. Relaxation and controlled breathing involve behavioral manipulation of the autonomic nervous system by systematically tensing and relaxing various muscle groups, both general and specific to the particular area of pain reported by patients. These skills are useful to reduce anxiety and stress responses associated with pain and improve sleep. It is important that patients understand that relaxation is an active process. Many people mistakenly believe that relaxation is a passive process where one rests and avoids working (eg, laying down in a couch and watching TV). Physiological effects of such active relaxation can be easily measured with a fingertip thermometer that tends to indicate a slight increase in finger temperature due to increased blood flow in the periphery during and after active relaxation [4,5]. Furthermore, it provides a simple demonstration to patients that their behaviors can alter their physiological states, and thereby substantiate the credibility of behavioral medicine approaches.

Another behavioral skill that is often used in CBT is attentional training. Attention plays a major role in any perceptual process. The pain experience tends to be exacerbated by increased attention to pain-related somatic signals [6]. Because our attentional resources are limited, by actively directing a patient's attention to nonpain stimuli, the available attentional resources directed toward pain should decrease. This can be achieved by having patients directly engage in overt behaviors (eg, breathing exercises, progressive muscle relaxation) or use mental imageries to situations that are typically ones unrelated to pain. Although imagery-based strategies (eg, refocusing attention on pleasant pain-incompatible scenes) have received much attention, the results have *not* consistently demonstrated that imagery strategies are uniformly effective for all patients [7]. The important component as to whether this intervention is effective seems to be the patient's imaginative ability, involvement, and degree of absorption in using specific images. Guided imagery training is given to patients to enhance their abilities to use all sensory modalities. The specifics of the images seem less important than the details of sensory modalities incorporated and the patient's involvement in these images. Patients also vary in their ability to use distraction techniques as well as what they find to be an adequate distraction target. The collaborative working relationship between a therapist and patient becomes essential during this part of training.

A variety of other behavioral skills training can be incorporated into the treatment plan to meet patients' clinical needs. For example, some patients experience interpersonal stress to be a major aggravating factor for their pain. Interpersonal relationships are a key component of an individual's environment. Basic interpersonal skills training in the areas of communication, assertiveness, and problem-solving skills may help patients better regulate their stress levels and increase their ability to actively manage their pain.

Cognitive skills training

Typical cognitive training for pain management begins with helping patients understand their own cognitive response system. Specifically, patients can learn to monitor situational factors that tend to trigger their pain/stress and what they actually experience emotionally, behaviorally, and physically when they have pain/stress (see Table 1). In the middle column, patients monitor and understand their own processes that may mediate the relationship between situational factors and the consequential experience. There are a number of potential processes that can be discussed; however, the focus is on cognitive processes that patients learn to monitor and regulate.

Effective self-regulation of pain depends on the individual's specific ways of dealing with pain, adjusting to pain, and reducing or minimizing pain and distress caused by pain through use of coping strategies. Coping strategies include positive self-talk focused on the intention to manage pain and the belief that one is able to execute necessary acts to do so effectively. Through the use of coping strategies, a person has an improved chance of successfully engaging in everyday activities, thereby reducing functional limitations and enhancing his or her sense of control over pain and associated symptoms. It is, however, important to note that effective coping largely depends on various personal (eg, self-efficacy beliefs), situational (eg, work, living arrangements), and psychosocial factors (eg, family history of pain, level of support). Interaction between coping strategies and personal and situational factors may be a critical factor in how coping strategies are implemented. Clinicians need to understand how patients interpret their world through the use of their cognitive systems (eg, self-talk, self-efficacy beliefs, instrumentality).

In cognitive skills training, self-efficacy beliefs are particularly important in treatment. Self-efficacy is defined as a personal conviction that one can effectively handle a situation by executing a course of action to produce a desired outcome [8]. The self-efficacy expectation is a critical mediator of therapeutic change for chronic pain patients [9]. Pain patients' self-efficacy beliefs are largely influenced by their own past success/failure at performing tasks to manage their pain; thus, it is imperative that a therapeutic process leads to an experience of effective performance. Such experience may be created by encouraging patients to undertake a relatively easy task in the beginning and gradually increasing the difficulty to match the difficulty of the desired behavioral repertoire. This developmental process allows self-efficacy to increase. In short, effective coping behaviors are essentially directed

Table 1
Cognitive behavioral framework for stress/pain management

Stressors	Processes	Stress response
What triggers stress/pain cycle	Modulating processes mediating between stressors and stress responses	What experientially happens to a person in response to stressors • Physiological • Behavioral • Emotional

by the individual's beliefs that situation demands do not exceed their coping resources.

Another important aspect in cognitive training is to understand specific patients' cognitive repertoires. Tendency to appraise situations negatively is known to deter treatment success [10,11]. Some of the common negative cognitions are listed in Box 2. In cognitive training, therapists help patients become aware of their own tendency for negative cognitions, and then to exercise the application of alternative ways of appraising the situations. A large number of self-help books and therapy manuals are available to help patients and clinicians go through the process in a step-by-step manner (eg, [12–14]).

Behavioral approach to improve compliance and motivation

One of the critical requirements for successful rehabilitation of chronic pain is that patients adopt an active, participatory role in their treatments. Literature repeatedly indicates that multidisciplinary pain care that includes an activating therapy to restore functioning is effective [2], requiring patients to modify lifestyles to incorporate various physical activities. Such adaptation is often difficult even for healthy individuals; a report to the surgeon general [15] shows that 50% of those who sign up with gyms at the beginning of a year drop out within 6 months. Thus, it is not surprising that

---

Box 2. Examples of common negative cognitive patterns

Polarizing pattern: Black-and-white thinking. If a patient's performance falls short of perfect, the patient sees himself or herself as a total failure, leading to high expectation that is often unattainable.

Overgeneralization pattern: A patient generalizes beyond the specific facts of a situation, and sees a single negative experience as a never-ending pattern of defeat.

Catastrophizing pattern: A patient consistently assumes the worst possible outcomes. The patient's understanding of his or her own plight is extremely negative and the patient tends to interpret relatively minor problems as major catastrophes.

Filtering pattern: A patient focuses on a single negative detail, rather than a whole picture, of the event and lets the single detail characterize the entire experience.

Emotional reasoning pattern: A patient assumes that his or her negative emotions reflect the reality. "I really feel it, therefore this must be true."

pain patients find it difficult to comply with regular physical activity regimens, even with the implementation of CBT to improve coping.

Therapeutic effort to help patients comply with their treatment regimen is of a growing interest. Long-term treatment success depends on regular adherence to recommended self-care regimens for people suffering from chronic pain conditions [16]. Historically, clinicians invest less energy in patients who show little commitment to therapies. However, as we increasingly face issues related to chronic illness that are closely tied with people's lifestyle issues, helping patients comply with functional regimens has become a critical clinical issue in pain management.

Motivation Enhancement Therapy

Motivation Enhancement Therapy (MET), developed by William Miller and his colleagues [17], is one of the therapeutic methods that targets patient motivation. MET is based on the assumption that people vary in their degree of readiness for change. Stated differently, patients are considered to be in a certain motivational stage of change. MET strategies are organized to help a patient move from a low level of motivation (or a lower level in the model) to increased motivation (or a higher level in the model) via therapist-patient interactions. Each of the motivational stages is presented in Box 3.

MET is a problem-focused, therapist-directed approach aiming to help patients enhance their commitment and motivation for treatment. MET offers a collection of therapeutic techniques to help patients (1) clearly recognize their problems, (2) perform a personal cost-benefit analysis of their therapeutic or countertherapeutic behaviors, (3) develop consistency between their therapy goals and motivation, and (4) internalize motivational thoughts via improved self-efficacy.

MET has been tested for facilitating change to reduce problem behaviors, such as smoking [18,19], problem drinking [20,21], problem gambling [22],

---

Box 3. Stages of change

1. **Precontemplative stage:** Patient does not perceive a need to change and actively resists change.
2. **Contemplation stage:** Patient begins to see a need for change and may consider making a change in the future
3. **Preparation stage:** Patient feels ready to change and takes a first concrete (behavioral) change
4. **Action stage:** Patient actively engages in behaviors consistent with regimen
5. **Maintenance stage:** Patient executes plans to sustain the changes made

eating disorders [23] and high risk sexual behaviors [24,25]. MET has also been shown to increase healthy behaviors such as promoting exercise with myocardial infarction patients [26], adherence to glucose control regimen in patients with diabetes [27], and mammography screening [28].

Motivation Enhancement Therapy for pain patients

MET is based on the assumption that people vary in their levels of commitment and motivation for complying with activating regimens. There are several key components in MET [29] that facilitate increased motivation to change maladaptive behavioral patterns and replace them with more adaptive ones. First, a clinician should refrain from judgmental attitudes and responses. Empathy and reflection of patients' feelings is useful at the early stage of MET. Rolling with resistance (ie, not pressuring the patient to change) is another essential interpersonal strategy used in MET. The clinician and patient should remain on the same side, thereby not increasing resistance to change. One of the easy pitfalls is for a clinician to push his or her agenda and as a consequence, let the patient present a counter-argument for why he or she should not engage in therapeutic effort. By going with the patient's resistance, the clinician facilitates the formation of a therapeutic alliance, which is critical to increase the patient's motivation to change. Second, the clinician helps patients to identify specific discrepancies between what they want from pain care (eg, "I want to get well and go out more often") and what they actually do (eg, "I can't do my exercise because I have no time and I don't feel well"). By focusing on the discrepancy, patients gain insight that their maladaptive behaviors and attitudes are actually preventing them from obtaining their goal of getting better. This insight promotes the patient's motivation to change. Similarly, patients benefit greatly from engaging in "decisional balance analysis" of their own behaviors. For example, patients list their "pros" for exercising, as well as for not exercising, and "cons" for exercising as well as for not exercising, which can be discussed and used to increase the discrepancy between the patient's goals and actions. The decisional balance analysis helps patients gain a better understanding of their behavior, in this case, why they do not want to exercise. Through this process, patients become more aware of their role in maintaining maladaptive behaviors as well as identifying strategies to engage in more adaptive behaviors.

Another essential feature of MET is to provide a supportive environment to nurture a sense of self-efficacy and ultimately a patient's ability to change his or her behaviors. By understanding that change is a process that the patient has control over, patients realize that change is possible. With increased self-efficacy beliefs comes a sense of responsibility and an awareness that it is patients themselves who will choose to engage in therapeutic efforts and execute them. MET is a clinician-directed approach that is heavily patient-centered. Detailed descriptions of the specific MET approach are beyond the scope of this paper. Interested readers may find a comprehensive book by Miller and Rollnick helpful [29].

Summary

Managing pain patients can be a challenging task for many clinicians because of the complexity of the condition. Pain by definition [30] is a multifactorial phenomenon for which biomedical factors interact with a web of psychosocial and behavioral factors. Behavioral medicine approaches for pain generally address specific cognitive and behavioral factors relevant to pain, thereby aiming to modify the overall pain experience and help restore functioning and quality of life in pain patients.

Behavioral medicine focuses on patients' motivation to comply with a rehabilitative regimen, particularly those with chronic, disabling pain. Since patients' own commitment and active participation in a therapeutic program are critical for the successful rehabilitation, the role that behavioral medicine can play is significant. It is not unreasonable to state that success outcomes of the rehabilitative approach depend on how effectively behavioral medicine can be integrated into the overall treatment plan. Past research in general supports this assertion, demonstrating clinical benefit and cost-effectiveness of multidisciplinary interventions that include behavioral medicine. Some of the approaches listed in this paper can be incorporated into clinicians' practice regardless of specialties, and such practice will likely provide helpful venues for managing pain patients.

References

[1] Gentry WD. Behavioral medicine: A new research paradigm. In: Gentry WD, editor. Handbook of behavioral medicine. New York: Guilford; 1984.
[2] Okifuji A. Interdisciplinary pain management with pain patients: evidence for its effectiveness. Sem Pain Med 2003;1(2):110–9.
[3] Turk DC. Clinical effectiveness and cost-effectiveness of treatments for patients with chronic pain. Clin J Pain 2002;18(6):355–65.
[4] Bacon M, Poppen R. A behavioral analysis of diaphragmatic breathing and its effects on peripheral temperature. J Behav Ther Exp Psychiatry 1985;16(1):15–21.
[5] Jacobson AM, Manschreck TC, Silverberg E. Behavioral treatment for Raynaud's disease: a comparative study with long-term follow-up. Am J Psychiatry 1979;136(6):844–6.
[6] McCabe C, Lewis J, Shenker N, et al. Don't look now! Pain and attention. Clin Med 2005; 5(5):482–6.
[7] Fernandez E, Turk DC. The utility of cognitive coping strategies for altering pain perception: a meta-analysis. Pain 1989;38(2):123–35.
[8] Bandura A. Self-efficacy: toward a unifying theory of behavioral change. Psychol Rev 1977; 84(2):191–215.
[9] Council JR, Ahern DK, Follick MJ, et al. Expectancies and functional impairment in chronic low back pain. Pain 1988;33(3):323–31.
[10] Cook AJ, Degood DE. The cognitive risk profile for pain: development of a self-report inventory for identifying beliefs and attitudes that interfere with pain management. Clin J Pain 2006;22(4):332–45.

[11] Tota-Faucette ME, Gil KM, Williams DA, et al. Predictors of response to pain management treatment. The role of family environment and changes in cognitive processes. Clin J Pain 1993;9(2):115–23.
[12] Caudill-Slosberg M. Managing pain before it manages you. Revised edition. New York: Guilford Press; 2001.
[13] Thorn B. Cognitive therapy for chronic pain: a step-by-step guide. New York: Guilford Press; 2004.
[14] Turk DC, Winter F. The pain survival guide: how to reclaim your life. Washington, DC: American Psychological Association; 2005.
[15] US Department of Health and Human Services. Physical activity and health: a report of the Surgeon General. Atlanta (GA): Centers for Disease Control and Prevention, National Center for Chronic Disease Prevention; 1996.
[16] Turk DC, Rudy TE. Neglected topics in the treatment of chronic pain patients—relapse, noncompliance, and adherence enhancement. Pain 1991;44(1):5–28.
[17] Miller W. Motivational interviewing with problem drinkers. Behav Psychother 1983;11: 147–72.
[18] Town GI, Fraser P, Graham S, et al. Establishment of a smoking cessation programme in primary and secondary care in Canterbury. N Z Med J 2000;113(1107):117–9.
[19] Velasquez MM, Hecht J, Quinn VP, et al. Application of motivational interviewing to prenatal smoking cessation: training and implementation issues. Tob Control 2000;9(Suppl 3): III36–40.
[20] Brown RL, Saunders LA, Bobula JA, et al. Remission of alcohol disorders in primary care patients. Does diagnosis matter? J Fam Pract 2000;49(6):522–8.
[21] Handmaker NS, Miller WR, Manicke M. Findings of a pilot study of motivational interviewing with pregnant drinkers. J Stud Alcohol 1999;60(2):285–7.
[22] Hodgins DC, Currie SR, el-Guebaly N. Motivational enhancement and self-help treatments for problem gambling. J Consult Clin Psychol 2001;69(1):50–7.
[23] Feld R, Woodside DB, Kaplan AS, et al. Pretreatment motivational enhancement therapy for eating disorders: a pilot study. Int J Eat Disord 2001;29(4):393–400.
[24] Carey MP, Braaten LS, Maisto SA, et al. Using information, motivational enhancement, and skills training to reduce the risk of HIV infection for low-income urban women: a second randomized clinical trial. Health Psychol 2000;19(1):3–11.
[25] Kalichman SC, Cherry C, Browne-Sperling F. Effectiveness of a video-based motivational skills-building HIV risk-reduction intervention for inner-city African American men. J Consult Clin Psychol 1999;67(6):959–66.
[26] Song R, Lee H. Managing health habits for myocardial infarction (MI) patients. Int J Nurs Stud 2001;38(4):375–80.
[27] Smith DE, Heckemeyer CM, Kratt PP, et al. Motivational interviewing to improve adherence to a behavioral weight-control program for older obese women with NIDDM. A pilot study. Diabetes Care 1997;20(1):52–4.
[28] Bernstein J, Mutschler P, Bernstein E. Keeping mammography referral appointments: motivation, health beliefs, and access barriers experienced by older minority women. J Midwifery Womens Health 2000;45(4):308–13.
[29] Miller W, Rollnick S. Motivational interviewing: preparing people for change. 2nd edition. New York: Guilford Press; 2002.
[30] International Association for the Study of Pain. Classification of chronic pain. Descriptions of chronic pain syndromes and definitions of pain terms. Pain 1986;3:S217.

ANESTHESIOLOGY
CLINICS

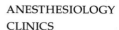

Anesthesiology Clin
25 (2007) 721–759

Physical Medicine Rehabilitation Approach to Pain

Steven P. Stanos, DO[a,b,*], James McLean, MD[a,c],
Lynn Rader, MD[a,b]

[a]Department of Physical Medicine and Rehabilitation, Northwestern University,
Feinberg School of Medicine, 303 East Chicago Ave., Chicago, IL 60611, USA
[b]Chronic Pain Care Center, Rehabilitation Institute of Chicago, 1030 N. Clark Street,
Suite 320, Chicago, IL 60610, USA
[c]Sports and Spine Rehabilitation Center, Rehabilitation Institute of Chicago,
1030 N. Clark Street, 5th Floor, Chicago, IL 60610, USA

The physiatric model of care is based on a fundamental understanding of the individuals' unique condition as it relates to the concept of (1) impairment, (2) disability, and (3) handicap [1]. Impairment is the psychologic, physical, or functional loss or abnormality. Disability is a restriction or lack of ability to perform activities due to related impairments. Handicap is the disadvantage that an individual possesses due to the impairment or disability that affects the patient's fulfillment of life roles in society (Box 1). A patient-centered approach is necessary to effectively address these important individual concepts. A team-centered approach focuses on helping patients to achieve individual goals, which enables them to improve physical and psychosocial function, decrease pain, and improve quality of life. By working together, the rehabilitation team is able to help patients achieve better outcomes than could be achieved by an individual practitioner. Treatment models include a continuum of care based on patient severity and needs, with increasing complexity of treatment philosophies and need for communication and decreasing individual team-member autonomy [2]. Focused treatment programs for acute conditions may involve individual physical therapy directed by the physiatrist, followed by a coordinated program including ongoing communication with the patient's case manager and therapist. With chronic pain conditions, more diverse assessment and treatment

A version of this article originally appeared in the 91:1 issue of Medical Clinics of North America.

* Corresponding author.
E-mail address: sstanos@ric.org (S.P. Stanos).

1932-2275/07/$ - see front matter © 2007 Elsevier Inc. All rights reserved.
doi:10.1016/j.anclin.2007.07.008

anesthesiology.theclinics.com

Box 1. World Health Organization definitions of impairment, disability, and handicap

Impairment: "Any loss or abnormality of psychological, physiological, or anatomic structure or function"

Disability: "Any restriction or lack (resulting from an impairment) of ability to perform an activity in the manner or within the range considered normal for a human being"

Handicap: "A disadvantage for a given individual, resulting from an impairment or a disability, that limits or prevents the fulfillment of a role that is normal (depending on age, sex, and social and cultural factors) for that individual"

---

teams include multi- and interdisciplinary programs. In the multidisciplinary model, patient care is planned and managed by a team leader. This model is often hierarchical, with one or two individuals directing the services of a range of team members, many with individual goals. Box 2 lists some of the specialists who are commonly part of a comprehensive pain rehabilitation team. Treatment may be delivered at different facilities or centers. Even more collaborative is the interdisciplinary model, involving team members working together toward a common goal. Team members are able to communicate and consult with other team members on an ongoing basis, facilitated by regular, face-to-face meetings. In this model, team members possess a combination of skills that no single individual demonstrates alone.

This article provides a description of the basic framework of approaching acute and chronic pain conditions with an important focus on the comprehensive functionally based history and physical examination that includes assessment of gait pattern, posture, strength, and balance. This approach helps to more clearly identify physical impairments and, in turn, lead to

---

Box 2. Members of a pain rehabilitation team

Physiatrists
Rehabilitation nurses
Physical therapists
Occupational therapists
Recreation therapists
Speech language pathologists
Psychologists
Nutritionists
Social workers
Vocational rehabilitation counselors

a more appropriate treatment plan. In addition, this article reviews individual team roles and treatment responsibilities. Various assessment techniques and treatment strategies are discussed. Finally, the application of the continuum of care is applied to acute and chronic pain conditions commonly encountered, including low back pain–related disorders, myofascial pain, and fibromyalgia (FM).

Management continuum for acute and chronic pain

In acute pain syndromes, the experience of pain is often directly linked to an underlying tissue injury. For example, an acute episode of low back pain may be due to a herniated fifth lumbar (L5) disc. Receptors in the outer annulus fibrosus of the disc and surrounding neural tissue transmit signals to the dorsal horn where the signals are first modulated [3] and then ascend to higher brain levels where the multidimensional experience of pain is perceived [4]. In treating patients who have acute pain syndromes, the three important goals are acute management, rehabilitation, and prevention of further, future injury. The acute pain and inflammation should initially be managed using the traditional acronym RICE: rest, ice, compression, and elevation. Oral medications, bracing, therapy, or injections can be used during the initial time following the injury to help alleviate symptoms and aid in the normal healing process. As symptoms begin to resolve, the next phase should focus on addressing factors that may have predisposed the patient to injury. Finally and most importantly, rehabilitation should be geared toward educating the patient about what they have to do to avoid incurring the same injury or similar injuries in the future.

For the patient who has an acute herniated L5 disc, initial management may include several days of relative rest, ice on the lower back, and possibly oral anti-inflammatory medications. Corticosteroid injections can be used to reduce inflammation in selected patients. Physical therapy focuses on normalizing range of motion (ROM) and emphasizing postures that will unload the herniated disc and facilitate healing. As symptoms resolve, biomechanical deficits that may have led to the disc herniation can be addressed. Some of these may include weakness in the core musculature; hamstring inflexibility; decreased hip ROM, causing increased stress on the lumbar spine; previous injury elsewhere in the kinetic chain, resulting in maladaptive adaptations; or poor lifting biomechanics. At the conclusion of treatment, the patient is given recommendations about exercises and lifestyle modifications to help reduce the likelihood of recurrence of the disc herniation.

Patients who fail to see a complete resolution of pain may continue to experience pain and develop psychologic and social distress. A more comprehensive approach is in order when dealing with patients who have persistent pain. In effectively managing chronic pain, the biomedical model of injury is inadequate due to its focus on biologic determinants of disease and illness while inherently ignoring psychologic and behavioral aspects of pain and pain-related suffering. A biopsychosocial approach, as described by Engel [5], equally embraces the physiologic, psychologic, and social determinants of illness and serves as the foundation of the multidisciplinary and interdisciplinary pain continuum [6,7].

The role of the physician

The first role of the physician in the management of patients who have pain is to establish a complete and accurate diagnostic assessment. Without a clear diagnosis or an understanding of contributing musculoskeletal impairments, rehabilitation is not likely to be effective and could possibly contribute to ongoing pain or re-injury. Arriving at this diagnosis involves a complete history, a comprehensive physical assessment, and appropriate use of laboratory and radiologic testing. After a diagnosis is reached, the physician develops a comprehensive plan of care, prioritizing short- and long-term goals. Individual treatment plans focus on a wide range of areas including a rational pharmacotherapy approach (ie, analgesia, improved mood, and restoring quality sleep); physical or occupational therapy; cognitive and behavioral treatments (ie, counseling and relaxation training); vocational rehabilitation; and patient education. The physiatric approach encourages a stepwise approach that starts with exercise and noninvasive means and progresses to more interventional procedures when necessary as a means of more aggressively controlling pain and helping the patient progress through active therapies. Finally, re-introduction of previous leisure and sport activities is pursued with progression guided by the therapist.

A physiatric history

A physiatric pain history starts like any standard evaluation of pain. This evaluation includes identifying the onset of the pain, precipitating events, location, character, quality, and relieving and exacerbating factors, with an additional focus on pain-related functional changes. Previous diagnostic tests and treatments are reviewed. The analysis of function may vary dramatically based on individual patient characteristics (ie, age, vocation, leisure interests, and medical comorbidities). For example, a treatment plan for a collegiate runner may focus entirely on returning the patient to a previous level of competitive running, whereas for a 70-year-old woman who has an acute thoracic compression fracture, her functional goals may include independently dressing herself and taking care of her home. A functional assessment may be done informally or by using a standardized scale. The Functional Independence Measure is commonly used by rehabilitation professionals (Box 3) [8]. Significant variability exists in chronic pain patients with regard to how one's individual pain condition affects function. For example, consider a 40-year-old male construction worker who has severe, progressive low back pain. He reports additional frustration with his

---

Box 3. Levels of functional independence by the Functional Independence Measure

Complete dependence
1. Total assistance: subject does <25% with assistance
2. Maximal assistance: subject does 25%–50% with assistance

Modified dependence
3. Moderate assistance: subject does 50%–75% with assistance
4. Minimal assistance: subject does 75%–100% with assistance
5. Supervision: subject does 100% without assistance but needs supervision

Independence
6. Modified independence: independent with assistive devices
7. Complete independence: independent without devices and performs tasks timely and safely

---

Scores are assessed for various activities of daily living including self-care, bowel and bladder management, transfers, ambulation, communication, and social integration.

---

inability to tolerate his normal required physical job demands and fears possible job termination. The assessment may include identifying more specific job demands, conditions at the workplace, and job-related stressors and work relationships (ie, patient–employer, coworkers). Another patient, an elderly woman who has progressive left hip osteoarthritic pain, reports having more difficulty caring for herself due to difficulty dressing herself and loss of mobility due to worsening walking tolerance. Her assessment may focus more on difficulty with specific tasks that she encounters on a daily basis. With that information, the physical examination may more specifically examine hip and lumbar ROM, functional mobility, balance, and ability to rise efficiently from a seating position. In turn, treatment may first focus on adaptive equipment for dressing, initiating gait training exercises, and providing the patient the necessary resources for assisting her with community transportation.

Finally and most importantly, the physiatric history assesses for the factors that will serve to motivate the patient to reach their goals. Consider a competitive runner who has an overuse injury. Runners, like many athletes, are often willing to accept a certain amount of pain or injury to continue training. Suggesting relative rest to this patient as a means of helping to limit injury may not be successful; however, emphasizing how a more balanced training regimen can improve the patient's long-term performance may allow for a paradigm shift, leading to a change in behavior and a successful rehabilitation outcome.

Comprehensive physical assessment

Physical examination

A physiatric musculoskeletal examination includes a complete examination of the painful area including bony structures, cartilage, joints, ligaments, tendons, bursa, nerves, and skin. Equally important is a more global evaluation of posture, core strength, balance, and gait. Performing a proficient physical examination is a fundamental part of identifying pain generators, diagnosing and identifying potential areas of dysfunction, narrowing the clinical differential diagnosis, and establishing a rational treatment plan. The following sections describe important aspects of a global musculoskeletal assessment and how the findings of this examination can help guide treatment.

Illness behavior

Although often overlooked or recorded in routine examinations and reports, patient "pain behaviors" ("illness behavior") are important parts of the comprehensive chronic pain assessment. Pain behaviors are based on operant contingency models of reinforcement and act as a means for the patient to communicate to the environment that he or she is experiencing pain or distress [9]. These behavioral manifestations of pain (ie, grimacing, complaining, and inactivity) may be positively reinforced, for example, by obtaining attention from family members and being excused from undesirable obligations such as work or pain-provoking activities. Many times, these reinforcement contingencies remain long after the precipitation injury (ie, tissue trauma) has resolved. Other pain behaviors include guarding, bracing, rubbing the painful area, facial grimacing, and sighing [10,11]. Pain behaviors have been found to correlate with self-report measures of pain intensity, pain disability, and self-efficacy [12] and may serve as targets for cognitive and behavioral treatment and, in turn, be "unlearned."

Waddell and Main [13] described illness behavior as "what people say and do to express and communicate they are ill." They classically described five general categories of nonanatomic signs (tenderness, simulation, distraction, regional complaints, and over-reaction) in patients who have low back pain and have what are commonly referred to as Waddell signs (WS) (Box 4) [11]. In their initial study, Waddell and Main [13] found that patients who displayed at least three signs were more likely to have evidence of psychosocial distress. These signs were not intended to be signs of, or a test for, malingering (the intentional production of false or grossly exaggerated physical or psychologic symptoms). It is unfortunate that WS have been routinely used in this regard in clinical practice, something that should be done with significant caution. Controlled studies have demonstrated no consistent evidence that WS are associated with malingering or secondary gain, which is defined as interpersonal advantages that one obtains as the result of injury or disease [14]. Pain behaviors should be described on an individual basis as

---

Box 4. Waddell symptoms and signs

Waddell symptoms
1. Pain at the tip of the tailbone
2. Whole leg pain
3. Whole leg numbness
4. Whole leg giving way
5. Complete absence of any spells with very little pain in the last year
6. Intolerance of, or reactions to, many treatments
7. Emergency admission to hospital with simple backache

Waddell signs
1. Tenderness: superficial or nonanatomic
2. Simulation tests: axial loading or simulated rotation
3. Distraction tests: physical examination finding is retested with the patient distracted (ie, straight leg raise, seated and supine)
4. Regional changes: weakness or sensory change
5. Over-reaction: exaggerated response to physical examination

---

observed during the physical examination. Of interest, Fishbain and colleagues [15] demonstrated that WS were not associated with physician perception of effort exaggeration and found evidence that WS decreased with comprehensive pain treatment.

Posture

Posture is defined as the position of the body at one point in time and is influenced by each of the joints of the body. Proper posture is achieved when the joints line up in such a way as to create the least amount of stress and muscle activation as possible. Poor or dysfunctional postures promote abnormal stresses on the joints and can lead to tissue trauma and eventually pain. For example, forward flexed lumbar posture has been found to correlate with amount of vertebral pain, muscular impairments, motor function, and disability in elderly women [16]. In standing, normal posture includes cervical and lumbar lordosis and a slight thoracic kyphosis. In addition, the examiner should assess the position of the head in relation to the shoulders and assess more global, side-to-side asymmetries. For example, one may observe a superiorly positioned (elevated) right shoulder and a superior (elevated) left iliac crest due to pelvic obliquity and malalignment. Posture may be observed indirectly during the patient interview or formally during the physical examination. Exaggeration or flattening of the relatively normal cervical, thoracic, and lumbar curves is often seen in chronic spine and soft tissue injury conditions. Pelvic asymmetry has been shown to alter body mechanics in sitting and standing, placing various segments under strain, contributing to musculoskeletal pain [17]. It is important to evaluate the patient in his or her normal sitting position. Poor sitting posture places excess strain on multiple structures including the lumbar discs, cervical discs, and the low back and cervical musculature. Postural training, worksite evaluations, lumbar rolls, core strengthening, and stretching of tight musculature can help to improve poor sitting posture. Fig. 1 shows examples of normal and abnormal sitting postures.

Range of motion and muscle imbalances

ROM, muscle strength, and balance should be assessed because deficits in this area can affect a patient's ability to perform the activities of daily living and achieve efficient functional mobility. Active ROM, active assistive ROM, and passive ROM can be assessed for each joint. The examiner should note general hypermobility or hypomobility, side-to-side differences in ROM, and which of the movements result in pain. The findings on ROM testing combined with the results of manual muscle testing may lead to

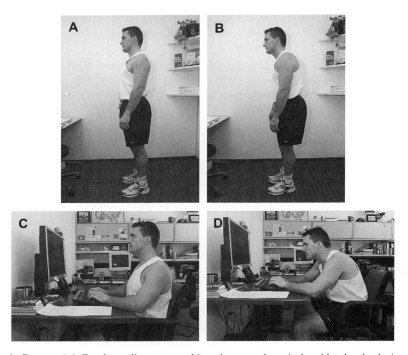

Fig. 1. Posture. (*A*) Good standing posture. Note the normal cervical and lumbar lordosis and thoracic kyphosis. (*B*) Poor standing posture. The shoulders are rounded forward. There is a loss of lumbar lordosis and an exaggeration of the thoracic kyphosis. (*C*) Good sitting posture. The normal cervical, thoracic, and lumbar curvatures are maintained. (*D*) Poor sitting posture. The shoulders are rounded forward. The there is a loss of the normal lumbar and thoracic curvatures. The neck is in compensatory hyperextension.

objective findings of muscle imbalances about a joint. This concept has been well described by Janda and colleagues [18–20] as the upper-crossed and pelvic-crossed syndromes. An upper-crossed syndrome is characterized by contracted and hypertonic postural muscles (pectoralis major and upper trapezius) and lengthened phasic muscles (rhomboids, serratus anterior, middle and lower trapezius), which may present with related neck and shoulder pain and headaches. Pelvic-crossed syndrome is characterized by contracted hip flexors and lumbar extensors and weak, lengthened phasic muscles (abdominals and gluteus maximus) and may present with chronic low back and buttock pain.

Core strength

The "core" has been likened to a box, with the abdominal muscles in the front, the diaphragm as the roof, and the pelvic floor and hip muscles as the bottom. It includes more than 20 pairs of muscle groups that stabilize spinal structures and the pelvis and coordinate movements during functional tasks such as bending, lifting, and squatting [21]. Efficient functioning of the core helps to distribute, absorb, and limit translational and shearing forces. The outer, more superficial group of muscles is composed of predominantly fast-twitch fibers. These muscles are therefore capable of producing large torque forces, greater speed, and larger arcs of motion (Box 5). The deeper muscles lay closer to the spine and are composed predominantly of slow twitch muscle fibers. These muscles help control segmental motion and help maintain mechanical stiffness of the spine. In one study, operative patients who had unilateral low back pain had evidence of ipsilateral multifidi atrophy (10%–30%) compared with the contralateral side [22]. Weakness of these deep core muscles has been implicated as a precipitator and contributor to the development of chronic low back pain.

There are several ways to assess for core strength. A commonly used test is assessing for Trendelenberg's sign during a single-leg stance (Fig. 2). The

---

Box 5. Core muscles

Superficial core musculature
Rectus abdominus
Erector spinae
External obliques

Deep core musculature
Transverse abdominus
Multifidi
Internal obliques
Deep transversospinalis
Pelvic floor musculature

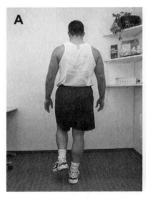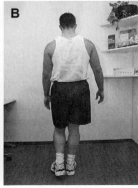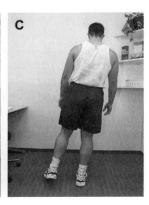

Fig. 2. Trendelenberg's sign. (*A*) Patients who do not have hip gluteus medius weakness are able to maintain the alignment of the hips during a single-leg stance. Note that the iliac crests are at the same level on the left and the right. (*B*) Note the subtle drop of the pelvis on the left. This drop occurs with right gluteus medius weakness and is called the Trendelenberg's sign. (*C*) Patients who have gluteus medius weakness often walk with a compensated Trendelenberg's gait. During stance phase of the affected side, the patient leans the trunk over the stance leg to gain stability and circumducts the contralateral leg.

examiner stands behind the patient and asks him or her to stand on the leg that is being assessed. In an individual who does not have hip weakness, the pelvis remains level. In a patient who has gluteus medius weakness, however, the contralateral hip drops because the ipsilateral hip abductor is not sufficiently strong to stabilize the pelvis. Another test that can be easily performed in the clinic is the "bridge" (Fig. 3). The patient lies supine with his or her knees and hips flexed and feet on the table. The patient then lifts the pelvis while keeping the upper back and feet stabilized on the examination table. The examiner looks for any unsteadiness or pelvic tilting. To make the test more difficult or to assess for more subtle weakness, the patient can additionally be asked to lift one leg off the table and maintain the leg in alignment with the contralateral femur.

Balance and stability

A closely related concept to core strength is balance and stability. Patients who have weak core musculature often demonstrate deficits in this area. These deficits may lead to increased stress in other parts of the body and an increased risk of injury. Tissue injury may then result in more core weakness and instability, resulting in a vicious cycle. In one study, patients who had low back pain demonstrated less balance and postural stability than those who did not have low back pain [23]. In addition, anticipatory postural adjustments, those that precede voluntary movements to stabilize the spine, are abnormally coordinated in patients who have chronic low back pain, primarily due to impaired deep trunk muscle strength [24,25].

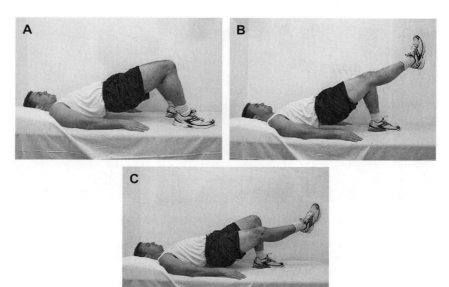

Fig. 3. The "bridge." (*A*) The patient lies supine with knees flexed and feet on the table. The patient elevates the pelvis while maintaining a neutral spine and pelvic alignment. (*B*) To make the exercise more difficult, the patient can alternatively elevate the right and left legs while maintaining the pelvic alignment. (*C*) When core weakness is present, the patient will not be able to maintain the neutral pelvic alignment.

Balance can be assessed in various ways. A simple method is to have the patient stand on one leg. A patient who has impaired balance may be unsteady, sway, or be unable to safely lift up one leg without losing balance. If the patient is able perform a single-leg stance without difficulty, then the exercise can be made more challenging by having the patient stand on one leg and perform a single-leg squat. Patients who have poor balance often flail their arms and go into excessive genu valgum (knee angles medial compared with foot) as they "corkscrew" through the ROM (Fig. 4). To detect differences in balance in athletes or well-conditioned individuals, the maneuver may be progressed to a more challenging level by having the patient extend the unsupported leg out into the frontal, sagittal, and transverse planes or by having the patient close his or her eyes.

Gait

Normal gait may be categorized into two phases and seven parameters (Box 6) [26]. Understanding the normal gait cycle helps the examiner identify gait deviations that occur in common pathologic conditions. For example, in a normal individual, stance phase represents 60% of the gait cycle, whereas swing phase represents 40% of the gait cycle. Often, with acute

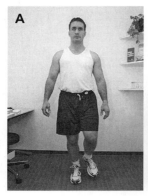 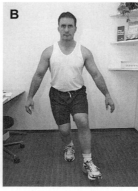 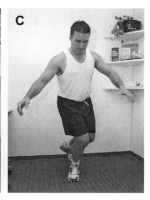

Fig. 4. Single-leg stance and single-leg squat. (*A*) Patients who have good balance will be able to perform the maneuver without falling and with minimal swaying. (*B*) To make the test more difficult, a single-leg squat can be performed. Note that the knee, foot, and hip alignment are maintained. (*C*) Patients who have poor core strength and impaired balance often "corkscrew" as they perform the squat. Notice the pronation, genu valgum, hip rotation, and flailing arms.

or chronic pain conditions in the lower extremity, an antalgic gait pattern is seen. On the affected side, less time is spent in stance phase as the patient shifts his or her weight to the contralateral side to avoid pain. This pain-avoidance pattern can cause problems in other areas including the

---

Box 6. Phases of gait and important gait parameters

Phases of gait
Stance: 60% of the walking cycle; shortened on the painful side
Swing: 40% of the walking cycle; lengthened on the painful side

Important parameters of gait
Width of support: distance between feet; normally 2–4 inches; larger when pathology of the dorsal columns or an ataxic gait is present
Step length: distance between sequential corresponding points of contact by opposite feet; normally 14–16 inches
Step length: shortened on the pain-free side
Stride length: distance between sequential corresponding points of contact by the same foot; normally 30 inches
Pelvic and trunk rotation: helps to elongate the leg, increasing step length and stride length
Cadence: number of steps per minute; normally 100 steps per minute
Center of gravity: 2 inches anterior to the second sacral vertebrae

compensated hip, knee, and ankle joint or related soft tissue structures. Another common gait deviation is the compensated Trendelenberg's gait. Consider a patient who has right gluteus medius weakness resulting in a positive Trendelenberg's sign and poor balance when performing a single-leg stance. To maintain the contralateral hip in alignment during stance phase, the patient often leans over the affected hip to compensate for the weak hip abductors. The patient may also circumduct or swing the contralateral leg to prevent dragging the foot (see Fig. 4).

When possible, gait should be assessed when the patient enters the examination room. Subsequently, a more detailed examination of gait can be performed with the formal examination, looking for inconsistencies. For a complete assessment of gait, the patient should be without shoes or socks and wearing minimal clothing, allowing the examiner to assess the shoulders, low back, hips, knees, ankles, and feet. Successive trials should be performed and the examiner should assess each of these joints independently. It is important to remember that gait deviations in one area usually affect other areas of the body. For example, a significant pes planus (flat foot) can affect the forces at the knee and at the hip during gait. A hip flexion contracture results in excessive lumbar lordosis (extension of the lumbar spine relative to the sacrum and pelvis) and can exacerbate painful low back pain conditions such as facet arthropathy due to increased forces and strain through the facet joints caused by relative hyperextension of the lumbar spine as a means of maintaining standing posture.

Kinetic chain

After the completion of the musculoskeletal examination, having a firm understanding of the kinetic chain helps the clinician to interpret the patient's deficits and to develop a treatment regimen. The kinetic chain concept is based on the fundamental premise that for functional movement in space, each link of the body must move in a coordinated manner. The sequence of the links and the inter-relationship of muscle activation and translation of forces within the body are referred to as the kinetic chain [27]. Each link of this system creates force and energy that are ultimately transferred from the proximal core stabilizing link to the distal peripheral link. When one link is weak or injured, other links compensate. Distal links typically compensate for proximal links, and the added stress and loads result in further injury. For instance, if a patient has weak hip abductors, the knee often has to absorb more of the forces during gait. If the patient also has a tendency to overpronate (flat-foot position), then the forces in the knee are increased. Malalignment of the foot may lead to changes at the knee such as excessive patellofemoral joint pressures and abnormal patellar tracking. Patellar tracking is described as dynamic movement of the kneecap, with its insertion to the tibia and muscle attachment to the quadriceps during extension and flexion of the knee. Hence, proper rehabilitation of patellofemoral joint pain must address factors along the kinetic chain—that is, proximally to the knee (strengthening of the quadriceps, gluteus muscle groups, and hip external rotators) and distally (correcting pronation at the foot) [28].

The role of the therapists

Physical and occupational therapy

Physical therapy is an indispensable part of the treatment continuum. Physical therapists (PTs) and occupational therapists (OTs) use therapeutic exercises, manual techniques, and passive physical modalities to address deficits in flexibility, strength, balance, neuromuscular control, posture, functional mobility, locomotion, and endurance. Both types of therapists also help patients to overcome fear of movement and activity-related pain. Although there is some crossover between the skill sets of PTs and OTs, they possess established core competencies that are fairly universal. PTs specialize in gait training and locomotion, core stability, and activities of daily living such as bed mobility and transfers. They are also experts in the development of aerobic conditioning programs aimed at improving cardiopulmonary health and endurance. OTs typically focus on educating patients regarding proper posture and ergonomics related to upper-limb functional activities such as lifting and computer usage. They address upper-extremity–related activities of daily living including feeding, hygiene, grooming, bathing, and dressing. PTs and OTs also play a primary role in the education of patients, family members, and other caregivers.

PTs and OTs involved in interdisciplinary chronic pain treatment programs must be adept in their ability to assess initial levels of functional ability and then monitor and progressively increase the level and complexity of therapeutic exercises. Most chronic pain patients have secondary impairments in addition to their primary pain-related diagnoses (ie, general inflexibility, deconditioning, myofascial pain, and other postural abnormalities), which are important focuses of treatment. OTs may instruct patients on proper pacing techniques, graded-activity tolerance training, and energy conservation techniques as they apply to physical demands of a task or job.

Recreation therapists

Therapeutic recreation specialists are important members of the rehabilitation team and key team members who help restore patients to previous levels of function that are often lost due to the development of chronic pain. A recreation therapist assessment examines previous patient interests and patient barriers to return to leisure activities. Within a formal program, recreation therapists evaluate and plan leisure activities that serve to promote mental and physical health. Recreation therapists help patients to incorporate strategies learned from various disciplines of multidisciplinary treatment into social and community functions. Application of these techniques in the community and at home (ie, correct biomechanics, pacing, relaxation techniques) leads to the reduction of stress, fear of movement, and depression while fostering a feeling of self-efficacy and confidence. In addition, therapeutic recreation specialists help patients to increase social awareness and promote integration of individuals back into the community.

Treatment modalities used by physical and occupational therapists

Exercise

An exercise regimen specifically tailored to the patient is at the core of a physical or occupational therapy program. Daily exercise is important in maintaining physical health and has been associated with 25% less self-reported musculoskeletal pain (compared with more sedentary control subjects) [29]. In addition, inactivity has been shown to be a predictor of future pain with injury [30]. The therapist usually starts with a prescription from the physician outlining the important diagnoses and the goals of treatment. The therapist then performs his or her own assessment and develops a plan of care. During each session, the therapist works closely with the patient to help alleviate pain and to address physiologic deficits. The goal of treatment is to provide the patient with a home exercise program that can be continued after completion of formal therapy.

Stretching

Until ROM is normalized or near normalized, movement patterns cannot be retrained and strengthening cannot be performed within the physiologic range. Stretching is a key component to restoring normal ROM. When done properly, stretching lengthens tissue including skin, fascia, muscle, and ligaments, thereby increasing overall ROM. Increased ROM decreases contracture, improves functional mobility, and allows the muscles and joints to function properly. ROM exercises vary from passive (in which there is no voluntary muscle contraction and with the application of total external force) to active assisted (in which there is partial contraction and external force) and active (in which there is complete contraction and no external force). In general, most ROM exercises increase blood flow and prevent contracture.

Muscle conditioning

After ROM is normalized, muscle conditioning is addressed because muscles around a joint impact stability, function, and pain. Muscle conditioning comprises three important areas: strength, endurance, and re-education.

Muscle strength is increased through isometric, isotonic, or isokinetic exercises. Isometric strengthening is characterized by contraction of the muscle without change in length or movement. Isometric exercises are typically used in acute pain states such as active inflammation or induced immobilization. Isotonic exercises are those in which muscles contract and the length and movement change but the load remains the same, such as doing a bicep curl with a dumbbell. In contrast, with isokinetic exercise, muscle contracts at a constant angular velocity, such as with a cybex or muscle pulley machine. Muscle strengthening depends on vascularization, energy metabolism, increase in number of myofibrils, and motor unit recruitment. Strengthening muscle tissue results from increasing the load, speed, number, frequency, form, or ROM of the exercise.

Muscle endurance—the ability to sustain and perform repeated contractions—is increased through aerobic activity. Aerobic activity is defined by low-intensity, high-repetition exercise. Walking, running, cycling, and swimming are some examples of aerobic activity used in physical therapy programs. The physiologic changes that occur with aerobic training are numerous and include an increased capillary density around muscle fibers, an increased number of mitochondria, increased activity of mitochondrial enzymes, and increased myoglobin content. Aerobic exercise is also associated with increased levels of endogenous endorphins [31] and enkephalins [32] and may be responsible for an additional antinociceptive or analgesic effect.

Motor re-education may also be simulated with exercise and is often co-ordinated by the therapist as the patient progresses in treatment. Motor re-education involves breaking down a motion into individual chronologic movements. The therapist assists the patient in identifying and then unlearning potentially abnormal movement patterns. Proper posture and retraining of movements are practiced and incorporated into the general strengthening, endurance, and flexibility program [28].

Aquatic therapy

Aerobic and anaerobic exercise can be performed in an aquatic environment. The physiologic advantages of water as a therapeutic medium include thermal conductive properties and high specific heat. The viscosity of water provides resistance for aerobic and strengthening exercises, compressive forces that help to decrease edema, and buoyancy that decreases weight bearing [33]. Therapeutically, aquatic therapy may help in decreasing muscle and joint stiffness and decreasing pain. Hydrostatic forces with immersion in water lead to cardiopulmonary benefits secondary to centralization of blood flow, resulting in increased venous return, stroke volume, cardiac output, and subsequent reflex bradycardia [34,35]. Patients participating in an aquatic therapy program more than 2 days per week as part of a long-term maintenance treatment program demonstrated reduction in pain and improved function [36]. Pool programs are often offered in group settings, providing an added social benefit for the patient.

Mind–body therapy

Mind–body therapy is defined by the National Institutes of Health as an intervention that may "use a variety of techniques designed to facilitate the mind's capacity to affect bodily function and symptoms." Various mind–body treatments may help to improve coordination, decrease abnormal movement patterns, and improve psychologic well-being and include tai chi, body awareness therapy (BAT), and Feldenkrais (FK).

Tai chi, a traditional Chinese mind–body relaxation exercise, consists of approximately 108 intricate exercise sequences performed in a slow, relaxed manner. Tai chi has been found to increase physical and mental health, including physical, social, and emotional function; decrease anxiety; decrease pain perception; and increase flexibility and balance [37–39]. In addition, this mind–body therapy combines the mind with movement to reprogram the nervous system, improve coordination, reduce abnormal motor patterns, and improve physical and emotional health.

BAT and FK are therapies that use patterns of movement to improve flexibility, posture, breathing, and overall function. BAT and FK have been shown to increase body awareness and decrease pain [40]. In addition, BAT and FK improve health-related quality of life and self-efficacy of pain to a higher degree than conventional physiotherapy [41].

Passive modalities

A modality describes any physical agent used to produce a physiologic response in a targeted tissue. Commonly prescribed passive physical modalities for the treatment of acute and chronic pain include cryotherapy, heat, and electrical stimulation. Modalities are initially incorporated into therapy sessions by PTs or OTs, with a goal of educating the patient on appropriate application and use at home. Depending on the specific pain complaint, modalities may be incorporated early in treatment in acute conditions as a means of decreasing local swelling, as analgesia, and to help progression and tolerance of therapies (Boxes 7 and 8, Tables 1 and 2) [42,43]. They are also used as part of a daily treatment regimen (eg, cryotherapy to osteoarthritic knee after exercise, electrical stimulation to low back region during prolonged upright postures) or as a "rescue" treatment for "flare ups."

Electrical stimulation

Transcutaneous electrical nerve stimulation (TENS) and interferential current therapy (ICT) involve the transmission of electrical energy to the peripheral nervous system by way of an external stimulator and conductive gel pads on the skin. TENS is based theoretically on the "gate control theory" proposed by Melzack [44]. TENS stimulates non-nociceptive large afferent A-β fibers "closing" the "gate" of facilitated sensory input, normally "opened" by small-diameter nociceptive C fibers. Electrical stimulation

Box 7. Cryotherapy

Indication
Acute injury
Muscle spasticity
Osteoarthritis
Minor burns
Arthritis
Bursitis
Acute/chronic pain
Myofascial pain
Contusion inflammation

Effect
Analgesia
Vasoconstriction
Decreases muscle spindle
Decreases nerve conduction
Decreases metabolism
Decreases enzymatic activity
Increases tissue stiffness
Increases viscosity

Example
Ice
Cold pack
Cryotherapy compression unit
Whirlpool bath
Vapo-coolant spray

Contraindication
More than 30 minutes
Ischemia/arterial insufficiency
Raynaud's disease
Impaired sensation
Burns
Cryoglobulinemia
Paroxysmal cold hemoglobinuria
Cold allergy or hypersensitivity

releases endogenous opioids and activates peripherally located α_{2A}-adrenergic receptors [45]. TENS has been shown to be beneficial in acute pain states, reducing the amount of analgesic medication consumed after surgical procedures, and in chronic pain conditions in which it helps to relieve pain and foster patient independence (see Table 2).

Box 8. Heat

Indication
Chronic inflammation
Arthritis
Myofascial pain
Collagen vascular disease
Strains
Sprains
Contracture thrombophlebitis

Effect
Analgesia
Vasodilation, increases blood flow
Increases oxygen and leukocytes
Muscle relaxation
Increases metabolism
Increases capillary permeability
Increases collage extensibility

Contraindication
Acute trauma, inflammation
Bleeding disorders
Edema, scars, impaired sensation
Malignancy
Multiple sclerosis

ICT is a variant of TENS that involves the mixing of two unmodulated sine waves with different frequencies (one at 4 kHz and a second within a variable range) to generate frequencies between 4 and 250 Hz. ICT allows for the stimulation of deeper tissues with decreased discomfort. The proposed mechanism of action involves the direct stimulation of muscle fibers, as opposed to nerve fibers, to achieve improved muscle blood flow and to promote the healing process. Variable frequency helps to prevent adaptation. There is less scientific evidence for the use of ICT compared with TENS.

Manual techniques

Manual techniques may include a number of different approaches for the treatment of acute and chronic pain such as massage, mobilization, and manipulation. Massage therapy has various physiologic effects. The effects of massage can be classified into reflexive and mechanical. Reflexive effects include vasodilatation, resulting in improvement in circulation, endogenous opioid release, and general relaxation. Mechanical effects include assisting

Table 1
Superficial and deep heat therapy

	Composition	Effect	Contraindication
Superficial heat[a]			
Hydrocollator packs	Bags of silicone dioxide heated in stainless steel containers in water 65–90°C	Increases temperature 3.3°C at 1 cm	—
	Applied to body part over towels	Increases temperature 1.3°C at 2 cm [42]	
Paraffin	Paraffin wax and mineral oil in 7:1 ratio heated to 52°C	Increases temperature 5.5°C in forearm subcutaneous tissue	—
	Body part dipped in bath, wax hardens, repeated 7–12 times, then wrapped in plastic and covered by towel	Increases temperature 2.4°C in brachioradialis muscle	
Hydrotherapy			
Whirlpool	Water heated to 40°C (body submersion)	Heats, messages, debrides	—
Hubbard tank	Water heated to 43°C (limb submersion)	Can elevate core temperature depending on surface area	
Fluidotherapy	Hot air blown through medium of dry powder or glass beads at a temperature of 46°C–49°C	Produces temperature of 42°C in hand and joint capsule	—
		Produces temperature of 39.5°C in foot and joint capsule [43]	
Deep heat[b]			
Ultrasound [c]	Electrical current applied to quartz crystal or ceramic	Produces acoustic vibration above the audible range	Heat contraindications
	Heat greatest at areas of impedance: bones > tendon > skin > muscle		Near brain or spine
			Near heart

Table 1 (*continued*)

	Composition	Effect	Contraindication
			Near reproductive organs
			Near pacemakers
			Near tumors
			Gravida or menstruating uterus
			Eyes
			Immature epiphysis
			Arthroplasty

[a] Depth of 0.5–2 cm; amount of heating depends on amount of adipose tissue present.

[b] Depth of 0.5–2 cm; amount of heating depends on amount of adipose tissue present. Heating is by conversion.

[c] Intensity of 0.8–3 W/cm^2; Frequency of 0.8–1 MHz.

venous return and lymphatic drainage, decreasing muscle tightness, and braking adhesions in muscles, tendons, and ligaments. In addition, there is likely a beneficial psychologic effect of massage, which can result in a general sense of well-being. Although massage can produce short-term results, studies have demonstrated mixed results with regard to long-term efficacy [46,47]. Various studies have demonstrated the magnitude of pain reduction as modest [48] and transient between sessions [49]. Diagnostic technique and treatment methods may vary among professional groups (ie, manual therapist, chiropractors, and osteopathic physicians), leading to a difference in treatment outcomes and results of clinical trials [50].

Mobilization involves passive movement of tissue within the limit of joint range. Manipulation may include similar soft tissue techniques in addition to high-velocity techniques whereby forces are generated at a particular joint level beyond physiologic barrier of joint restriction and is more commonly

Table 2
Transcutaneous electrical nerve stimulation

Tens type	Amplitude/ frequency	Indication	Duration	Setting changes
Conventional (low-intensity, high-frequency)	1–2 mA/ 50–100 Hz	Acute pain state	1–20 min for rapid relief 30 min to 2 h for short duration of analgesia Repeat as needed	Increase amplitude or pulse width to avoid adaptation and maintain analgesia
Dense-disperse/ acupuncture-like (high-intensity, low-frequency)	15–20 mA/ 1–5 Hz	Chronic pain state	30 min for short duration 2–6 h for long duration Once daily	Minimal adaptation

practiced by chiropractic practitioners and osteopathic physicians [51]. Geisser and colleagues [52] found manual therapy with specific adjuvant exercise to be beneficial in treating chronic low back pain with no significant change in function. Others have demonstrated efficacy of spinal manipulation in short-term studies, although the effect size was small compared with active therapies [53] and placebo [54]. Osteopathic manipulation in a study of subacute low back pain patients demonstrated similar results compared with standard medical care but also used less physical therapy and medications [55].

Pain psychologists

Psychologic factors have been shown to predict long-term disability and contribute to the transition of acute pain to chronic pain [56]. One's cognitions may also impact mood, behavior, and function [57]. Pain psychology assessment and intervention focuses on cognitive and behavioral factors related to pain.

Psychologic interventions are focused on unlearning maladaptive responses and reactions to pain while fostering wellness, improving coping and perceived control, and decreasing catastrophizing. In addition, cognitive interventions focus on fear-avoidance beliefs, a construct that has been closely linked to self-reported disability and physical performance in chronic pain [58,59]. The benefits of cognitive behavioral therapy (CBT) in treating multiple dimensions of chronic pain have been supported by numerous reviews and meta-analyses [60–62]. Coping skills training can be integrated into CBT, focusing on attention-diversion techniques, altering activity patterns, and altering negative-related emotions [63]. The pain psychologists also can contribute to the team as a facilitator of group education classes related to pain and as a guide in relaxation training classes. Formal multidisciplinary and interdisciplinary psychologic treatment may also incorporate family counseling and help to coordinate ongoing psychologic treatment with community counselors at the completion of formal program treatment.

Clinical conditions

This section reviews theoretic issues related to underlying mechanisms of common pain conditions (osteoarthritis [OA], low back pain, myofascial pain, and FM) and principles guiding active physical medicine approaches. In many cases, theses same principles can be applied to other acute and chronic pain conditions.

Osteoarthritis

OA is characterized by an ongoing pathophysiologic cycle. Here, compensatory guarding and pain lead to a loss of ROM, decreased strength and endurance, increasing joint contracture and subsequent development of abnormal posture and motor patterns, joint overload, further joint destruction, and pain. Active therapy is aimed at unloading the joint, improving local muscle condition, and increasing joint and muscle flexibility. Because muscles provide the "dynamic" joint stability during movement, signs of OA, such as osteophytes and capsular thickening, may develop to increase stability when there is muscle dysfunction and dynamic instability. For example, although controversial, it has been proposed that quadriceps dysfunction and weakness may be a risk factor for progression of knee OA [64]. It was found that independent of body weight, knee extensor strength was 18% lower at baseline in women who developed knee OA compared with controls [65]. Studies have shown that exercise programs resulting in increased quadriceps strength and joint position sense reduced pain and improved function. In addition, improvements in quadriceps sensorimotor function resulted in decreased disability in patients who had knee OA and who followed a standard daily exercise regime. In addition to strength, alignment is equally important for dynamic stability and proper functioning. Sharma and colleagues [66] found that quadriceps weakness was not related to progression of knee OA, except in lax and malaligned knees.

A knee orthosis may be helpful when malalignment or instability is present. An orthosis is any externally applied device used to modify structural and functional characteristics of the neuromuscular system [67]. Braces, neoprene sleeves, and foot orthotics have been found to be helpful in increasing stability and in decreasing pain of the knee. Braces and neoprene sleeves have been found to be better than medical treatment alone. Furthermore, braces are more effective than neoprene sleeves in improving stiffness, pain, and function [68]. Dynamic fluoroscopic imaging of braced knees has demonstrated clinically significant distraction between the tibial and femoral condyles [69]. In addition, proprioception, which is commonly reduced in those who have knee OA, is increased with the use of braces [70]. In addition, heel wedges and medial wedge insoles can improve abnormal biomechanics at the foot, ankle, and knee [71]. In addition to foot orthotics, walking aids such as canes, forearm crutches, and walkers are used in those who have OA and gait disturbances. Devices help to unload the joint, improve body mechanics, and decrease pain [72].

Strengthening and endurance exercise relieves symptoms in patients who have mild and moderate OA [73]. Studies have shown that aerobic walking and home-based quadriceps strengthening exercise reduce pain and disability from knee OA [74]. Aerobic exercise only, not strengthening, was found to significantly lower depressive symptoms in high- and low-depressive symptomatology subgroups. Intensity of the aerobic exercise was not a factor. Aerobic cycling at high and low intensities was found to be equally effective in improving functional status, gait, pain, and aerobic capacity with OA of the knee [75]. Thus, exercise appears to moderately decrease pain, increase quadriceps strength, and increase physical function [76]. Exercise has been shown to increase self-efficacy. Self-efficacy is the belief that one has the capabilities to execute the courses of action required to manage prospective situations [77]. In one study, when persons stopped exercising, self-efficacy beliefs declined—only to increase later after resuming exercise [78].

Although exercise is beneficial, it must be actively maintained. Long-term follow-up and compliance of patients who participated in a randomized 3-month intervention showed that the beneficial effects declined with time and disappeared during the 6-month follow-up period [79]. In another study [73], however, significant differences were found in measures of disability, physical performance, and pain after 18 months of exercise in patients who had knee OA. Exercise is also beneficial when combined with the manual therapy or passive movements the therapist uses to increase ROM. A randomized trial [80] compared manual therapy to the knee, hip, foot and ankle, or lumbar spine combined with exercises for lower-extremity strengthening, ROM, and endurance with placebo ultrasound treatment. Significant improvements in pain, the 6-minute walk test, and self-reported function scores were found in the manual therapy plus exercise group compared with the control group. Treatment effects remained at 1-year follow-up.

TENS use and aquatic therapy are also beneficial. TENS use had a positive effect that was greatest with high-intensity burst modes, repeated treatments, and when used for at least 4 weeks [81]. Aquatic therapy has been found to improve aerobic capacity, walk time, physical activity level, and depression in those who have OA [82]. In addition, those who have OA and rheumatoid arthritis have been able to reduce the amount of postural sway (a risk factor for fall) from 18% to 30% with a 6-week aquatic exercise program [33].

Low back pain

Physical therapy approaches for spine-related disorders

A number of active physical therapy treatments for spine-related conditions have demonstrated efficacy in decreasing pain and improving function [83]. The heterogeneous nature of underlying spinal conditions poses a challenge for determining the specific or multiple pain generators involved (ie, disc degeneration, herniation, nerve root compression, facet arthropathy, or sacroiliac dysfunction). From a more mechanical view of low back pain, several subgroups of low back pain exist and may benefit from different exercise treatments. Treatment approaches include cervical and lumbar ROM, stabilization exercises [84], flexion-based exercises (ie, Williams), specific directional preference exercises (ie, McKenzie-based treatment), and neurodynamic techniques. These techniques and underlying theories are reviewed briefly in the following sections, with the understanding of significant overlap and variability between deliveries by therapists.

Stabilization exercises

The concept of lumbar stability has been an area of extensive research for over 30 years. Initial theory was based on an understanding that pain in the spine was the result of gradual degeneration of joints and related soft tissue as a result of microtrauma and poor control of spinal structures, a dynamic process involving static positions and controlled movements [85]. Biomechanical changes of spine stability include postural and motor control that help to reduce tissue strain and provide efficient muscle action [86]. Panjabi [87] classically described a three-component, interdependent system comprising bone and ligamentous structures, muscles, and the neural control system. An important focus of spine stability for low back pain includes assessment and strengthening of core muscle groups, controlling intersegmental stability, and restoring motion [88].

A basic individualized physical therapy approach includes stretching tight or contracted muscles, activating inhibited muscles, and improving core strength. Exercises are commonly targeted on retraining the multifidus (back muscle) and transverses abdominus (a deep abdominal muscle) along with supplemented exercises for the pelvic floor and breathing control [21]. Therapists help to train patients to contract these muscles independently from more superficial muscles. As the patient progresses through core strengthening, balance and conditioning are incorporated into the exercise program. These exercises can be facilitated with the use of an exercise or medicine ball, balance boards, theraband elastic strips, and an air-filled plastic disc with adjustable inflations [89]. Research has suggested that stability exercises may prevent recurrence of pain and improve function in patients compared with control groups [84,90].

Directional preference

The concept of centralization, recognized and popularized by McKenzie [91], is based on the concept by which pain radiating from the cervical, thoracic, or lumbar spine is sequentially abolished, neurologic symptoms are decreased [92], or a reduction of symptoms is noted [93,94] distally to proximally in the affected limb or body region in response to spinal positions or maneuvers (ie, extension, flexion, side bending). Centralization phenomena can be reliably assessed, and because of its association with more favorable clinical outcomes (physical therapy and lumbar surgery), it can be used to guide treatment in selected patients [95–97].

Peripheralization, the opposite response, involves the distal spread of pain into the limb with similar positioning. Noncentralization has been shown to be a more reliable predictor of poorer outcomes in physical therapy and surgery. In the sole trial involving subacute pain [98], those who underwent a graded-activity program returned to work more quickly, had fewer absences during the next 2 years, and had improved back mobility and fitness.

Neurodynamic therapy

Neurodynamic therapy is based on the concept of altered mechanosensitivity of the damaged neurogenic tissue. It is based on a more comprehensive functional understanding of the peripheral and central nervous system plasticity. Classically, this is represented clinically by a positive straight-leg raise, identifying the possible presence of perineuritis. Maitland [99] more formally described this as the slump test (or seated straight-leg raise), which incorporates cervical flexion and ankle dorsiflexion as a means of assessing mechanosensitivity of neural structures within the spinal vertebral canal. Peripheral nerves may become pain generators due to related innervated connective tissue or injury processes along the nerve myelin sheath. Butler [100] described abnormal impulse-generating sites as areas of injury along the central nervous system where ion channels accumulate, leading to abnormal firing. Therapy is focused peripherally at decreasing the firing of abnormal impulse-generating sites by improving mobility of the nerve by decreasing tension or pressure along the perineural structures.

Exercise

Exercise benefits in low back pain treatment have been demonstrated with regard to improved muscle performance, strength, and endurance [59,101]. General exercise guidelines may be useful in developing an individual treatment program for acute and chronic pain conditions. The American College of Sports Medicine proposed three areas of focus, including (1) muscle strengthening, (2) flexibility training, and (3) cardiovascular endurance as discussed earlier in this article [102]. Exercise-based treatments may help to promote wellness rather than illness behavior [103] and empower patients to take a more active role in their progress toward improved function [59,104]. Meta-analysis and reviews have shown exercise-based treatment to be more effective at decreasing pain and improving function with chronic low back pain [105] compared with reviews of acute low back pain [106]. Of interest, a systematic review of exercise therapy concluded that specific back exercises should not be recommended for acute or chronic pain but that exercise in general may be beneficial as part of an active rehabilitation program [106]. Keller and colleagues [107] examined lumbar paraspinal muscle density—an indication of muscle strength—in patients who underwent lumbar fusion compared with a nonsurgical group. The nonsurgical group participated in a low-intensity exercise and cognitive behavioral interventional program. The exercise and cognitive intervention group demonstrated significant improvement in lumbar strength (increased by 30%) at 1 year compared with surgical counterparts. Lumbar fusion patients demonstrated a 10% reduction in muscle density, whereas the exercise group's muscle density remained unchanged. Other studies have also suggested that activity in general may itself be therapeutic in reducing pain and improving psychosocial functioning [108,109].

Myofascial pain syndrome

Myofascial pain syndrome (MPS) is characterized by tenderness in the muscle, characteristic pain referral patterns, and restriction of motion

[110]. MPS may be a primary source of pain or be present as part of a more complicated multifactorial pain condition. Trigger points are discrete, focal, hyperirritable spots located in a taut band of skeletal muscle that are painful on compression and may produce referred pain, referred tenderness, motor and or autonomic dysfunction, and autonomic dysfunction. Myofascial trigger points (MTrPs) may be classified as active or latent. Latent trigger points are tender to palpation and may be associated with restricted ROM and stiffness but are not associated with spontaneous complaints of pain. MTrPs are commonly found in postural muscles including the neck, shoulders, and pelvic girdle and in the upper trapezius, scalene, levator scapulae, quadratus lumborum, and lumbosacral muscles. MTrP may develop or be aggravated by acute tissue trauma, repetitive microtrauma, muscle deconditioning, postural abnormalities, poor sleep, or metabolic abnormalities (ie, vitamin deficiencies, hypothyroidism [111]). Occupational and recreational activities often precipitate or aggravate MPS. Common workplace activities such as holding a telephone receiver between the ear and shoulder, prolonged bending over a table, sitting in chairs with poor back support, improper height of arm rests and computer work stations, and moving boxes using improper body mechanics [112] may lead to musculoskeletal dysfunction and MPS (Table 3).

Diagnosis of MPS is primarily based on clinical findings. Clinically, confirmation of MPS is not related to any specific laboratory tests (eg, imaging studies, electromyography, or muscle biopsy). Assessment of posture, body mechanics, dynamic joint function, and palpation of MTrPs may help to confirm the diagnosis. In assessing active MTrPs, one palpates across muscle fibers, and feels for a "rope like" nodularity of tight muscle. These

Table 3
Soft tissue pain

Characteristic	Myofascial pain	Fibromyalgia
Clinical sign	Local tenderness	Local tenderness or diffuse pain
	Referred pain pattern	for 3 mo
	Trigger points	Tender points
	Pain in taut band of muscle	11 of 18 symmetric tender points
	Local twitch response	are positive
	"Jump sign"	
Sex predominance	Male = female	Female > male
Location	Occur in any muscle	Specific locations: fat pad,
	Asymmetric	epicondyle, joint, muscle
		insertion site, muscle
		Symmetric
Associated factors	Acute tissue trauma	Insidious cause of pain
	Repetitive microtrauma	Increase in pain sensitivity
	Muscle deconditioning	Sleep disturbance
	Postural abnormalities	Increase in catastrophizing
	Sensitized nerve foci	Decreased serotonin production

discrete areas may reproduce characteristic pain-referral patterns usually traveling in a proximal to distal direction. There may be a local "twitch response," characterized by a palpable and visible reflex contraction of involved muscle. A "jump sign" is a pain-related withdrawal reflex secondary to applied pressure to a painful MTrP.

Although the physical examination is sensitive and specific in diagnosing MPS, research has demonstrated fine-needle electromyographic findings characteristic of the disorder and may help to develop mechanistic strategies for pharmacologic and nonpharmacologic treatment. Abnormal acetylcholine release at the motor end plate, and end plate noise is more frequent in MTrPs than at end plates outside of the zone or MTrPs. End plate noise is characteristic but not diagnostic of MTrPs and may be increased in any situation in which there is a mechanical, chemical, or other noxious stimuli. With sustained acetylcholine release, sarcomeres shorten, which produces a "contraction knot." This increase in sarcomere activity results in an increase in energy consumption and a relative reduction in circulation, creating localized hypoxia and ischemia. Pronociceptive substances such as bradykinin, serotonin, and histamine are in turn released, sensitizing afferents and producing local tenderness. Central convergence and facilitation at the level of the dorsal horn leads to referred pain in adjacent myotomes and to expansion of receptive fields. Increased neuronal excitability at the level of the dorsal horn leads to the release of substance P and glutamate key players in the development and maintenance of central sensitization.

The autonomic nervous system may also be activated by neurovasoreactive substances (ie, bradykinin, substance P, serotonin, and histamine). With autonomic nervous system activation, more acetylcholine is released. Audette and colleagues [37], in a study of dry-needle treatment of MTrPs, found that bilateral motor unit activation was produced with unilateral needle stimulation of the symptomatic MTrP. Contralateral or mirror-image electromyographic activity may support the concept of abnormal central nervous system processing of sensory input at the level of the spinal cord as a key perpetuator of pain and muscle dysfunction. Clinically, ongoing psychologic stress, maladaptive posture, and elevated muscle tension may also contribute to the muscle pain dysfunction cycle [113].

Effective treatment of MPS focuses on pharmacologic and nonpharmacologic treatments including physical and occupational therapy, exercise, ergonomic assessment, relaxation and stress reduction training. Physical and occupational treatment goals include reducing pain, restoring ROM, and improving function. MTrP muscles fatigue more rapidly and recover more slowly. Therapies involve a graded stabilization and strengthening program. When strengthening is done too early, there is the risk for overload and compensation of other muscles, which may develop MTrP. In addition, physical and occupational therapy are important in helping to reduce fear of movement and are incorporated in a gradually progressive submaximal exercise program, helping the patient to gain confidence in independent movements. Muscle-release techniques and other self-management approaches are commonly included. Overall, stretching is the basis of all exercise programs for MPS because it is vital to reset the muscle fiber length. Aerobic exercises have been found to increase endogenous pain control, improve mood, have additive effects with physical therapy, and prevent recurrence of MPS.

Modalities, such as the spray and stretch technique, involve the therapist passively stretching the target muscle while simultaneously applying a local soft tissue coolant. Chemicals such as dichlorodifluoromethane-trichloromonofluoromethane or ethyl chloride spray produce a drop in skin temperature and temporary anesthesia, theoretically blocking the spinal stretch reflex and sensation of pain centrally. The muscle may then be passively stretched toward its normal length, inactivating trigger points, relieving spasm, and reducing referred pain.

Another commonly used modality, TENS, may be used for acute or chronic myofascial pain; see the earlier section "Electrical stimulation." High-frequency, high-intensity TENS has been shown to reduce pain in MPS. High-power ultrasound applied to the trigger points before stretching was found to be more effective than conventional ultrasound and to significantly decrease the length of therapy [114]. One study looked at the immediate effects of various physical therapeutic modalities on cervical myofascial pain and trigger-point sensitivity and found that hot pack plus active ROM plus ICT plus myofascial release technique was more effective for easing MTrP pain and increasing cervical ROM [115] than hot pack plus active ROM plus stretch and spray plus TENS, which was more effective than hot pack plus active ROM plus stretch and spray.

Interventional treatments such as trigger point injections and acupuncture have been found to be effective in treating MTrP. In comparative studies, dry needling was found to be as effective as injecting an anesthetic solution such as procaine or lidocaine. Postinjection soreness, however, was more intense and of longer duration than the soreness with lidocaine. In one study, 58% of subjects reported verbal rating scores (VRS) of 0 on a 0 to 10 scale immediately after trigger-point injection; 42% had minimal pain scores (1 to 2 on a 10-point VRS) [116]; however, overall pain relief did not differ, supporting the theory that mechanical disruption of the muscle fibers and the increase in blood flow is important in relieving pain. Porta [117], in a single-center randomized study, reported a greater reduction in pain in patients who had chronic MPS injected with botulinum toxin type A (BTX-A) compared with steroid. Pain-reduction gains continued at 60 days in the BTX-A group but decreased in the steroid-treated patients. BTX-A has been studied in other MPS-related disorders, showing efficacy in cervicogenic pain [118] and mixed outcomes with headache disorders [119–121]. BTX-A has been compared with dry needling and lidocaine trigger-point injections and has not been found to be cost-effective [63].

Fibromyalgia

FM syndrome (FMS), another common musculoskeletal pain disorder, may share some common characteristics with MPS and may coexist in patients; however, these disorders may remain distinct, although there may be significant sign and symptom overlap (see Table 3). FMS is characterized by widespread musculoskeletal pain (at least 3 months) and stiffness, with symmetrically distributed tender points (TPs) and associated symptoms (ie, irritable bowel/bladder syndrome, dysautonomia, cognitive and endocrine dysfunction, dizziness, cold intolerance, or mood disorder) [122].

Recent studies support evidence of central changes in brain processing [123] and neurochemical abnormalities (elevated excitatory neurotransmitter substance P [124], nitric oxide [125], and amino acids [126]) as possible mediators of peripheral and central sensitization.

TPs, distinguished from MTrPs associated with MPS, are characterized by eliciting pain with at least 4 kg of pressure to at least 11 or 18 muscle tendon sites, based on common research criteria [127]. Reported prevalence rates of FM are approximately 2% in the United States, including 3.4% of women and 0.5% of men [127]. FMS patients may have lowered mechanical and thermal pain thresholds and psychologic factors including increased levels of catastrophizing [128].

The comprehensive treatment of FM involves a balance between rational pharmacologic treatments, exercise, physical and occupational therapy, and patient education. This multidisciplinary approach has demonstrated successful treatment outcomes such as decreased depression, self-reported pain behaviors, observed pain behaviors, and myalgia scores [129].

FM was once considered a "nonrestorative sleep syndrome," and evidence exists that patients who have FM do not obtain adequate amounts of restorative non–rapid eye movement sleep [130], which may result from disorders of serotonin metabolism. Thus, encouraging proper sleep hygiene and restoring proper levels of serotonin and non–rapid eye movement sleep is important in reducing pain and fatigue.

Physical medicine approaches to managing FMS include a comprehensive program incorporating a range of pharmacologic and nonpharmacologic strategies including active physical therapy, exercise, cognitive and behavioral treatments, and patient education (Box 9) [131]. A recent study identified clusters of patients based on severity of TP tenderness, affective distress (depression and anxiety), and psychologic traits (sense of self-efficacy and catastrophizing) and may help to individually classify the level of clinical intervention needed [132].

Pharmacologic management is an important aspect in the treatment of FM and focuses on decreasing pain, improving mood, and restoring quality sleep. Medicines are focused on modulating levels of serotonin, norepinephrine, and substance P. The tricyclic antidepressants amitriptyline and cyclobenzaprine, taken at night [133], and tramadol [134] have been found to be

---

Box 9. Stepwise fibromyalgia management

Step 1
- Confirm the diagnosis.
- Explain the condition.
- Evaluate and treat comorbid illnesses such as mood disturbance and primary sleep disturbances.

Step 2
- Initiate trial of low-dose tricyclic antidepressant or cyclobenzaprine.
- Begin cardiovascular fitness exercise program.
- Refer patient for CBT or combine with exercise.

Step 3
- Make a specialty referral (eg, rheumatologist, physiatrist, psychiatrist, pain management).
- Conduct trials with selective serotonin reuptake inhibitor, serotonin and norepinephrine reuptake inhibitor, or tramadol.
- Consider a combination-medication trial or anticonvulsant.

---

effective. Selective serotonin reuptake inhibitors are helpful, and fluoxetine has been found to decrease fatigue, depression, and pain [135]. Newer pharmacologic agents that include serotonin norepinephrine dual-reuptake inhibitors, including venlafaxine and duloxetine, and pregabalin, an anticonvulsant and calcium channel modulator, may help to decrease central sensitization and have demonstrated efficacy in decreasing pain and improving sleep [131,136,137].

The pain and fatigue reported by individuals who have FM results in a relative sedentary lifestyle and, hence, a decrease in the fitness level of skeletal muscles. Low-intensity aerobic exercise regimens are effective in reducing the number of TPs in total myalgic scores and reducing TP tenderness, and improving aerobic capacity, physical function, subjective well-being, and self-efficacy. Aerobic exercise also has been found to be better than stretching in decreasing depression, pain, and the emotional aspects and mental health domains of the Medical Outcomes Study Short Form Survey (SF-36) [138].

FMS patients may have difficulty tolerating general exercise programs due to fatigue and muscle sensitivity. Gowans and deHueck [139] recommended that (1) exercise be initiated below the patient's capacity and increased gradually, (2) patients be aware of tolerable short-term increase in pain and fatigue after initiating exercise, and (3) capacity to exercise be increased over time, with similar or lower levels of pain.

Pool therapy has been found to improve cardiovascular capacity, walking time, number of days of feeling good, self-reported physical impairment, pain, anxiety, depression, and daytime fatigue in those who have FM [140].

CBT has been found to improve pain, fatigue, mood, and function in FMS [141]. In general, CBT includes three treatment components (educational phase, skills training, and application phase) focusing on changes in negative perceptions of pain, improved coping and relaxation strategy training, and relapse prevention [142]. Greater benefits of CBT may be found when used adjunctively with exercise and other active treatments [143].

Multidisciplinary tertiary center-based outpatient programs have also been found to be beneficial in patients who have FM by incorporating structured multimodal treatment (pharmacologic management, physical therapy and exercise, psychologic treatment, and education) [144]. A recent review found that multidisciplinary approaches were effective for decreasing pain, decreasing impact of FMS, and increasing self-efficacy and walk time [145]. Pfeiffer and colleagues [146] examined a 1.5-day multidisciplinary treatment program that incorporated educational and self-management sessions, physical and occupational therapy, and medical management and demonstrated a positive effect on impact of illness in FMS patients who did and did not have concomitant depression. In general, compared with pharmacologic treatment, nonpharmacologic treatment appears to be more efficacious in improving self-report of FMS symptoms than pharmacologic treatment alone [141].

Summary

A physical medicine and rehabilitation approach to acute and chronic pain syndromes includes a wide spectrum of treatment focus. Whether assessing or treating acute or chronic pain syndromes, management should include a biopsychosocial approach. Assessment may include a focused joint and functional examination including more global areas of impairment (ie, gait, balance, and endurance) and disability. More complicated multidimensional chronic pain conditions may require the use of a more collaborative continuum of multidisciplinary and interdisciplinary treatment approaches. Regardless of the scope of care that each individual patient requires, treatment options may include active physical therapy, rational polypharmacy, CBT, and the use of passive modalities. Treatment goals generally emphasize achieving analgesia, improving psychosocial functioning, and reintegration of recreational or leisure pursuits (ie, community activities and sports). Progress in all therapies necessitates close monitoring by the health care provider and necessitates ongoing communication between members of the treatment team. Although this article focuses on diagnoses related to acute and chronic low back pain, OA, and musculoskeletal disorders, assessment and treatment recommendations may be generalized to most other pain conditions.

References

[1] World Health Organization. International classification of impairments, disabilities, and handicaps. Geneva (Switzerland): WHO; 1980.

[2] Boon H, Verhoef M, O'Hara D, et al. From parallel practice to integrative health care: a conceptual framework. BMC Health Serv Res 2004;4:1–5.

[3] Wolf CJ, Costigan M. Transcriptional and posttranslational plasticity and the generation of inflammation. Proc Natl Acad Sci U S A 1999;96:7723–30.

[4] Price DD. Psychological and neural mechanisms of the affective dimension of pain. Science 2000;288:1769–72.

[5] Engel GL. The need for a new medical model: a challenge for biomedical science. Science 1977;196:129–36.

[6] Frey SG, Fordyce WE. Behavioral rehabilitation of the chronic pain patient. Annu Rev Rehabil 1983;3:32–63.

[7] Turk DC, Meichenbaum D, Genest M. Pain and behavioral medicine: a cognitive-behavioral perspective. New York: Guildford Press; 1983.

[8] Anonymous. Guide for the uniform data set for medical rehabilitation (adult FIM). Version 4.0. Buffalo (NY): State University of New York at Buffalo; 1993.

[9] Fordyce WE. Behavioral methods for chronic pain and illness. St. Louis (MO): Mosby; 1976.

[10] Keefe FJ, Block AR, Williams RB Jr, et al. Behavioral treatment of chronic low back pain: clinical outcome and individual differences in pain relief. Pain 1981;11(2):221–31.

[11] Turk DC, Wack JT, Kerns RD. An empirical examination of the "pain-behavior" construct. J Behav Med 1985;8:119–30.

[12] McCahon S, Strong J, Sharry R, et al. Self-report and pain behavior among patients with chronic pain. Clin J Pain 2005;21(3):223–31.

[13] Waddell G, Main CJ. Illness behavior. Edinburgh (UK): Churchill Livingstone; 1998.

[14] Fishbain DA, Rosomoff HL, Cutler RB, et al. Secondary gain concept: a review of the scientific evidence. Clin J Pain 1995;11:6–21.

[15] Fishbain DA, Cutler RB, Rosomoff HL, et al. Is there a relationship between nonorganic physical findings (Waddell Signs) and secondary gain/malingering? Clin J Pain 2004;20(6): 399–408.

[16] Balzini L, Vannucchi L, Benvenuti F, et al. Clinical characteristics of flexed posture in elderly women. J Am Geriatr Soc 2003;51(10):1419–26.

[17] Al-Eisa E, Egan D, Deluzio K, et al. Effects of pelvic asymmetry and low back pain on trunk kinematics during sitting: a comparison with standing. Spine 2006;31:E135–43.

[18] Jull GA, Janda V. Muscles and motor control in low back pain: assessment and management. New York: Churchill Livingstone; 1987.

[19] Janda V. Physical therapy of the cervical and thoracic spine. New York: Churchill Livingstone; 1998.

[20] Janda V. Muscles and motor control in cervicogenic disorders: assessment and management. New York: Churchill Livingstone; 1994.

[21] Richardson CG. Therapeutic exercises for spinal stabilization and low back pain: scientific bases and clinical approach. Edinburgh (UK): Churchill Livingstone; 1999.

[22] Laasonen EM. Atrophy of sacrospinal muscle groups in patients with chronic, diffusely radiating lumbar back pain. Neuroradiology 1984;26(1):9–13.

[23] Bergmark A. Stability of the lumbar spine. A study in mechanical engineering. Acta Orthop Scand Suppl 1989;230:1–54.

[24] Radebold A, Cholewicki J, Polzhofer GK, et al. Impaired postural control of the lumbar spine is associated with delayed muscle response times in patients with chronic idiopathic low back pain. Spine 2001;26:724–30.

[25] Hodges PW, Richardson CA. Inefficient muscular stabilization of the lumbar spine associated with low back pain: a motor control evaluation of transverse abdominis. Spine 1996; 80:1005–12.

[26] Esquenazi A, Hirai B. Assessment of gait and orthotic prescription. Phys Med Rehabil Clin N Am 1991;2:473–85.

[27] Kibler WB. Determining the extent of the functional deficit. In: Herring SA, Press JM, editors. Functional rehabilitation of sports and musculoskeletal injuries. 1st edition. Gaithersburg (MD): Aspen Publication; 1998. p. 16–9.

[28] Brukner P, Kahn K. Clinical sports medicine. 2nd edition. McGraw Hill; 2001.

[29] Bruce B, Fries JF, Lubeck DP. Aerobic exercise and its impact on musculoskeletal pain in older adults: a 14 year prospective, longitudinal study. Arthritis Res Ther 2005;7(6): R1263–70.

[30] Taimela S, Diederich C, Hubsch M, et al. The role of physical exercise and inactivity in pain recurrence and absenteeism from work after active outpatient rehabilitation for recurrent or chronic low back pain: a follow-up study. Spine 2000;25(14):1809–16.

[31] Farrell PA, Gates WK, Maksud MG, et al. Increases in plasma beta-endorphin/beta-lipotropin immunoreactivity after treadmill running in humans. J Appl Physiol 1982;52(5): 1245–9.

[32] Grossman A, Sutton JR. Endorphins: what are they? How are they measured? What is their role in exercise? Med Sci Sports Exerc 1985;17(1):74–81.

[33] Suomi R, Collier D. Effects of arthritis exercise programs on functional fitness and perceived activities of daily living measures in older adults with arthritis. Arch Phys Med Rehabil 2003;84(11):1589–94.

[34] Choukroun M, Kays C, Varene P. Effects of water temperature on pulmonary volumes in immersed human subjects. Respir Physiol 1989;75:255–66.

[35] Anstey K, Roskell C. Hydrotherapy: detrimental or beneficial to the respiratory system? Physiotherapy 2000;86:5–12.

[36] Ariyoshi M, Sonoda K, Nagata K, et al. Efficacy of aquatic exercises for patients with low-back pain. Kurume Med J 1999;46(2):91–6.

[37] Audette J, Wang F, Smith HS. Bilateral activation of motor unit potentials with unilateral needle stimulation of active myofascial trigger points. Am J Phys Med Rehabil 2004;83: 368–74.

[38] Ross MC, Bohannon AS, Davis DC, et al. The effects of a short-term exercise program on movement, pain, and mood in the elderly. Results of a pilot study. J Holist Nurs 1999;17(2): 139–47.

[39] Song R, Lee EO, Lam P, et al. Effects of tai chi exercise on pain, balance, muscle strength, and perceived difficulties in physical functioning in older women with osteoarthritis: a randomized clinical trial. J Rheumatol 2003;30(9):2039–44.

[40] Gard G. Body awareness therapy for patients with fibromyalgia and chronic pain. Disabil Rehabil 2005;27(12):725–8.

[41] Malmgren-Olsson EB, Branholm IB. A comparison between three physiotherapy approaches with regard to health-related factors in patients with non-specific musculoskeletal disorders. Disabil Rehabil 2002;24(6):308–17.

[42] Lehmann JF, Silverman DR, Baum BA, et al. Temperature distributions in the human thigh, produced by infrared, hot pack and microwave applications. Arch Phys Med Rehabil 1966;47(5):291–9.

[43] Borrell RM, Parker R, Henley EJ, et al. Comparison of in vivo temperatures produced by hydrotherapy, paraffin wax treatment, and fluidotherapy. Phys Ther 1980;60(10): 1273–6.

[44] Melzack R, Wall P. Pain mechanisms: a new theory. Sci Justice 1965;150:971–9.

[45] King EW, Audette K, Athman GA, et al. Transcutaneous electrical nerve stimulation activates peripherally located alpha-2A adrenergic receptors. Pain 2005;115(3):364–73.

[46] Ernst E. Massage therapy for low back pain. J Pain Symptom Manage 1999;17:65–9.

[47] Furlan A, Brosseau L, Imamura M, et al. Massage for low back pain. A systematic review. Cochrane Database Syst Rev 2002;2:CD001929.

[48] Cherkin DC, Eisenberg D, Sherman KJ, et al. Randomized trial comparing traditional Chinese medical acupuncture, therapeutic massage, and self-care education for chronic low back pain. Arch Intern Med 2001;161(8):1081–8.

[49] Hernandez-Reif M, Field T, Krasnegor J, et al. Lower back pain is reduced and range of motion increased after massage therapy. Int J Neurosci 2001;106:131–45.

[50] Van de Veen E, De Vet H, Pool J, et al. Variance in manual treatment of nonspecific low back pain between orthomanual physicians, manual therapists, and chiropractors. J Manipulative Physiol Ther 2005;28:108–16.

[51] Greenman P. Principles of manual medicine. 2nd edition. Baltimore (MD): Williams and Wilkins; 1996.

[52] Geisser M, Wiggert E, Haig A, et al. A randomized, controlled trial of manual therapy and specific adjuvant exercise for chronic low back pain. Clin J Pain 2005;21:463–70.

[53] Assendelft WJ, Morton SC, Yu EI, et al. Spinal manipulative therapy for low back pain. A meta-analysis of effectiveness relative to other therapies. Ann Intern Med 2003;138(11): 871–81.

[54] Ferreira ML, Ferreira PH, Latimer J, et al. Does spinal manipulative therapy help people with chronic low back pain? Aust J Physiother 2002;48(4):277–84.

[55] Andersson GB, Lucente T, Davis AM, et al. A comparison of osteopathic spinal manipulation with standard care for patients with low back pain. N Engl J Med 1999;341(19): 1426–31.

[56] Burton AK, Battie MC, Main CJ. The relative importance of biomechanical and psychosocial factors in low back injuries. In: Karwowski W, Marras W, editors. The occupational ergonomics handbook. Boca Raton (FL): CRC Press; 1999. p. 1127–38.

[57] Linton SJ. A review of psychological risk factors in back and neck pain. Spine 2000;25(9): 1148–56.

[58] Crombez G, Vlaeyen JWS, Heuts PH. Pain-related fear is more disabling than pain itself: evidence on the role of pain-related fear in chronic back pain disability. Pain 1999;80:920–9.

[59] Mannion AF, Junge A, Taimela S, et al. Active therapy for chronic low back pain: part 3. Factors influencing self-rated disability and its change following therapy. Spine 2001;26(8): 920–9.

[60] McCracken LM, Turk D. Behavioral and cognitive behavioral treatment for chronic pain: outcome, predictors of outcome, and treatment process. Spine 2002;22:2564–73.

[61] Morley S, Eccleston C, Williams A. Systematic review and meta-analysis of randomized trials of cognitive behavior therapy and behavior therapy for chronic pain in adults, excluding headache. Pain 1999;80:1–13.

[62] van Tulder MV, Ostelo R, Vlaeyen JW, et al. Behavioral treatment for low back pain: a systematic review within the framework of the Chochrane Back Review Group. Spine 2001;26: 270–81.

[63] Kamanli A, Kaya A, Ardicoglu O, et al. Comparison of lidocaine injection, botulinum toxin injection, and dry needling to trigger points in myofascial pain syndrome. Rheumatol Int 2005;25(8):604–11.

[64] Slemenda C, Brandt KD, Heilman DK, et al. Quadriceps weakness and osteoarthritis of the knee. Ann Intern Med 1997;127(2):97–104.

[65] Slemenda C, Heilman DK, Brandt KD, et al. Reduced quadriceps strength relative to body weight: a risk factor for knee osteoarthritis in women? Arthritis Rheum 1998;41(11): 1951–9.

[66] Sharma L, Song J, Felson DT, et al. The role of knee alignment in disease progression and functional decline in knee osteoarthritis. JAMA 2001;286(2):188–95.

[67] Redford J, Basmajian J, Trautman P. Orthotics: clinical practice and rehabilitation technology. New York: Churchill Livingstone; 1995.

[68] Brouwer RW, Jakma TS, Verhagen AP, et al. Braces and orthoses for treating osteoarthritis of the knee. Cochrane Database Syst Rev 2005;1:CD004020.

[69] Komistek RD, Dennis DA, Northcut EJ, et al. An in vivo analysis of the effectiveness of the osteoarthritic knee brace during heel-strike of gait. J Arthroplasty 1999;14(6):738–42.

[70] Birmingham TB, Kramer JF, Kirkley A, et al. Knee bracing after ACL reconstruction: effects on postural control and proprioception. Med Sci Sports Exerc 2001;33(8):1253–8.

[71] Ogata K, Yasunaga M, Nomiyama H. The effect of wedged insoles on the thrust of osteoarthritic knees. Int Orhop 1997;21(5):308–12.

[72] Van der Esch M, Heijmans M, Dekker J. Factors contributing to possession and use of walking aids among persons with rheumatoid arthritis and osteoarthritis. Arthritis Rheum 2003;49(6):838–42.

[73] Ettinger WHJ, Burns R, Messier SP, et al. A randomized trial comparing aerobic exercise and resistance exercise with a health education program in older adults with knee osteoarthritis. The Fitness Arthritis and Seniors Trial (FAST). JAMA 1997;277(1):25–31.

[74] Roddy E, Zhang W, Doherty M. Aerobic walking or strengthening exercise for osteoarthritis of the knee? A systematic review. Ann Rheum Dis 2005;64(4):544–8.

[75] Mangione KK, McCully K, Gloviak A, et al. The effects of high-intensity and low-intensity cycle ergometry in older adults with knee osteoarthritis. J Gerontol A Biol Sci Med Sci 2000; 54(4):M184–90.

[76] Van Baar ME, Dekker J, Oostendorp RA, et al. The effectiveness of exercise therapy in patients with osteoarthritis of the hip or knee: a randomized clinical trial. J Rheumatol 1998; 25(12):2432–9.

[77] Baron RA, Byrne D, Branscombe NR. Social psychology. 11th edition (MyPsychLab Series). Boston: Allyn & Bacon; 2005.

[78] McAuley E, Lox C, Duncan TE. Long-term maintenance of exercise, self-efficacy, and physiological change in older adults. J Gerontol A Biol Sci Med Sci 1993;48(4):218–24.

[79] Van Baar ME, Dekker J, Oostendorp RA, et al. Effectiveness of exercise in patients with osteoarthritis of hip or knee: nine months' follow up. Ann Rheum Dis 2001;60(12): 1123–30.

[80] Deyle GD, Henderson NE, Matekel RL, et al. Effectiveness of manual physical therapy and exercise in osteoarthritis of the knee. A randomized, controlled trial. Ann Intern Med 2000; 132(3):173–81.

[81] Osiri M, Welch V, Brosseau L, et al. Transcutaneous electrical nerve stimulation for knee osteoarthritis. Cochrane Database Syst Rev 2000;4:CD002823.

[82] Bunning RD, Materson RS. A rational program of exercise for patients with osteoarthritis. Semin Arthritis Rheum 1991;21(3 Suppl):33–43.

[83] Malmivaara A, Hakkinen U, Aro T, et al. The treatment of acute low back pain—bed rest, exercises, or ordinary activity? N Engl J Med 1995;332:351–5.

[84] O'Sullivan PB, Phyty GD, Twomey LT, et al. Evaluation of specific stabilizing exercise in the treatment of chronic low back pain with radiologic diagnosis of spondylolysis or spondylolisthesis. Spine 1997;22(24):2959–67.

[85] Barr KP, Griggs M, Cadby T. Lumbar stabilization: core concepts and current literature, part 1. Am J Phys Med Rehabil 2005;84(6):473–80.

[86] Sahrman SA. Does postural assessment contribute to patient care? J Orthop Sports Phys Ther 2002;32(8):376–9.

[87] Panjabi MM. The stabilizing system of the spine. Part I. Function, dysfunction, adaptation, and enhancement. J Spinal Disord 1992;5(4):383–9 [discussion: 397].

[88] Cholewicki J, McGill SM. Lumbar posterior ligament involvement during extremely heavy lifts estimated from fluoroscopic measurements. J Biomech 1992;25(1):17–28.

[89] Akuthota V, Nadler SF. Core strengthening. Arch Phys Med Rehabil 2004;85(3, Suppl 1): S86–92.

[90] Hides J. Paraspinal mechanism and support of the lumbar spine. Edinburgh (UK): Churchill Livingstone; 2004.

[91] McKenzie R. The lumbar spine. Mechanical diagnosis and therapy. Waikanae (New Zealand): Spinal Publications; 1981.

[92] Fritz JM, Delitto A, Vignovic M, et al. Interrater reliability of judgments of the centralization phenomenon and status change during movement testing in patients with low back pain. Arch Phys Med Rehabil 2000;81(1):57–61.

[93] Delitto A, Cibulka MT, Erhard RE, et al. Evidence for use of an extension-mobilization category in acute low back syndrome: a prescriptive validation pilot study. Phys Ther 1993;73(4):216–28.

[94] Erhard RE, Delitto A, Cibulka MT. Relative effectiveness of an extension program and a combined program of manipulation and flexion and extension exercises in patients with acute low back syndrome. Phys Ther 1994;74(12):1093–100.

[95] Werneke M, Hart DL. Centralization phenomenon as a prognostic factor for chronic low back pain and disability. Spine 2001;26(7):758–64 [discussion: 765].

[96] Wetzel FT, Donelson R. The role of repeated end-range/pain response assessment in the management of symptomatic lumbar discs. Spine 2003;3(2):146–54.

[97] Aina A, May S, Clare H. The centralization phenomenon of spinal symptoms—a systematic review. Man Ther 2004;9(3):134–43.

[98] Lindstrom I, Ohlund C, Eek C, et al. Mobility, strength, and fitness after a graded activity program for patients with subacute low back pain. A randomized prospective clinical study with a behavioral therapy approach. Spine 1992;17(6):641–52.

[99] Maitland G. The slump test: examination and treatment. Aust J Physiother 1985;31:215–9.

[100] Butler D. Sensitive nervous system. Adelaide (Australia): Noigroup Publications; 2000.

[101] Liddle SD, Baxter GD, Gracey JH. Exercise and chronic low back pain: what works? Pain 2004;107(1–2):176–90.

[102] American College of Sports Medicine. American College of Sports Medicine (ACSM) guidelines for exercise testing and prescription. 6th edition. Philadelphia: Lippincot Williams and Wilkins; 2000.

[103] Cohen I, Rainville J. Aggressive exercise as treatment for chronic low back pain. Sports Med 2002;32(1):75–82.

[104] Rainville J, Ahern DK, Phalen L. Altering beliefs about pain and impairment in a functionally oriented treatment program for chronic low back pain. Clin J Pain 1993;9(3):196–201.

[105] Hayden JA, van Tulder MW, Malmivaara A, et al. Exercise therapy for treatment of nonspecific low back pain. Cochrane Database Syst Rev 2005;3:CD000335.

[106] Van Tulder M, Malmivaara A, Esmail R, et al. Exercise therapy for low back pain: a systematic review within the framework of the Cochrane Collaboration Back Review Group. Spine 2000;25(21):2784–96.

[107] Keller A, Brox JI, Gunderson R, et al. Trunk muscle strength, cross-sectional area, and density in patients with chronic low back pain randomized to lumbar fusion or cognitive intervention and exercises. Spine 2003;29:3–8.

[108] Abenhaim L, Rossignol M, Valat J, et al. The role of activity in the therapeutic management of back pain. Spine 2002;25(4 Suppl):1S–33S.

[109] Hurwitz EL, Morgenstern H, Chiao C. Effects of recreational physical activity and back exercises on low back pain and psychological distress: findings from the UCLA Low Back Pain Study. Am J Public Health 2005;95(10):1817–24.

[110] Simons D, Travell J. Myofascial pain and dysfunction: the trigger point manual. 2nd edition. Baltimore (MD): Williams & Wilkins; 1999.

[111] Han SC, Harrison P. Myofascial pain syndrome and trigger-point management. Reg Anesth 1997;22(1):89–101.

[112] Rachlin E. Trigger points. In: Rachlin E, editor. Myofascial pain and fibromyalgia: trigger point management. St. Louis (MO): Mosby; 1994. p. 145–57.

[113] McNulty WH, Gevirtz RN, Hubbard DR, et al. Needle electromyographic evaluation of trigger point response to a psychological stressor. Psychophysiology 1994;31(3):313–6.

[114] Majlesi J, Unalan H. High-power pain threshold ultrasound technique in the treatment of active myofascial trigger points: a randomized, double-blind, case-control study. Arch Phys Med Rehabil 2004;85(5):833–6.

[115] Hou CR, Tsai LC, Cheng KF, et al. Immediate effects of various physical therapeutic modalities on cervical myofascial pain and trigger-point sensitivity. Arch Phys Med Rehabil 2002;83(10):1406–14.

[116] Hong C. Lidocaine injection versus dry needling to myofascial trigger point. The importance of the local twitch response. Am J Phys Med Rehabil 1994;73:256–63.

[117] Porta M. A comparative trial of botulinum toxin type A and methylprednisolone for the treatment of myofascial pain syndrome and pain from chornic muscle spasm. Pain 2000; 85:101–5.

[118] Wheeler A, Goolkasian P, Gretz S. A randomized, double-blind, prospective pilot study of botulinum toxin injection for refractory, unilateral, cervicothoracic, paraspinal, myofascial pain syndrome. Spine 1998;23:1662–6.

[119] Blumenfeld A. Botulinum toxin type A as an effective prophylactic treatment for primary headache disorders. Headache 2003;42:853–60.

[120] Padberg M, De Haan R, Tavy D. Treatment of chronic tension-type headache with botulinum toxin: a double-blind, placebo-controlled clinical trial. Cephalgia 2004;24: 675–80.

[121] Sundaraj R, Ponciano P, Johnstone C, et al. Treatment of chronic refractory intractable headache with botulinum toxin type A: a retrospective study. Pain Pract 2004;4:229–34.

[122] Larsen J. Current considerations in pain management for the patient with fibromylagia syndrome. Pharm Times 1999;66:2HPT–6HPT.

[123] Bradley L, Sotolongo A, Alberts K, et al. Abnormal regional cerebral blood flow in the caudate nucleus among fibromylagia patients and non-patients is associated with insidious symptom onset. J Musculoskeletal Pain 1999;7:285–92.

[124] Russell I, Orr MD, Littman B, et al. Elevated cerebrospinal fluid levels of substance P in patients with the fibromyalgia syndrome. J Bacteriol Virol Immunol [Microbiol] 1994;37: 1593–601.

[125] Bradley L, Weigent D, Sotolongo A, et al. Blood serum levels of nitric oxide (NO) are elevated in women with fibromyalgia (FM): possible contributions to central and peripheral sensitization. Arthrits Rheum 2000;43:S173.

[126] Larson A, Giovengo S, Russell I, et al. Changes in the concentrations of amino acids in the cerebrospinal fluid that correlate with pain in patients with fibromyalgia; implications for nitric oxide pathways. Pain Headache 2000;87:201–11.

[127] Wolfe F, Smythe H, Yunus M, et al. The American College of Rheumatology 1990 criteria for the classification of fibromyalgia: report of the Mutlicenter Criteria Committee. Arthritis Rheum 1990;33:160–72.

[128] Geisser ME, Casey KL, Brucksch CB, et al. Perception of noxious and innocuous heat stimulation among healthy women and women with fibromyalgia: association with mood, somatic focus, and catastrophizing. Pain 2003;102(3):243–50.

[129] Nicassio PM, Radojevic V, Weisman MH, et al. A comparison of behavioral and educational interventions for fibromyalgia. J Rheumatol 1997;24(10):2000–7.

[130] Moldofsky H, Scarisbrick P, England R, et al. Musculosketal symptoms and non-REM sleep disturbance in patients with "fibrositis syndrome" and healthy subjects. Psychosom Med 1975;37(4):341–51.

[131] Goldenberg D, Burchardt C, Crofford L. Management of fibromyalgia syndrome. JAMA 2004;292:2916–22.

[132] Giesecke T, Williams D, Harris R, et al. Subgrouping of fibromyalgia patients on the basis of pressure-pain thresholds and psychological factors. Arthritis Rhuem 2003;48:2916–22.

[133] Carette S, Bell MJ, Reynolds WJ, et al. Comparison of amitriptyline, cyclobenzaprine, and placebo in the treatment of fibromyalgia. A randomized, double-blind clinical trial. Arthritis Rheum 1994;37(1):32–40.

[134] Biasi G, Manca S, Manganelli S, et al. Tramadol in the fibromyalgia syndrome: a controlled clinical trial versus placebo. Int J Clin Pharmacol Res 1998;18(1):13–9.

[135] Arnold LM, Hess EV, Hudson JI, et al. A randomized, placebo-controlled, double-blind, flexible-dose study of fluoxetine in the treatment of women with fibromyalgia. Am J Med 2002;112(3):191–7.

[136] Arnold LM, Lu Y, Crofford LJ, et al. A double-blind, multicenter trial comparing duloxetine with placebo in the treatment of fibromyalgia patients with or without major depressive disorder. Arthritis Rheum 2004;50(9):2974–84.

[137] Sayar K, Aksu G, Ak I, et al. Venlafaxine treatment of fibromyalgia. Ann Pharmacother 2003;37:1561–5.

[138] Valim V, Oliveira L, Suda A, et al. Aerobic fitness effects in fibromyalgia. J Rheumatol 2003;30(5):1060–9.

[139] Gowans S, DeHueck A. Effectiveness of exercise in management of fibromyalgia. Curr Opin Rheumatol 2004;16:138–42.

[140] Jentoft ES, Kvalvik AG, Mengshoel AM. Effects of pool-based and land-based aerobic exercise on women with fibromyalgia/chronic widespread muscle pain. Arthritis Rheum 2001; 45(1):42–7.

[141] Rossy LA, Buckelew SP, Dorr N, et al. A meta-analysis of fibromyalgia treatment interventions. Ann Behav Med 1999;21(2):180–91.

[142] Keefe F. Cognitive behavioral therapy for managing pain. Clin Psychol 1996;49:4–5.

[143] Williams D. Psychological and behavioral therapies in fibromyalgia and related syndromes. Best Pract Res Clin Rheum 2003;17:649–65.

[144] Buckelew SP, Conway R, Parker J, et al. Biofeedback/relaxation training and exercise interventions for fibromyalgia: a prospective trial. Arthritis Care Res 1998;11(3):196–209.

[145] Burckhardt C. Multidisciplinary approaches for management of fibromyalgia. Curr Pharm Des 2006;12:59–66.

[146] Pfeiffer A, Thompson J, Nelson A, et al. Effects of a 1.5-day multidisciplinary outpatient treatment program for fibromyalgia: a pilot study. Am J Phys Med Rehabil 2003;82: 186–91.

ELSEVIER
SAUNDERS

Anesthesiology Clin
25 (2007) 761–774

ANESTHESIOLOGY
CLINICS

Nonopioid Analgesics

Muhammad A. Munir, MD*, Nasr Enany, MD,
Jun-Ming Zhang, MSc, MD

*Department of Anesthesiology, University of Cincinnati College of Medicine,
231 Albert Sabin Way, PO Box 67031, Cincinnati, OH 45267-0531, USA*

Drug therapy is the mainstay of management for acute, chronic, and cancer pain in all age groups, including neonates, infants, and children. The analgesics include opioids, nonopioid analgesics, and adjuvants or coanalgesics. In this article we will overview various nonopioid analgesics including salicylates, acetaminophen, traditional nonselective nonsteroidal anti-inflammatory drugs (NSAIDs), and cyclooxygenase-2 (COX-2) inhibitors. Unless contraindicated, any analgesic regimen should include a nonopioid drug, even when pain is severe enough to require the addition of an opioid [1].

Nonopioid analgesics

Acetaminophen and NSAIDs are useful for acute and chronic pain resulting from a variety of disease processes including trauma, arthritis, surgery, and cancer [2,3]. NSAIDs are indicated for pain that involves inflammation as an underlying pathologic process because of their ability to suppress production of inflammatory prostaglandins. NSAIDs are both analgesic and anti-inflammatory, and may be useful for the treatment of pain not involving inflammation as well [4].

Nonopioid analgesics differ from opioid analgesics in certain important regards. These differences should be realized to provide the most effective care to acute pain patients and include the following:

1. There is a ceiling effect to the dose response curve of NSAIDs, therefore after achieving an analgesic ceiling, increasing the dose increases the side effects but additional analgesia does not result.

A version of this article originally appeared in the 91:1 issue of Medical Clinics of North America.

This work was partly supported by Grant No. NS45594 from the National Institutes of Health.

* Corresponding author.

E-mail address: munirma@ucmail.uc.edu (M.A. Munir).

doi:10.1016/j.anclin.2007.07.007   ***anesthesiology.theclinics.com***

2. NSAIDs don't produce physical or psychological dependence and therefore sudden interruption in treatment doesn't cause drug withdrawals.
3. NSAIDs are antipyretic.

Nonopioid analgesics are underrated for the treatment of chronic pain and unnecessarily omitted for patients with chronic pain and patients unable to take oral medications. Parenteral, topical, and rectal dosage forms are available for some NSAIDs that are often underused.

All NSAIDs, including the subclass of selective COX-2 inhibitors, are anti-inflammatory, analgesic, and antipyretic. NSAIDs are a chemically heterogeneous group of compounds, often chemically unrelated, which nevertheless share certain therapeutic actions and adverse effects. Aspirin also inhibits the COX enzymes but in a manner molecularly distinct from the competitive, reversible, active site inhibitors and is often distinguished from the NSAIDs. Similarly, acetaminophen, which is antipyretic and analgesic but largely devoid of anti-inflammatory activity, also is conventionally segregated from the group despite its sharing NSAID activity with other actions relevant to its clinical action in vivo.

Mechanism of action

All NSAIDs inhibit the enzyme cyclooxygenase (COX), thereby inhibiting prostaglandin synthesis [5]. In addition to peripheral effects, NSAIDs exert a central action at the brain or spinal cord level that could be important for their analgesic effects [6]. More than 30 years ago, multiple isoforms of COX were hypothesized. In 1990s, the second form (COX-2) was isolated. COX-1, the originally identified isoform, is found in platelets, the gastrointestinal (GI) tract, kidneys, and most other human tissues. COX-2 is found predominantly in the kidneys and central nervous system (CNS), and is induced in peripheral tissues by noxious stimuli that cause inflammation and pain. The inhibition of COX-1 is associated with the well-known gastrointestinal bleeding and renal side effects that can occur with NSAID use. The anti-inflammatory therapeutic effects of NSAIDs are largely due to COX-2 and not the COX-1 inhibition. Until recently all available NSAIDs nonselectively inhibited the COX-1 and COX-2 isoforms. Drugs that do so are termed nonselective or traditional NSAIDs. Most NSAIDs inhibit both COX-1 and COX-2 with little selectivity, although some conventionally thought of as nonselective NSAIDs, diclofenac, etodolac, meloxicam, and nimesulide, exhibit selectivity for COX-2 in vitro. Indeed, meloxicam acts as a preferential inhibitor of COX-2 at relatively low doses (eg, 7.5 mg daily).

COX-2 selective NSAIDs that first became available in the late 1990s provide all of the beneficial effects of nonselective NSAIDs but fewer adverse effects on bleeding and the GI tract. COX-2 selective NSAIDs are no safer to the kidneys than nonselective NSAIDs. As of mid-2003, three members of the initial class of COX-2 inhibitors, the coxibs, were approved for use in the United States and Europe. Both rofecoxib and valdecoxib have now been withdrawn from the market in view of their potential cardiovascular adverse event profile. None of the coxibs have established greater clinical efficacy over NSAIDs.

Aspirin covalently modifies COX-1 and COX-2, irreversibly inhibiting cyclooxygenase activity. This is an important distinction from all the NSAIDs because the duration of aspirin's effects is related to the turnover rate of cyclooxygenases in different target tissues. The duration of effect of nonaspirin NSAIDs, which competitively inhibit the active sites of the COX enzymes, relates more directly to the time course of drug disposition. The importance of enzyme turnover in relief from aspirin action is most notable in platelets, which, being anucleate, have a markedly limited capacity for protein synthesis. Thus, the consequences of inhibition of platelet COX-1 last for the lifetime of the platelet. Inhibition of platelet COX-1-dependent thromboxane (TX)A2 formation therefore is cumulative with repeated doses of aspirin (at least as low as 30 mg/day) and takes roughly 8 to 12 days, the platelet turnover time, to recover once therapy has been stopped.

Acetaminophen is a nonsalicylate that may produce similar analgesic and antipyretic potency as aspirin, but has no antiplatelet effects, lacks clinically useful peripheral anti-inflammatory effects, and does not damage the gastric mucosa. A proposed mechanism of acetaminophen is inhibition of a third isoform of cyclooxygenase (COX-3) that was identified recently [7]. COX-3 is only found within the CNS, which would account for the analgesic and antipyretic, but not anti-inflammatory, action of acetaminophen. However, the significance of COX-3 remains uncertain, and the mechanism(s) of action of acetaminophen has yet to be defined.

Clinical uses

All NSAIDs, including selective COX-2 inhibitors, are antipyretic, analgesic, and anti-inflammatory, with the exception of acetaminophen, which is antipyretic and analgesic but is largely devoid of anti-inflammatory activity.

Analgesic

When employed as analgesics, these drugs usually are effective only against pain of low-to-moderate intensity, such as dental pain. Although their maximal efficacy is generally much less than the opioids, NSAIDs lack the unwanted adverse effects of opiates in the CNS, including respiratory depression and the development of physical dependence. NSAIDs do not change the perception of sensory modalities other than pain. Chronic postoperative pain or pain arising from inflammation (eg, somatic pain) is controlled particularly well by NSAIDs.

Antipyretics

NSAIDs reduce fever in most situations, but not the circadian variation in temperature or the rise in response to exercise or increased ambient temperature. It is important to select an NSAID with rapid onset for the management of fever associated with minor illness in adults. Due to the association with Reye's syndrome, aspirin and other salicylates are contraindicated in children and young adults less than 12 years old with fever associated with viral illness.

Anti-inflammatory

NSAIDs have their key application as anti-inflammatory agents in the treatment of musculoskeletal disorders, such as rheumatoid arthritis and osteoarthritis. In general, NSAIDs provide only symptomatic relief from pain and inflammation associated with the disease, and do not arrest the progression of pathological injury to tissue.

Other clinical uses

In addition to analgesic, antipyretic and anti-inflammatory effects, NSAIDs are also used for closure of patent ductus arteriosus in neonates, to treat severe episodes of vasodilatation and hypotension in systemic mastocytosis, treatment of biochemical derangement of Bartter's syndrome, chemoprevention of certain cancers such as colon cancer, and prevention of flushing associated with use of niacin.

Adverse reactions of NSAID treatment

Adverse effects of aspirin and NSAIDs therapy are listed in Table 1 and are considerably common in elderly patients and caution is warranted in choosing an NSAID for pain management in the elderly.

Gastrointestinal

The most common symptoms associated with these drugs are gastrointestinal, including anorexia, nausea, dyspepsia, abdominal pain, and diarrhea. These symptoms may be related to the induction of gastric or intestinal ulcers, which is estimated to occur in 15% to 30% of regular users. The risk is further increased in those with *Helicobacter pylori* infection, heavy alcohol consumption, or other risk factors for mucosal injury, including the concurrent use of glucocorticoids. All of the selective COX-2 inhibitors have been shown to be less prone than equally efficacious doses of traditional NSAIDs to induce endoscopically visualized gastric ulcers [8].

Table 1
Side effects of NSAID therapy

Gastrointestinal	Nausea, anorexia, abdominal pain, ulcers, anemia, gastrointestinal hemorrhage, perforation, diarrhea
Cardiovascular	Hypertension, decreased effectiveness of anti-hypertensive medications, myocardial infarction, stroke, and thromboembolic events (last three with selective COX-2 inhibitors); inhibit platelet activation, propensity for bruising and hemorrhage
Renal	Salt and water retention, edema, deterioration of kidney function, decreased effectiveness of diuretic medication, decreased urate excretion, hyperkalemia, analgesic nephropathy
Central nervous system	Headache, dizziness, vertigo, confusion, depression, lowering of seizure threshold, hyperventilation (salicylates)
Hypersensitivity	Vasomotor rhinitis, asthma, urticaria, flushing, hypotension, shock

Gastric damage by NSAIDs can be brought about by at least two distinct mechanisms. Inhibition of COX-1 in gastric epithelial cells depresses mucosal cytoprotective prostaglandins, especially PGI_2 and PGE_2. These eicosanoids inhibit acid secretion by the stomach, enhance mucosal blood flow, and promote the secretion of cytoprotective mucus in the intestine. Another mechanism by which NSAIDs or aspirin may cause ulceration is by local irritation from contact of orally administered drug with the gastric mucosa.

Co-administration of the PGE_1 analog, misoprostol, or proton pump inhibitors (PPIs) in conjunction with NSAIDs can be beneficial in the prevention of duodenal and gastric ulceration [9].

Cardiovascular

Selective inhibitors of COX-2 depress PGI_2 formation by endothelial cells without concomitant inhibition of platelet thromboxane. Experiments in mice suggest that PGI_2 restrains the cardiovascular effects of TXA_2, affording a mechanism by which selective inhibitors might increase the risk of thrombosis [10,11]. This mechanism should pertain to individuals otherwise at risk of thrombosis, such as those with rheumatoid arthritis, as the relative risk of myocardial infarction is increased in these patients compared with patients with osteoarthritis or no arthritis. The incidence of myocardial infarction and stroke has diverged in such at-risk patients when COX-2 inhibitors are compared with traditional NSAIDs [12]. Placebo-controlled trials have now revealed that there may be an increased incidence of myocardial infarction and stroke in patients treated with rofecoxib [13], valdecoxib [14], and celecoxib [15], suggesting potential for a mechanism-based cardiovascular hazard for the class, ie, selective COX-2 inhibitors (although not equal for all agents) [16].

Blood pressure, renal, and renovascular adverse events

Traditional NSAIDs and COX-2 inhibitors have been associated with renal and renovascular adverse events [17]. NSAIDs have little effect on renal function or blood pressure in normal human subjects. However, in patients with congestive heart failure, hepatic cirrhosis, chronic kidney disease, hypovolemia, and other states of activation of the sympathoadrenal or renin-angiotensin systems, prostaglandin formation and effects in renal blood flow/renal function becomes significant in both model systems and in humans [18].

Analgesic nephropathy

Analgesic nephropathy is a condition of slowly progressive renal failure, decreased concentrating capacity of the renal tubule, and sterile pyuria. Risk factors are the chronic use of high doses of combinations of NSAIDs and frequent urinary tract infections. If recognized early, discontinuation of NSAIDs permits recovery of renal function.

Hypersensitivity

Certain individuals display hypersensitivity to aspirin and NSAIDs, as manifested by symptoms that range from vasomotor rhinitis with profuse watery secretions, angioedema, generalized urticaria, and bronchial asthma to laryngeal edema, bronchoconstriction, flushing, hypotension, and shock. Aspirin intolerance is a contraindication to therapy with any other NSAID because cross-sensitivity can provoke a life-threatening reaction reminiscent of anaphylactic shock. Despite the resemblance to anaphylaxis, this reaction does not appear to be immunological in nature.

Although less common in children, this syndrome may occur in 10% to 25% of patients with asthma, nasal polyps, or chronic urticaria, and in 1% of apparently healthy individuals.

Pharmacokinetics and pharmacodynamics

Most of the NSAIDs are rapidly and completely absorbed from the gastrointestinal tract, with peak concentrations occurring within 1 to 4 hours. Aspirin begins to acetylate platelets within minutes of reaching the presystemic circulation. The presence of food tends to delay absorption without affecting peak concentration. Most NSAIDs are extensively protein-bound (95% to 99%) and undergo hepatic metabolism and renal excretion. In general, NSAIDs are not recommended in the setting of advanced hepatic or renal disease due to their adverse pharmacodynamic effects (Tables 2 and 3).

Selected nonopioid analgesics: clinical pearls

Salicylates

Salicylates include acetylated aspirin (acetylsalicylic acid) and the modified salicylate diflunisal, which is a diflurophenyl derivative of salicylic acid. Aspirin was invented in 1897; it is one of the oldest nonopioid oral analgesics. Gastric disturbances and bleeding are common adverse effects with therapeutic doses of aspirin. Because of the possible association with Reye's syndrome, aspirin should not be used for children younger than the age of 12 with viral illness, particularly influenza.

Salicylate salts (nonacetylated)

Salicylate salts such as choline magnesium trisalicylate and salsalate are effective analgesics and produce fewer GI side effects than aspirin [19]. Unlike aspirin and other nonselective NSAIDs, therapeutic doses do not greatly affect bleeding time or platelet aggregation tests in patients without prior clotting abnormalities [20].

Acetaminophen

Acetaminophen is a nonsalicylate that may produce similar analgesic and antipyretic potency as aspirin, but has no antiplatelet effects, lacks clinically useful peripheral anti-inflammatory effects, and does not damage the gastric mucosa. Although acetaminophen is well tolerated at recommended doses of up to 4000 mg/day, acute overdoses can cause potentially fatal hepatic necrosis. Patients with chronic alcoholism and liver disease and patients who are fasting can develop severe hepatotoxicity, even at usual therapeutic doses [21]. The Food and Drug Administration (FDA) now requires alcohol warnings for acetaminophen as well as all other nonprescription analgesics [22]. Acetaminophen overdoses are common because acetaminophen is a frequent ingredient in many nonprescription and prescription analgesic formulations. Acetaminophen has a reduced risk of ulcers and ulcer complications when compared with nonselective NSAIDs and is rarely associated with renal toxicity. Acetaminophen is an underrecognized cause of over-anticoagulation with warfarin in the outpatient setting [23].

Pyrrolacetic acids

Ketorolac is a pyrrolacetic acid, which is available in injection form. An initial dose of 30 mg followed by 10 to 15 mg intravenously (IV) every 6 hours is equianalgesic to 6 to 12 mg of IV morphine. Ketorolac may precipitate renal failure especially in elderly and hypovolemic patients. It is therefore recommended to limit use of Ketorolac to 5 days only. Also, clinicians should try to use the lowest dose felt to be needed.

Phenylacetic acid

Diclofenac potassium has been shown to be superior in efficacy and analgesic duration to aspirin and also inhibits selectively more COX-2 then COX-1.

Table 2
Nonopioid analgesics: comparative pharmacology

Drug	Proprietary names (not all-inclusive)	Average oral analgesic dose, mg	Dose interval, h	Maximal daily dose, h mg	Analgesic efficacy compared to standards	Plasma half-life, h	Comments
Acetaminophen	Numerous	500–1,000	4–6	4000	Comparable to aspirin	2–3	Rectal suppository available for children and adults. Sustained-release preparation available, >2g/day may increase INR in patients receiving Warfarin.
Salicylates	Numerous	500–1000	4–6	4000		0.25	Because of risk of Reye's syndrome, do not use in children under 12 with possible viral illness. Rectal suppository available for children and adults. Sustained-release preparation available.
Acetylated Aspirin							
Modified Diflunisal	Dolobid	1000 initial, 500 subsequent	8–12	1500	500 mg superior to aspirin 650 mg, with slower onset and longer duration; an initial dose of 1000 mg significantly shortens time to onset	8–12	Dose in elderly 500–1000 mg/day
							Does not yield salicylate

Drug	Brand name(s)	Dose (mg)	Duration (hr)	Max dose (mg)	Comparison	Half-life	Comments
Salicylate salts							
Choline magnesium	Trilisate	1000–1500	12	2000–3000	Longer duration of action than aspirin 650 mg	9–17	Unlike aspirin and NSAIDs, does not increase bleeding time
Trisalicylate	Tricosal						
NSAIDs							
Propionic acids							
Ibuprofen	Motrin, Rufen, Nuprin, Advil, Medipren, others	200–400	4–6	2400	Superior at 200 mg to aspirin 650 mg	2–2.5	Most commonly used NSAID in US. Available without prescription.
Naproxen	Naprosyn	500 initial, 250 subsequent	6–8	1500	—	12–15	Better tolerated than indomethacin and aspirin.
Naproxen sodium	Naprolan, Anaprox	550 initial, 275 subsequent	6–8	1650	275 mg comparable to aspirin, 650 mg, with slower onset and longer duration; 550 mg superior to aspirin 650 mg		
Naproxen sodium	Aleve	220 mg	8–12	—	Comparable to aspirin	2–3	—
Fenoprofen	Nalfon	200	4–6	3200	Superior at 25 mg to aspirin 650 mg	1.5	Sustained-release preparation available
Ketoprofen	Orudis	25–50	6–8	300			
Ketoprofen OTC	Actron, Orudis-K+	12.5–25	4–6	—			
Oxaprozin	Daypro	600	12–24	1200		24–69	
Indolacetic acids							
Indomethacin	Indocin, Indocin SR, Indochron E-R				Comparable to aspirin 650 mg	2	Not routinely used because of high incidence of gastrointestinal and Central nervous system side effects; rectal and sustained-release oral forms available for adults

Table 3
Selected nonopioid analgesics: analgesic dosage and comparative efficacy to standards

Drug	Proprietary names (not all-inclusive)	Average oral analgesic dose, mg	Dose interval, h	Maximal daily dose, mg	Analgesic efficacy compared to standards	Plasma half-life, h	Comments
Sulindac	Clinoril	150	12	400		7.8 Activemeta = 16	
Etodolac	Lodine	300–400	8–12	1000	More potent than sulindac and naproxen, but less potent than indomethacin		
Pyrrolacetic acids							
Ketorolac	Toradol	30 or 60 mg IM or 30 mg IV initial, 15 or 30 mg IV or IM subsequent	6	150 first day, 120 thereafter	In the range of 6–12 mg of morphine	6	Limit treatment to 5 days; may precipitate renal faiure in dehydrated patients, average dose in elderly 10–15 mg IM/IV Q6 h
Tolmetin	Tolectin	200–600	8	1800		5	
Anthramilic acids							
Mefenamic acid	Ponstel	500 initial, 250 subsequent	6	1500	Comparable to aspirin 650 mg	2	In US use is restricted to interval of 1 week

Phenylacetic acids							
Diclofenac potassium	Cataflam	50 mg	8	150	Superior in efficacy and analgesic duration to aspirin 650 mg		More selective for COX-2 than COX-1
Enolic acids							
Meloxicam	Mobic	7.5–15	24	15		15–20	Ten-fold selective for COX-2
Piroxicam	Feldene	20–40	24	40		50	
Naphthylalkanone							
Nabumetone	Relafen	1000 initial 500–750 subsequent	8–12	2000	Pain relief equal to aspirin, indomethacin, naproxen, and sulindac	24	Fewer gastrointestinal side effects
Cox-2 selective							
Celecoxib	Celebrex	200–400	12–24	400	Anti-inflammatory and analgesic effect similar to naproxen	11	
Rofecoxib	Vioxx	12.5–50	24	25 50 up to 5 days		17	
Valdecoxib	Bextra	10–20	12–24	40		8–11	

Enolic acids

Meloxicam has long half-life and roughly 10-fold COX-2 selectivity on average in ex vivo assays [24]. There is significantly less gastric injury compared with piroxicam (20 mg/d) in subjects treated with 7.5 mg/d of meloxicam, but the advantage is lost with 15 mg/d [25].

Naphthylalkanone

Nabumetone is a prodrug; it is absorbed rapidly and is converted in the liver to one or more active metabolites, principally 6-methoxy-2-naphtylacetic acid, a potent nonselective inhibitor of COX [26]. The incidence of gastrointestinal ulceration appears to be lower than with other NSAIDs [27] (perhaps because of its being a prodrug or the fact that there is essentially no enterohepatic circulation).

Propionic acids

Ibuprofen and naproxen are the most commonly used NSAIDs in the United States. These are available without a prescription in the United States. The relative risk of myocardial infarction appears unaltered by ibuprofen, but it is reduced by around 10% with naproxen, compared with a reduction of 20% to 25% by aspirin. Ibuprofen and naproxen are better tolerated than aspirin and indomethacin and have been used in patients with a history of gastrointestinal intolerance to other NSAIDs.

Indolacetic acids

Indomethacin is a more potent inhibitor of the cyclooxygenase than is aspirin, but patient intolerance generally limits its use to short-term dosing. A very high percentage (35% to 50%) of patients receiving usual therapeutic doses of indomethacin experience untoward symptoms. CNS side effects, indeed the most common side effects, include severe frontal headache, dizziness, vertigo, and light-headedness; mental confusion and seizure may also occur, severe depression, psychosis, hallucinations, and suicide have also been reported. Caution must be exercised when starting indomethacin in elderly patients, or patients with history of epilepsy, psychiatric disorders, or Parkinson's disease, because they are greater risk of CNS adverse effects.

COX-2 selective inhibitors

Three members of the initial class of COX-2 inhibitors, the coxibs, were approved for use in the United States. Both rofecoxib and valdecoxib have now been withdrawn from the market in view of their adverse event profile. Valdecoxib has been associated with a threefold increase in cardiovascular risk in two studies of patients undergoing cardiovascular bypass graft surgery [28]. Based on interim analysis of data from the Adenomatous Polyp

Prevention on Vioxx (APPROVe) study, which showed a significant (two-fold) increase in the incidence of serious thromboembolic events in subjects receiving 25 mg of rofecoxib relative to placebo [13], rofecoxib was withdrawn from the market worldwide [29]. The FDA advisory panel agreed that rofecoxib increased the risk of myocardial infarction and stroke and that the evidence accumulated was more substantial than for valdecoxib and appeared more convincing than for celecoxib. Effects attributed to inhibition of prostaglandin production in the kidney (hypertension and edema) may occur with nonselective COX inhibitors and also with celecoxib. Studies in mice and some epidemiological evidence suggest that the likelihood of hypertension on NSAIDs reflects the degree of inhibition of COX-2 and the selectivity with which it is attained. Thus, the risk of thrombosis, hypertension, and accelerated atherogenesis may be mechanistically integrated. The coxibs should be avoided in patients prone to cardiovascular or cerebrovascular disease. None of the coxibs has established clinical efficacy over NSAIDs. While selective COX-2 inhibitors do not interact to prevent the antiplatelet effect of aspirin, it now is thought that they may lose some of their gastrointestinal advantage over NSAIDs alone when used in conjunction with aspirin.

Summary

NSAIDs are useful analgesics for many pain states, especially those involving inflammation. Their use is frequently overlooked in patients with postoperative and chronic pain. Unless there is a contraindication, the use of an NSAID should be routinely considered to manage acute pain, chronic cancer, and noncancer pain.

References

[1] Acute Pain Management Guideline Panel. Acute pain management: operative or medical procedures and trauma: clinical practice guidelines. Rockville (MD): Agency for Healthcare Policy and Research, Public Health Service, US Department of Health and Human Services; 1992.

[2] Carr D, Goudas L. Acute pain. Lancet 1999;353:2051–8.

[3] Zuckerman L, Ferrante F. Nonopioid and opioid analgesics. In: Ashburn M, Rice L, editors. The management of pain. Philadelphia (PA): Churchill-Livingstone; 1998. p. 111–40.

[4] McCormack K. Non-steroidal anti-inflammatory drugs and spinal nociceptive processing. Pain 1994;59:9–43.

[5] Vane J. Inhibition of prostaglandin synthesis as a mechanism of action for aspirin-like drugs. Nature 1971;234:231–8.

[6] Malmberg A, Yaksh T. Hyperalgesia mediated by spinal glutamate or substance P receptor blocked by spinal cyclooxygenase inhibition. Science 1992;257:1276–9.

[7] Chandrasekharan N, Dai H, Roos K, et al. COX-3, a cyclooxygenase-1 variant inhibited by acetaminophen and other analgesic/antipyretic drugs: cloning, structure, and expression. Proc Natl Acad Sci U S A 2002;99:13926–31.

[8] Deeks JJ, Smith LA, Bradley MD. Efficacy, tolerability, and upper gastrointestinal safety of celecoxib for treatment of osteoarthritis and rheumatoid arthritis: systematic review of randomised controlled trials. BMJ 2002;325:619–26.

[9] Rostom A, Dube C, Wells G, et al. Prevention of NSAID-induced gastroduodenal ulcers. Cochrane Database Syst Rev 2002;4:CD002296.

[10] McAdam BF, Catella-Lawson F, Mardini IA, et al. Systemic biosynthesis of prostacyclin by cyclooxygenase (cox)-2: the human pharmacology of a selective inhibitor of COX-2. Proc Natl Acad Sci U S A 1999;96:272–7.

[11] Catella-Lawson F, McAdam B, Morrison BW, et al. Effects of specific inhibition of cyclooxygenase-2 on sodium balance, hemodynamics, and vasoactive eicosanoids. J Pharmacol Exp Ther 1999;289:735–41.

[12] FitzGerald GA. COX-2 and beyond: approaches to prostaglandin inhibition in human disease. Nat Rev Drug Discov 2003;2:879–90.

[13] Bresalier RS, Sandler RS, Quan H, et al. Cardiovascular events associated with rofecoxib in a colorectal adenoma chemoprevention trial. N Engl J Med 2005;352:1092–102.

[14] Nussmeier NA, Whelton AA, Brown MT, et al. Complications of COX-2 inhibitors parecoxib and valdecoxib after cardiac surgery. N Engl J Med 2005;352:1081–91.

[15] Solomon SD, McMurray JV, Pfeffer MA, et al. Cardiovascular risk associated with celecoxib in a clinical trial for colorectal adenoma prevention. N Engl J Med 2005;352: 1071–80.

[16] Pitt B, Pepine C, Willerson JT. Cyclooxygenase-2 inhibition and cardiovascular events. Circulation 2002;106:167–9.

[17] Cheng HF, Harris RC. Cyclooxygenases, the kidney, and hypertension. Hypertension 2004; 43:525–30.

[18] Patrono C, Dunn MJ. The clinical significance of inhibition of renal prostaglandin synthesis. Kidney Int 1987;32:1–12.

[19] Ehrlich G. Primary drug therapy: aspirin vs. the nonsteroidal anti-inflammatory drugs. Postgrad Med 1983;May Spec:9–17.

[20] Stuart JJ, Pisko EJ. Choline magnesium trisalicylate does not impair platelet aggregation. Pharmatherapeutica 1981;2(8):547–51.

[21] Whitcomb D, Block G. Association of acetaminophen hepatotoxicity with fasting and ethanol use. JAMA 1994;272:1845–50.

[22] Food and Drug Administration. Over-the-counter drug products containing analgesic/antipyretic active ingredients for internal use; required alcohol warning; final rule; compliance date. Food and Drug Administration, HHS. Fed Regist 1999;64(51):13066–7.

[23] Hylek E, Heiman H, Skates S, et al. Acetaminophen and other risk factors for excessive warfarin anticoagulation. JAMA 1998;279:657–62.

[24] Panara MR, Renda G, Sciulli MG, et al. Dose-dependent inhibition of platelet cyclooxygenase-1 and monocyte cyclooxygenase-2 by meloxicam in healthy subjects. J Pharmacol Exp Ther 1999;290:276–80.

[25] Patoia L, Santucci L, Furno P, et al. A 4-week, double-blind, parallel-group study to compare the gastrointestinal effects of meloxicam 7.5 mg, meloxicam 15 mg, piroxicam 20 mg and placebo by means of faecal blood loss, endoscopy and symptom evaluation in healthy volunteers. B Brit J Rheumatol 1996;35:61–7.

[26] Patrignani P, Panara MR, Greco A, et al. Biochemical and pharmacological characterization of the cyclooxygenase activity of human blood prostaglandin endoperoxide synthases. J Pharmacol Exp Ther 1994;271:1705–12.

[27] Scott DL, Palmer RH. Safety and efficacy of nabumetone in osteoarthritis: emphasis on gastrointestinal safety. Aliment Pharmacol Ther 2000;14:443–52.

[28] Furberg CD, Psaty BM, FitzGerald GA. Parecoxib, valdecoxib and cardiovascular risk. Circulation 2005;111:249.

[29] FitzGerald GA. Coxibs and cardiovascular disease. N Engl J Med 2004;351:1709–11.

ANESTHESIOLOGY
CLINICS

Anesthesiology Clin
25 (2007) 775–786

Adjuvant Analgesics

Helena Knotkova, PhD[a],*, Marco Pappagallo, MD[b]

[a]Department of Pain Medicine and Palliative Care, 353 E 17th Street, Gilman Hall,
Unit 4C, Beth Israel Medical Center, New York, NY 10003, USA
[b]Department of Anesthesiology, Mount-Sinai Hospital, One Gustave L. Levy Place,
1190 Fifth Avenue, New York, NY 10029, USA

Adjuvant analgesics are a diverse group of drugs that were originally developed for a primary indication other than pain. Many of these medications are currently used to enhance analgesia under specific circumstances [1]. Of interest, a few of these agents are currently used as primary analgesics for specific pain conditions as well as adjuvants in some other pain conditions.

The proper use of adjuvant drugs is one of the keys to success in effective pain management. Since adjuvant analgesics are typically administered to patients who take multiple medications, decisions regarding administration and dosage must be made with a clear understanding of the stage of the disease and the goals of care [2,3]. Since adjuvants cause their own side effects, they are better be used when a patient cannot obtain satisfactory pain relief from a primary pain medication (ie, acetaminophen, nonsteroidal anti-inflammatory drugs, opioids). As a general recommendation, adjuvants should not be used only to lower the opioid dose in functional patients whose pain is well controlled with minimum side effects.

Antidepressants

Antidepressants play an important role in the treatment of chronic pain, as they display a wide variety of interactions with the neuraxis nociceptive pathways: monoamine modulation, opioid interactions, descending inhibition, and ion-channel blocking [4,5]. Tricyclic antidepressants (TCAs),

---

A version of this article originally appeared in the 91:1 issue of Medical Clinics of North America.

There is no funding related to this chapter.

* Corresponding author.

E-mail address: HKnotkov@chpnet.org (H. Knotkova).

such as amitriptyline, nortriptyline, and desipramine, inhibit both serotonin and norepinephrine reuptake to varying degrees, and are effective for most neuropathic conditions [5]. The use of TCAs should be closely monitored for relatively frequent, poorly tolerated adverse effects, including cardiotoxicity, confusion, urinary retention, orthostatic hypotension, nightmares, weight gain, drowsiness, dry mouth, and constipation.

Serotonin and noradrenaline reuptake inhibitors (SNRIs), eg, duloxetine and venlafaxine lack the anticholinergic and antihistamine effects of the TCAs [6–8]. Venlafaxine has been shown to modulate allodynia and pinprick hyperalgesia in human experimental models and to relieve neuropathic pain in breast cancer, perhaps by broadening its monoamine coverage by inhibiting the presynaptic uptake of both serotonin, norepinephrine, and, to a lesser extent, dopamine. Duloxetine has recently been approved by the Food and Drug Administration (FDA) for the treatment of pain secondary to diabetic neuropathy. Another antidepressant, *bupropion*, which inhibits the reuptake of dopamine, has also shown evidence to be effective for the treatment of neuropathic pain [9].

Selective serotonin reuptake inhibitors (SSRIs), such as paroxetine and fluoxetine, are effective antidepressants, but relatively ineffective analgesics. While being used for the management of comorbidities such as anxiety, depression, and insomnia, which frequently affect patients with chronic neuropathic pain, SSRIs have not shown the same efficacy as the TCAs in the treatment of neuropathic pain [10].

Anticonvulsants

Antiepileptic drugs (AEDs) are becoming the most promising agents for the management of neuropathic pain, given their propensity to dampen neuronal excitability. These qualities have made some AEDs first-line treatment in neuropathic conditions. The application of AEDs for pain stems from the shared pathophysiology of neuropathic pain and epilepsy. Neuronal hyperexcitability characterizes both conditions. The hyperexcitable state of neuropathic pain is characterized by reduced thresholds (sensitization) and ectopic discharges at the spinal dorsal horn or dorsal root ganglion (DRG) pain-signaling neurons due to, for example, the up-regulation of Na^+ and Ca^{++} membrane channels [11].

The gabapentinoid AEDs, gabapentin and pregabalin, have both established efficacy for neuropathic pain. Gabapentin and pregabalin act on neither gamma-aminobutyric acid (GABA) receptors nor sodium channels. In fact, they modulate cellular calcium influx into nociceptive neurons by binding to voltage-gated calcium channels, in particular to the alpha-2-delta subunit of the channel [12,13]. Gabapentin has been regarded as the first-line treatment for neuropathic pain syndromes, likely because of its favorable toxicity profile and lack of major drug interactions [14,15]. Therefore, when used specifically for neuropathic pain, gabapentinoid AEDs should be considered primary analgesics and not adjuvants any longer [15–18]. In a recent randomized, double-blind, active placebo-controlled, crossover trial [19], patients with neuropathic pain received either active placebo (lorazepam) or controlled-release morphine, gabapentin, and a combination of gabapentin and morphine, each treatment given orally for 5 weeks. The study indicated that the best analgesia was obtained from the gabapentin/morphine combination, with each medication given at a lower dose than when given as a single agent [19]. Additionally, other studies [20–22] have demonstrated that the concomitant administration of gabapentin reduces opioid requirements in the postoperative setting [20,21]. Side effects of gabapentin tend to occur early in treatment. The most common adverse events include somnolence, dizziness, ataxia, fatigue, impaired concentration, and edema. Pregabalin is also known to cause weight gain.

Another AED, carbamazepine, is very effective in the treatment of trigeminal neuralgia (a neuropathic condition characterized by brief excruciating lancinating pains), however the side effects and the need to monitor hematologic function are significant drawbacks that have often persuaded physicians to use other drugs, especially oxacarbamazepine, which is the keto-analog of carbamazepine. Oxacarbamazepine binds to sodium channels in their inactive state, increases potassium channel conductance, and modulates high-voltage activated calcium channels [23]. Oxacarbamazepine has been used at times successfully in the treatment of neuropathic pain syndromes. The most commonly observed adverse events are dizziness, somnolence, diplopia, fatigue, nausea, abnormal vision, and hyponatremia. Thus, Na^+ level should be monitored.

Lamotrigine has shown some efficacy for carbamazepine-resistant trigeminal neuralgia [24]. The benefit of lamotrigine may be from its blocking tetrodotoxin-resistant Na^+ channels [25] and from an inhibition of glutamate release from presynaptic neurons [26]. Lamotrigine has been widely studied in both animals and humans with some evidence pointing toward effectiveness in pain control. Preliminary observations and study have suggested the potential usefulness of lamotrigine for pain associated with diabetic neuropathy, multiple sclerosis, spinal cord injury, central poststroke pain, polyneuropathy, complex regional pain syndrome, and trigeminal neuralgia [27–30].

Several new AEDs, eg, levetiracetam, zonisamide, and tiagabine, along with topiramate, may have analgesic effect in primary headaches [13,30]. Topiramate has also been used anecdotally in the treatment of complex regional pain syndrome (CRPS) type 1 [31].

Alpha-2-adrenergic agonists

Alpha-2 adrenergic agonists are known to have a spinal antinociceptive effect via alpha-2 receptor subtypes [32]. Clonidine, a well-known alpha-2 adrenergic agonist, produces a synergistic antinociceptive effect with opioids [33]. In addition to being a primary analgesic when given intrathecally in the postoperative period, clonidine potentiates the analgesic benefit of opioids [34].

Tizanidine is a relatively short-acting, oral alpha-2 adrenergic agonist with a much lower hypotensive effect than clonidine. Tizanidine has been mostly used for the management of spasticity. However, animal studies and clinical experience indicate some usefulness of tizanidine for a variety of painful states, including neuropathic pain disorders [35–37].

Corticosteroids

Corticosteroids, eg, prednisone and dexamethasone, are effective as adjuvants for patients with inflammatory neuropathic pain from peripheral nerve injuries. In addition, corticosteroids have been used successfully to treat bone pain, pain from bowel obstruction, pain from lymphedema, and headache pain associated with intracranial pressure. Analgesic effect has been described for prednisone and dexamethasone in a broad range of doses. However, no analgesic studies have been performed about the relative potency among corticosteroids, long-term efficacy, and dose-response relationship. Short-term use of high doses of steroids is mainly recommended for patients whose pain rapidly escalates with functional impairment. The risk of adverse events increases with the dose and with the duration of therapy, and involves edema, dyspeptic symptoms, candidiasis, and occasional gastrointestinal bleeding.

Local anesthetics

The local anesthetics operate on the principle of decreasing neuronal excitability at the level of Na^+ channels that propagate action potentials. This channel blockade has an effect on both spontaneous pain and evoked pain [38]. An interesting point about these analgesic properties is that they occur at subanesthetic doses—lidocaine suppresses the frequency rather than the duration of Na^+ channel opening [39,40]. In addition, animal models suggest that both topical and central anesthetics may exhibit synergism with morphine [41,42].

Transdermal lidocaine shows a good efficacy for postherpetic pain [43]. In a controlled clinical trial, the transdermal form of 5% lidocaine relieved pain associated with post herpetic neuralgia (PHN) without significant adverse effects [44]. There are also observations that suggest some benefit for other neuropathic pain states [45], including diabetic neuropathy [46], CRPS, postmastectomy pain, and HIV-related neuropathy [47]. Intravenous lidocaine has also been used in patients with neuropathic pain [48].

The anti-arrhythmic local anesthetic mexiletine is a sodium channel blocker with analgesic properties for neuropathic pain similar to those of some AEDs (eg, lamotrigine, carbamazepine). Mexiletine is contraindicated in the presence of second- and third-degree atrium-ventricular conduction blocks. In addition, the incidence of gastrointestinal side effects (eg, diarrhea, nausea) is quite high in patients taking mexiletine.

Topical agents

A typical topical agent is capsaicin. Capsaicin, the natural substance in hot chili peppers, activates the recently cloned vanilloid neuronal membrane receptor [49,50]. After an initial depolarization, a single administration of a large dose of capsaicin appears to produce a prolonged deactivation of capsaicin-sensitive nociceptors [51,52]. The analgesic effect is dose-dependent and may last for several weeks. Studies at low capsaicin concentrations (0.075% or less) have shown mixed results, possibly a result of noncompliance. At the present time, preparations of injectable capsaicin and local anesthetics are being developed for site-specific, moderate to severe pain. These preparations should provide pain relief in patients with postsurgical, neuropathic, and musculoskeletal pain conditions for weeks or months after a single treatment.

NMDA antagonists

Animal experiments have shown that central and peripheral N-methyl-D-aspartate (NMDA) receptors play an important role in hyperalgesia and chronic pain [53]. NMDA antagonists dextromethorphan, methadone, memantine, amantadine, and ketamine seem to be effective in the management of hyperalgesic neuropathic states poorly responsive to opioid analgesics [53]. Ketamine when used as an adjuvant to opioids appears to increase pain relief by 20% to 30% and allows opioid dose reduction by 25% to 50% [54,55]. However, ketamine has a narrow therapeutic window and can cause intolerable side effects, such as hallucinations and memory impairment.

Of interest is the possibility that NMDA antagonists, such as D-methadone, memantine, and dextromethorphan, may prevent or counteract opioid analgesic tolerance [56,57].

Cannabinoids

Delta(9)-trans-tetrahydrocannabinol (Δ-9-THC) is the most widely studied cannabinoid. Evidence from animal studies and clinical observations indicate that cannabinoids have some analgesic properties [56,58,59]. Analgesic sites of action have been identified in brain areas, in the spinal cord, and in the periphery. Cannabinoids appear to have a peripheral anti-inflammatory action, and induce antinociception at lower doses than those obtained from effective central nervous system (CNS) concentrations.

In contrast to the strong preclinical data, good clinical evidence on the efficacy of cannabinoids is lacking. CNS depression seems to be the predominant limiting adverse effect. In chronic neuropathic pain, 1', 1'-dimethylheptyl-Δ8-tetrahydrocannabinol-11-oic acid (CT-3), a THC-11-oic acid analog, at a dose of 40 mg/d, has shown to be more effective than placebo and to produce no major unfavorable side effects [59].

Interestingly, the addition of inactive doses of cannabinoids to low doses of opioid mu agonists appears to potentiate opioid antinociception. Moreover, cannabinoids appear to have a predominant anti-allodynic/antihyperalgesic effect [56,58–60].

Bisphosphonates and calcitonin

Bisphosphonate therapy has proven highly valuable in the management of numerous bone-related conditions, including hypercalcemia, osteoporosis, multiple myeloma, and Paget's disease. Bisphosphonates, synthetic analogs of pyrophosphate, bind with a high affinity to the bone hydroxyapatite crystals and reduce bone resorption by inhibiting osteoclastic activity. Earlier bisphosphonates, such as etidronate, have been largely replaced by the use of second-generation bisphosphonates, including pamidronate, as well as third-generation bisphosphonates, including zolendronic acid and ibandronate. Multiple studies have demonstrated the efficacy of second- and third-generation bisphosphonates in pain reduction for bone metastases [61–64]. Zolendronic acid and ibandronate provide significant and sustained relief from metastatic bone pain, improving patient functioning and quality of life.

Bisphosphonates have been reported to be efficacious not only in bone cancer pain, but also in the treatment of CRPS, a neuropathic inflammatory pain syndrome [65,66]. However, the underlying mechanism of bisphosphonate analgesic effect is poorly understood. It may be related to the inhibition and apoptosis of activated phagocytic cells such as osteoclasts and macrophages. This leads to a decreased release of proinflammatory cytokines in the area of inflammation. In animal models of neuropathic pain (sciatic nerve ligature), bisphosphonates reduced the number of activated macrophages infiltrating the injured nerve, reduced Wallerian nerve fiber degeneration, and decreased experimental hyperalgesia [67]. One adverse event that has recently emerged in a number of oncology patients treated with the most potent bisphosphonates is osteonecrosis of the jaw. The disorder affects patients with cancer on bisphosphonate treatment for multiple myeloma or bone metastasis from breast, prostate, or lung cancer. Risk factors include prolong duration of bisphosphonate treatment (ie, monthly intravenous administration for more than 1 to 2 years), poor oral hygiene, and a history of recent dental extraction.

Calcitonin may have several pain-related indications in patients who have bone pain, including osseous metastases. The most frequent routes of absorption are intranasal and subcutaneous injection. Calcitonin reduces resorption of bone by inhibiting osteoclastic activity and osteolysis [68].

GABA agonists

Baclofen is an analog of the inhibitory neurotransmitter gamma-amino-butyric acid (GABA) and has a specific action on the GABA-B receptors. It has been used for many years as an effective spasmolytic agent. Baclofen also has shown anecdotal evidence of effectiveness in the treatment of trigeminal neuralgia [69]. Clinical experience supports the use of low-dose baclofen to potentiate the antineuralgic effect of carbamazepine for trigeminal neuralgia. Baclofen also has been used intrathecally to relieve intractable spasticity, and it may have a role as an adjuvant when added to spinal opioids for the treatment of intractable neuropathic pain and spasticity. The most common side effects of baclofen are drowsiness, weakness, hypotension, and confusion. It is important to note that discontinuation of baclofen always requires a slow tapering to avoid the occurrence of seizures and other severe neurological manifestations.

Neuroimmunomodulatory agents

Several lines of evidence indicate that tumor necrosis factor (TNF)-alpha, as well as other proinflammatory interleukins, may play a key role in the mechanism of inflammatory neuropathic pain. Neutralizing antibodies to TNF-alpha and interleukin-1 receptor may become an important therapeutic approach for severe inflammatory pain resistant to nonsteroidal anti-inflammatory drugs (NSAIDs), as well as for certain forms of neuropathic inflammatory pain [70–72]. Thalidomide has been shown to prevent hyperalgesia caused by nerve constriction injury in rats [73,74] and thalidomide is known to inhibit TNF-alpha production. TNF-alpha antagonists or newly developed thalidomide analogs with a better safety profile may play a relevant role in the prevention and treatment of otherwise intractable painful disorders [75]. Finally, inhibitors of microglia activation and of the transcription factor known as NF-κB are being explored and these lines of research may open new exciting treatment avenues.

Summary

Chronic pain, whether arising from viscera, bone, or any other tissue or structure, is, more often than commonly thought, the result of a mixture of pain mechanisms, and therefore there is no simple formula available to manage chronic complex pain states. Box 1 summarizes a pharmacological algorithm for difficult-to-treat chronic pain, which merely introduces the medication aspect of the treatment. In effect, any comprehensive algorithm should call for an interdisciplinary approach that would include rehabilitation, as well as psychosocial, and when indicated, interventional techniques.

The major rationale for introducing adjuvants is to better balance efficacy and adverse effects. The following scenarios should prompt the use of adjuvants in clinical practice:

- The toxic limit of a primary analgesic has been reached.
- The therapeutic benefit of a primary analgesic has plateaued, eg, treatment has reached its true efficacy limit or pharmachodynamic tolerance has developed.
- The primary analgesic is contraindicated, eg, substance abuse, aberrant behavior, organ failure, allergy, and so forth.

Box 1. Analgesic algorithm for difficult-to-treat pain syndromes

Pharmacological Interventions[1]
Moderate to severe pain/functional impairment; pain with a score of > 4 on the on the brief pain inventory [76]
1. Gabapentinoid (gabapentin, pregabalin) ± Opioid/opioid rotation **or**
2. *Antidepressant* (TCA, duloxetine, venlafaxine) ± *Opioid/opioid rotation* **or**
3. *Gabapentinoid + antidepressant + Opioid/opioid rotation*; in addition, may consider trials of one or more of the following adjuvants when clinically appropriate:
   Topical therapies for cutaneous allodynia/hyperalgesia[2]
   Anti-inflammatory drugs (corticosteroids for acute inflammatory neuropathic pain)
   IV bisphosphonates for cancer bone pain or CRPS/RSD
   Non-gabapentinoid AEDs such as carbamazepine or oxcarbazepine or lamotrigine ± baclofen for intermittent lancinating pain due to cranial neuralgias
   NMDA antagonists
   Mexiletine

---

[1] On a compassionate basis, according to the patient's clinical condition and pain mechanism, the physician may want to consider an empirical trial of one or more of the emergent topical, oral or parenteral/intrathecal therapies as discussed in the text.
[2] If SMP, consider topical clonidine and sympatholytic interventions; if clinically feasible, trials of topical therapies, eg, lidocaine 5% patch, may be considered for a variety of pain states and features.

- Subjective and qualitative symptoms demand broader coverage. Patients often convey that different medications will impart distinct analgesic benefits.
- Presence of disabling nonpainful complaints and need to manage symptoms such as insomnia, depression, anxiety, and fatigue that all cause worsening of the patient's quality of life and function.

Physicians have also been drawn to the adjuvants secondary to new realities of clinical practice. Moreover, aversion to addiction and diversion remains a potent force that shapes prescribing profiles.

References

[1] Wallenstein DJ, Portenoy RK. Nonopioid and adjuvant analgesics. In: Berger AM, Portenoy RK, Weissman DE, editors. Principles and practice of palliative care and supportive oncology. New York: Lippincott; 2002. p. 435–55.

[2] Banning A, Sjogren P, Henriksen H. Pain causes in 200 patients referred to a multidisciplinary cancer pain clinic. Pain 1991;45:45–8.

[3] Black DR, Sang CN. Advances and limitations in the evaluation of analgesic combination therapy. Neurology 2005;65(12, Suppl 4):S3–6.

[4] Sindrup SH, Otto M, Finnerup NB, et al. Antidepressants in the treatment of neuropathic pain. Basic Clin Pharmacol Toxicol 2005;96(6):399–409.

[5] Saarto T, Wiffen PJ. Antidepressants for neuropathic pain. Cochrane Database Syst Rev 2005;3:CD005454.

[6] Marchand F, Alloui A, Pelissier T, et al. Evidence for an antihyperalgesic effect of venlafaxine in vincristine-induced neuropathy in rat. Brain Res 2003;980:117–20.

[7] Grothe DR, Scheckner B, Albano D. Treatment of pain syndromes with venlafaxine. Pharmacotherapy 2004;24:621–9.

[8] Rowbotham MC, Goli V, Kunz NR, et al. Venlafaxine extended release in the treatment of painful diabetic neuropathy: a double-blind, placebo-controlled study. Pain 2004;110: 697–706.

[9] Semenchuk MR, Sherman S, Davis B. Double-blind, randomized trial of bupropion SR for the treatment of neuropathic pain. Neurology 2001;57:1583–8.

[10] Max MB, Lynch SA, Muir J, et al. Effects of desipramine, amitriptyline, and fluoxetine on pain in diabetic neuropathy. N Engl J Med 1992;326:1250–6.

[11] Han HC, Lee DH, Chung JM. Characteristics of ectopic discharges in a rat neuropathic pain model. Pain 2000;84(2–3):253–61.

[12] Matthews EA, Dickenson AH. Effects of spinally delivered N- and P-type voltage-dependent calcium channel antagonists on dorsal horn neuronal responses in a rat model of neuropathy. Pain 2001;92:235–46.

[13] Shi W, Liu H, Zhang Y, et al. Design, synthesis, and preliminary evaluation of gabapentin-pregabalin mutual prodrugs in relieving neuropathic pain. Arch Pharm (Weinheim) 2005; 338:358–64.

[14] Bennett M, Simpson K. Gabapentin in the treatment of neuropathic pain. Palliat Med 2004; 18:5–11.

[15] Rowbotham M, Harden N, Stacey B, et al. Gabapentin for the treatment of postherpetic neuralgia: a randomized controlled trial. JAMA 1998;280:1837–42.

[16] Backonja M, Beydoun A, Edwards KR, et al. Gabapentin for the symptomatic treatment of painful neuropathy in patients with diabetes mellitus: a randomized controlled trial. JAMA 1998;280:1831–6.

[17] Rice AS, Maton S. Gabapentin in postherpetic neuralgia: a randomized, double blind, placebo-controlled study. Pain 2001;94:215–24.

[18] Wiffen P, Collins S, McQuay H, et al. Anticonvulsant drugs for acute and chronic pain [systematic review]. Cochrane Pain, Palliative and Supportive Care Group. Cochrane Database Syst Rev 2005;4:CD001133.

[19] Gilron I, Bailey JM, Tu D, et al. Morphine, gabapentin, or their combination for neuropathic pain. N Engl J Med 2005;352:1324–34.

[20] Eckhardt K, Ammon S, Hofmann U, et al. Gabapentin enhances the analgesic effect of morphine in healthy volunteers. Anesth Analg 2000;91(1):185–91.

[21] Turan A, Karamanlioglu B, Memis D, et al. Analgesic effects of gabapentin after spinal surgery. Anesthesiology 2004;100(4):935–8.

[22] Tallarida RJ. Drug synergism: its detection and applications. J Pharmacol Exp Ther 2001; 298(3):865–72.

[23] Ichikawa K, Koyama N. Inhibitory effect of oxacarbamazepine on high-frequency firing in peripheral nerve fibers. Eur J Pharmacol 2001;42:119–22.

[24] Zakrzewska JM, Chaudhry Z, Nurmikko TJ, et al. Lamotrigine (lamictal) in refractory trigeminal neuralgia: results from a double-blind, placebo controlled, crossover trial. Pain 1997;73:223–30.

[25] Brau ME, Dreimann M, Olschewski A, et al. Effect of drugs used for neuropathic pain management on tetrodotoxin-resistant NaC currents in rat sensory neurones. Anesthesiology 2001;94:137–44.

[26] McNamara J. Drugs acting on the central nervous system. In: Harman G, Limbird LE, Morinoff PB, et al, editors. Goodman and Gilman's the pharmacological basis of therapeutics. 9th edition. New York: McGraw-Hill; 1996. p. 461–86.

[27] Vestergaard K, Andersen G. Lamotrigine for central poststroke pain: a randomized controlled trial. Neurology 2001;56:184–90.

[28] Webb J, Kamali F. Analgesic effect of lamotrigine and phenytoin on cold-induced pain: a cross-over placebo conrolled study in healthy volunteers. Pain 1998;76:357–63.

[29] Steiner TJ, Findley LJ, Yuen AW. Lamotrigine versus placebo in the prophylaxis of migraine with and without aura. Cephalgia 1997;17:109–12.

[30] Pappagallo M. Newer antiepileptic drugs: possible uses in the treatment of neuropathic pain and migraine. Clin Ther 2003;25:2506–38.

[31] Pappagallo M. Preliminary experience with topiramate in the treatment of chronic pain syndromes. Presented at the 17th Annual Meeting of the American Pain Society, San Diego, 1998.

[32] Khasar SG, Green PG, Chou B, et al. Peripheral nociceptive effects of alpha 2-adrenergic receptor agonists in the rat. Neuroscience 1995;66(2):427–32.

[33] Yaksh Tl, Malmberg AB. Pharmacological approaches to the treatment of chronic pain: new concepts and critical issues. Progress in pain research and management. Vol 1. Interaction of spinal modulatory receptor systems. Seattle: IASP Press; 1994. p. 151–71.

[34] Goudas LC, Carr DB, Filos KS, et al. The spinal clonidine-opioid analgesic interaction: from laboratory animals to the postoperative ward. A review of preclinical and clinical evidence. Analgesia 1998;3:277–90.

[35] Fogelholm R, Murros K. Tizanidine in chronic tension-type headache: a placebo controlled double-blind cross-over study. Headache 1992;32:509–13.

[36] Fromm GH, Aumentado D, Terrence CF. A clinical and experimental investigation of the effects of tizanidine in trigeminal neuralgia. Pain 1993;53:265–71.

[37] Semenchuk MR, Sherman S. Effectiveness of tizanidine in neuropathic pain: an open-label study. J Pain 2000;1(4):285–92.

[38] Cummins TR, Waxman SG. Downregulation of tetrodotoxin-resistant sodium currents and upregulation of a rapidly repriming tetrodotoxin-sensitive sodium current in small spinal sensory neurons after nerve injury. J Neurosci 1997;17(10):3503–14.

[39] Rowbotham MC, Reisner-Keller LA, Fields HL. Both intravenous lidocaine and morphine reduce the pain of postherpetic neuralgia. Neurology 1991;41(7):1024–8.

[40] Lai J, Hunter JC, Porreca F. The role of voltage-gated sodium channels in neuropathic pain. Curr Opin Neurobiol 2003;13:291–7.

[41] Saito Y, Kaneko M, Kirihara Y, et al. Interaction of intrathecally infused morphine and lidocaine in rats (part I): synergistic antinociceptive effects. Anesthesiology 1998;89:1455–63.

[42] Kolesnikov YA, Chereshnev I, Pasternak GW. Analgesic synergy between topical lidocaine and topical opioids. J Pharmacol Exp Ther 2000;295(2):546–51.

[43] Galer BS, Rowbotham MC, Perander J, et al. Topical lidocaine patch relieves postherpetic neuralgia more effectively than a vehicle topical patch: results of an enriched enrollment study. Pain 1999;80:533–8.

[44] Rowbotham MC, Davies PS, Verkempinck C, et al. Lidocaine patch: double-blind controlled study of a new treatment method for post-herpetic neuralgia. Pain 1996;65:39–44.

[45] Devers A, Galer BS. Topical lidocaine patch relieves a variety of neuropathic pain conditions: an open-label study. Clin J Pain 2000;16:205–8.

[46] Hart-Gouleau S, Gammaitoni A, Galer B, et al. Open label study of the effectiveness and safety of lidocaine patch 5% (Lidoderm) in patients with painful diabetic neuropathy [abstract]. Pain Medicine 2005;6:379–84.

[47] Berman SM, Justis JV, HO M, et al. Lidocaine patch 5% (Lidoderm) significantly improves quality of life (QOL) in HIV-associated painful periperal neuropathy [abstract 205]. Program and abstracts of the IASP 10th World Congress of Pain. Seattle: IASP; 2002.

[48] Wallace MS. Calcium and sodium channel antagonists for the treatment of pain. Clin J Pain 2000;16:S80–5.

[49] Caterina MJ, Schumacher MA, Tominaga M, et al. The capsaicin receptor: a heat-activated ion channel in the pain pathway. Nature 1997;389:816–24.

[50] Knotkova H, Pappagallo M. Pharmacology of pain transmission and modulation: peripheral mechanisms. In: Pappagallo M, editor. The neurological basis of pain. New York: McGraw-Hill; 2005. p. 53–61.

[51] Robbins WR, Staats PS, Levine J, et al. Treatment of intractable pain with topical large-dose capsaicin: preliminary report. Anesth Analg 1998;86:579–83.

[52] Vyklicky L, Knotkova H, Vitaskova Z, et al. Inflammatory mediators at acidic pH activate capsaicin receptor in cultured sensory neurons from newborn rats. J Neurophysiol 1998;79:670–6.

[53] Bennett GJ. Update on the neurophysiology of pain transmission and modulation: focus on the NMDA-receptor. J Pain Symptom Manage 2000;9:S2–6.

[54] Fitzgibbon EJ, Viola R. Parenteral ketamine as an analgesic adjuvant for severe pain: development and retrospective audit of a protocol for a palliative care unit. J Palliat Med 2005;8:49–57.

[55] Lossignol DA, Obiols-Portis M, Body JJ. Successful use of ketamine for intractable cancer pain. Support Care Cancer 2005;13:188–93.

[56] Davis AM, Inturrisi CE. d-Methadone blocks morphine tolerance and N-methyl-D-aspartate-induced hyperalgesia. J Pharmacol Exp Ther 1999;289:1048–53.

[57] Price DD, Mayer DJ, Mao J, et al. NMDA-receptor antagonists and opioid receptor interactions as related to analgesia and tolerance. J Pain Symptom Manage 2000;19:S7–11.

[58] Richardson JD. Cannabinoids modulate pain by multiple mechanisms of action. J Pain 2000;1(1):2.

[59] Karst M, Salim K, Burstein S, et al. Analgesic effect of the synthetic cannabinoid CT-3 on chronic neuropathic pain: a randomized controlled trial. JAMA 2003;290:1757–62.

[60] Richardson JD, Aanonsen L, Hargreaves KM. Antihyperalgesic effects of spinal cannabinoids. Eur J Pharmacol 1998;345(2):145–53.

[61] Smith MR. Osteoclast-targeted therapy for prostate cancer. Curr Treat Options Oncol 2004;5:367–75.

[62] Mystakidou K, Katsouda E, Stathopoulou E, et al. Approaches to managing bone metastases from breast cancer: the role of bisphosphonates. Cancer Treat Rev 2005;31:303–11.

[63] Wardley A, Davidson N, Barrett-Lee P, et al. Zoledronic acid significantly improves pain scores and quality of life in breast cancer patients with bone metastases: a randomized, crossover study of community vs hospital bisphosphonate administration. Br J Cancer 2005;92: 1869–76.

[64] Lerner UH. Neuropeptidergic regulation of bone resorption and bone formation. J Musculoskelet Neuronal Interact 2002;2:440–7.

[65] Cortet B, Flipo RM, Coquerelle P, et al. Treatment of severe, recalcitrant reflex sympathetic dystrophy: assessment of efficacy and safety of the second generation bisphosphonate pamidronate. Clin Rheumatol 1997;16:51–6.

[66] Varenna M, Zucchi F, Ghiringhelli D, et al. Intravenous clodronate in the treatment of reflex sympathetic dystrophy syndrome. A randomized, double blind, placebo controlled study. J Rheumatol 2000;27:1477–83.

[67] Liu T, van Rooijen N, Tracey DJ. Depletion of macrophages reduces axonal degeneration and hyperalgesia following nerve injury. Pain 2000;86:25–32.

[68] Szanto J, Ady N, Jozsef S. Pain killing with calcitonin nasal spray in patients with malignant tumors. Oncology 1992;49:180–2.

[69] Sindrup SH, Jensen TS. Pharmacotherapy of trigeminal neuralgia. Clin J Pain 2002;18(1): 22–7.

[70] Schafers M, Brinkhoff J, Neukirchen S, et al. Combined epineurial therapy with neutralizing antibodies to tumor necrosis factor-alpha and interleukin-1 receptor has an additive effect in reducing neuropathic pain in mice. Neurosci Lett 2001;310:113–6.

[71] Pedersen LH, Nielsen AN, Blackburn-Munro G. Anti-nociception is selectively enhanced by parallel inhibition of multiple subtypes of monoamine transporters in rat models of persistent and neuropathic pain. Psychopharmacology (Berl) 2005;182(4):551–61.

[72] Sevcik MA, Ghilardi JR, Peters CM, et al. Anti-NGF therapy profoundly reduces bone cancer pain and the accompanying increase in markers of peripheral and central sensitization. Pain 2005;115:128–41.

[73] Sommer C, Marziniak M, Myers RR. The effect of thalidomide treatment on vascular pathology and hyperalgesia caused by chronic constriction injury of rat nerve. Pain 1998; 74:83–91.

[74] Ribeiro RA, Vale ML, Ferreira SH, et al. Analgesic effect of thalidomide on inflammatory pain. Eur J Pharmacol 2000;391:97–103.

[75] George A, Marziniak M, Schafers M, et al. Thalidomide treatment in chronic constrictive neuropathy decreases endoneurial tumor necrosis factor-alpha, increases interleukin-10 and has long-term effects on spinal cord dorsal horn met-enkephalin. Pain 2000;88:267–75.

[76] Cleeland CS, Salek S. Compendium of QL instruments. Brief pain inventory. Chichester (West Sussex): Wiley; 1998. p. 1–5.

ELSEVIER
SAUNDERS

Anesthesiology Clin
25 (2007) 787–807

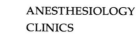

ANESTHESIOLOGY
CLINICS

Opioids for Persistent Noncancer Pain

Gary McCleane, MD, FFARCSI[a],*,
Howard S. Smith, MD, FACP[b]

[a]Rampark Pain Centre, 2 Rampark Dromore Road, Lurgan BT66 7JH,
Northern Ireland, UK
[b]Albany Medical College, Department of Anesthesiology, 47 New Scotland Avenue,
MC 131 Albany, New York 12208, USA

No discussion of analgesia would be possible without mention of the opioid analgesics. These agents, both "mild" and "strong," are extensively used in the management of all types of pain—acute, chronic, neuropathic, non-neuropathic, that arising from cancer, and that not arising from cancer—and their use is underpinned by extensive trial evidence and an abundance of practical experience. Indeed, a single journal issue, let alone a single article, could hardly be adequate for an in-depth discussion of the pharmacologic and clinical aspects of opioid use. Therefore, it would be simplistic to try to discuss the concept of opioid use in this article and hope that it would be in any way comprehensive. On the other hand, despite the 200 years that have passed since the chemical isolation of morphine, every year brings new understanding of the mode of action, propensity to cause side effects, and appropriate clinical use of opioids. This article concentrates on this "new" evidence as disclosed by recent publications.

Despite long experience with opioid use, prescribing habits are changing. Olsen and colleagues [1] have assessed opioid use by American primary care physicians and found that opioids were prescribed in 5% of all visits between 1992 and 2001. The rate was 4.1% in 1992 through 1993 and rose to 6.3% in 1998 through 1999. Possession of Medicaid or Medicare and receiving a nonsteroidal anti-inflammatory drug (NSAID) increased the chances of receiving an opioid, while being of Hispanic origin, being in a health maintenance organization, or living in the northeast or Midwest mitigated against opioid prescription. Undoubtedly, with the increasing availability of modified strong opioid preparations, either in transdermal

---

A version of this article originally appeared in the 91:2 issue of Medical Clinics of North America.

* Corresponding author.

E-mail address: gary@mccleane.freeserve.co.uk (G. McCleane).

1932-2275/07/$ - see front matter © 2007 Elsevier Inc. All rights reserved.
doi:10.1016/j.anclin.2007.08.002   *anesthesiology.theclinics.com*

or oral formulations, and the increased advertising of their use by the pharmaceutical industry, there is an increased pressure to prescribe accompanied by an increased willingness to use opioids, particularly those that are classified as strong (eg, clinically "pure" mu opioid agonists for severe pain).

With such use of strong opioids, particularly in the long term, questions of their effects with protracted use arise. At least some of the evidence is conflicting. Won and colleagues [2], in their study of 10,372 nursing home residents who had persistent pain, found that 18.9% were taking short-acting opioids, whereas 3.3% were taking long-acting opioids. They found no changes in cognitive status, mood status, or increased risk of depression with use of opioid analgesics. Furthermore, they found a decreased risk of falls with opioid use. In contrast, Vestergaard and colleagues [3] performed a nationwide survey of all patients sustaining a fracture in Denmark in 2000. This included 124,655 patients. Controls (373,962) were drawn from the background population. Morphine and other opiates were taken by 8.0% of the fracture subjects and by 3.2% of the control population. The odds ratio for sustaining a fracture were 1.47 with morphine, 2.23 with fentanyl, 1.39 with methadone, 1.36 with oxycodone, 1.54 with tramadol, 1.16 with codeine, and 0.86 with buprenorphine. Therefore, in this extensive review, the use of almost all opioids was association with an increased risk of fracture.

Aspects of the mode of action of opioids

A brief summary of the mode of action of opioids suggests that they achieve analgesia by interaction at four principle sites:

- Activating opioid receptors in the midbrain and turning on the descending inhibitory systems
- Activating opioid receptors on the second order pain transmission cells to prevent the ascending transmission of the pain signal
- Activating opioid receptors at the central terminals of C-fibers in the spinal cord
- Activating opioid receptors in the periphery to inhibit the activation of the nociceptors and to inhibit cells that may release inflammatory mediators

The now well-known opioid receptors (mu, delta, and kappa) belong to the G-protein–coupled receptor family. Agonist binding causes conformational changes that result in intracellular protein activation and inhibition of the activity of adenylyl cyclase. Adenylyl cyclase exists in 10 known forms. Kim and colleagues [4] have shown that, at least in mice, adenylyl cyclase type 5 is crucial for producing the analgesic and other effects of opioids. Specifically, they have shown that, in mice without genetic adenylyl cyclase type 5, the behavioral effects of selective mu and delta opioid receptor agonists are lost, whereas the effects of selective kappa agonists are unaffected.

Under resting conditions, adenylate cyclase converts adenosine triphosphate into cyclic adenosine monophosphate (cAMP). CAMP acts as a second messenger within the cell, resulting in several events, including the activation of protein kinases and gene transcription proteins. The inhibition of the activity of adenylyl cyclase induces a decrease in cAMP, which indirectly results in the inhibition of voltage-dependent calcium channels on presynaptic neurons. Those neurons are important in the release of neurotransmitters and transduction of neuronal communication (Fig. 1). Opioid receptors located on the presynaptic terminals of the nociceptive C-fibers and Aδ-fibers, when activated by an opioid agonist, indirectly inhibit these voltage-dependent calcium channels by way of decreasing cAMP levels, hence blocking the release of pain neurotransmitters, such as glutamate, substance P, and calcitonin gene-related peptide from the nociceptive fibers, resulting in analgesia.

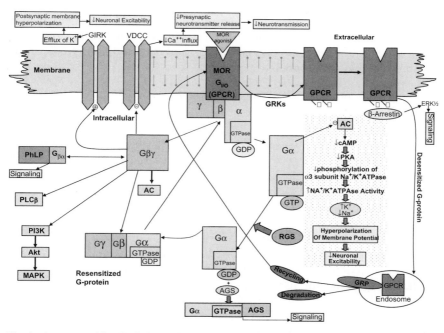

Fig. 1. Acute morphine (MOR) agonist-mediated signaling. AC, adenylate cyclase; AGS, activators of G-protein signaling; Akt, protein kinase B; ATPase, adenosine triphosphatase; ERK1/2, extra-cellular signal regulated kinase 1/2; GDP, guanosine diphosphate; GIRK, G-protein-activated inwardly rectifying potassium (K+) channels; GPCR, G-protein–coupled receptor; GRKs, G-protein–coupled receptor kinases; GRP, G-protein–coupled phosphatase; GTP, guanine triphosphate; MAPK, mitogen-activated protein kinase; PhLP, phosducin-like protein; PI3K, phosphatidyl inositol-3-kinase; PKA, protein kinase A; PLC, phospholipase C; RGS, regulator G protein; VDCC, voltage-dependent calcium channels. (*From* Smith HS. Mechanism and modulation of Mu-opioid receptor agonist signaling. Journal of Cancer Pain and Symptom Palliation 2006;1:3–13, copyright 2006, © The Haworth Press, Inc.; with permission.)

Unfortunately, our understanding of the multitude of effects induced by opioid administration is clouded by the presence of species variations. Berger and colleagues [5] have compared the presynaptic opioid receptors on noradrenergic and serotinergic neurons in human and rat neocortices. They have shown that in rats, mu opioid receptors modulate noradrenaline release, but serotonin release is only weakly affected by mu and kappa opioids. In contrast, noradrenaline release in the human neocortex is modulated by way of delta opioid receptors, but serotonin release mainly by way of kappa opioid receptors.

It is now clear that opioids exert an influence in many areas of the central nervous system either to inhibit or influence nociceptive impulses or to adapt physiologic responses to them. It may be possible that different opioid receptors in particular areas of the central nervous system differently influence pain or the symptoms and signs exhibited along with pain. For example, Wang and colleagues [6] examined the role of different types of opioid receptors in the thalamic nucleus submedius on allodynia in rats that had a spinal nerve ligation. The investigators showed that this particular brain area is involved in the antiallodynic effect of opioids and that this action is mediated by mu-opioid but not delta- and kappa-opioid receptors in this neuropathic pain model.

Clinical effects of opioids

The last few years have seen the publication of several systematic reviews concerning various aspects of the effects of opioids. To a large extent, these offer no surprises, but rather give reassurance that the widespread use of opioids in clinical practice is based on hard scientific evidence (Table 1 [7–21]).

What is lacking is any firm indication that any particular opioid has demonstrable superiority to others. One is therefore left to select an opioid for clinical use based on personal experience and familiarity of the various drugs and their formulations in different clinical circumstances.

This has led to more accepting attitudes from mainstream American medicine regarding the use of opioids for persistent noncancer pain [22]. However, the "opioid controversy" continues. Portenoy [23] has illustrated various "opiophobic" versus "opiophilic" views in his comments predicting responses of American physicians to the recommendation for the appropriate use of opioids published by the British Pain Society, the Royal College of Anaesthetists, the Royal College of General Practitioners, and the Royal College of Psychiatrists in the United Kingdom [24]. Kalso and colleagues [25] and Trescot and colleagues [26] have also published recommendations for using opioids in chronic noncancer pain.

Practicing in the "middle of the road" by employing the appropriate use of opioids in the context of good medical practice, as well as appropriate attention to the risk assessment and management of opioid abuse (ie, being cognizant of potential abuse, addiction, and diversion), has become known as "balance" [27–29].

The initiation (or maintenance) phase of long-term opioid therapy (LTOT) for persistent noncancer pain (PNCP) may involve the use of one or more of a number of tools, tests, and documents. These include opioid "contracts" or agreements, goal-directed therapy agreements [30,31], substance-abuse histories or "screening tools" for substance misuse, urine tests, unscheduled pill counts, and, optimally, some form of psychologic assessment (which could be an assessment by the provider), and documentation tools (see related article in this issue by Kirsh). Also, the nature and quality of the doctor–patient relationship may become an issue. That relationship should be well established and documented. Each clinic or clinician may use different items or tools in the practice—and there currently are no requirements for what some investigators call risk-management plans.

Perhaps one of the most important principles as a clinician in initiating and maintaining LTOT for PNCP is to "know where you are and where you are going." Goal-directed therapy agreements (GDTA) may be helpful when initiating LTOT for PNCP [30]. Clinicians are sometimes faced with patients who were started on opioids to achieve analgesia, or whose opioid medications were stopped, without clearly defined endpoints. Some such patients may remain in severe pain despite administration of high-dose opioids. To clarify patient and clinician expectations and attempt to make expected treatment outcomes more finite and concrete, some form of GDTAs may be useful. As with opioid treatment agreements, GDTAs are not necessarily advocated for all patients or all practices, but are merely suggested in situations in which clinicians deem them appropriate.

GDTAs should be tailored to each patient, should be clear and concise, and should have goals that are reasonable for the patient to attain over a finite period of time. Examples of specific issues in a GDTA may include increases in daily ambulation, social activities, or recreational activities by defined amounts. By using GDTAs before instituting opioid therapy, clinicians can set defined criteria that need to be met to continue opioid therapy. In this manner, patients may be expected to reach certain functional goals that are reasonable to attain and that may need to be documented by their physical or behavioral therapist to continue opioid therapy. The defined goals should be clearly stated in the GDTA. It's best to institute the GDTA before instituting opioid therapy. The GDTA is essentially a contract that requires the patient to meet a realistic translational analgesia target [30] in return for continued therapy.

Before LTOT there may not be any specific need for psychologic or psychiatric evaluations or psychologic testing. Even so, it seems prudent that clinicians should "know" a patient, and have an established provider–patient relationship before initiating LTOT for PNCP. Wasan and colleagues [31] reported that high levels of psychopathology (comprised mainly of depression, anxiety, and high neuroticism) are associated with diminished opioid analgesia in patients who have discogenic low-back pain.

Table 1
Recent systematic reviews concerning opioid use (published in 2004–2006)

Clinical scenario	No. of trials analyzed	No. of patients	Outcomes
NSAIDs +/− opioids in cancer pain [7,8]	42	3084	NSAID + opioid: no difference (4 of 14 papers); statistically insignificant benefit (1 of 14 papers); slight but statistically significant benefit (9 of 14 papers)
Oxycodone for cancer pain [9]	4	—[a]	Efficacy and tolerability of oxycodone similar to morphine
Oral transmucosal fentanyl for breakthrough pain in cancer [10]	4	393	Effective for cancer breakthrough pain
Efficacy of epidural	31	1343	72% of patients obtain "excellent" pain relief
Subarachnoid	28	722	62% of patients obtain "excellent" pain relief
Intracerebroventricular opioids in pain due to cancer [11]	13	337	73% of patients obtain "excellent" pain relief
Long-term oral opioid for chronic noncancer pain [12]	16	1427	No studies of good quality; insufficient evidence to produce conclusion
Opioids for chronic noncancer pain [13]	41	6019	Weak and strong opioids outperform placebo for all types of chronic noncancer pain
Tramadol for neuropathic pain [14]	5	161	NNT of tramadol compared with placebo: 3.5; NNH of tramadol compared with placebo: 7.7
Opioids for noncancer pain [35]	15	1145	Short-term good efficacy of opioids for both neuropathic and musculoskeletal pain; 80% of patients experienced at least one adverse event with opioid use; 44% of 388 patients on open-label treatment were still taking the opioid 7–24 months after commencement

Analgesia in postherpetic neuralgia [15]	31	—[a]	Strong opioids and tramadol effective; codeine ineffective
Opioids in neuropathic pain treatment [34]	22	—[a]	Opioids effective; high incidence of adverse effects
Mu agonists in treatment of evoked neuropathic pain [16]	9	—[a]	Dynamic allodynia significantly reduced; no consistent effect on static allodynia; small number of studies hinders interpretation
NSAIDs and opioids for renal colic [17]	20	1613	NSAIDs more effective than opioids in reducing pain; higher incidence of adverse events with opioids compared with NSAIDs
Intra-articular morphine after knee arthroscopy [18]	46	—[a]	Few well-controlled studies; no added analgesic effect of intra-articular morphine compared with saline
Opioid switching [19]	—[a]	—[a]	Opioid switching results in improvement in more than 50% of patients who have chronic pain and poor response to one opioid
Opioid side effects in chronic nonmalignant pain [20,21]	34	5546	Dry mouth: 25% of patients; nausea: 21%; constipation: 15%; 22% withdraw from opioid therapy because of side effects

Abbreviations: NNH, numbers needed to harm; NNT, numbers needed to treat.

[a] Number of patients not indicated in review paper.

Furthermore, clinicians have available brief assessment tools (eg, Screener and Opioid Assessment for Pain (SOAPP) [32]), Opioid Risk Tool (ORT) [33]) that attempt to screen risk potential for opioid-related aberrant behaviors among patients with PNCP.

Eisenberg and colleagues [34] published a systematic review and meta-analysis of trials evaluating the safety and efficacy of opioid agonists in the treatment of neuropathic pain of nonmalignant origin. Eisenberg and colleagues examined 22 studies that met inclusion criteria and were classified as short-term (<24 hours; n = 14) or intermediate-term (median 28 days; range 8–56 days; n = 8) trials. They reported that the short-term trials had contradictory results. However, all 8 intermediate-term trials demonstrated opioid efficacy for spontaneous neuropathic pain. A fixed-effects model meta-analysis of 6 intermediate-term trials showed mean posttreatment visual analog scale scores of pain intensity after opioids to be 14 units lower on a scale from 0 to 100 than after placebo (95% CI, -18-10, $P<.001$). The mean initial pain intensity recorded from 4 of the intermediate-term trials ranged from 46 to 69. This 14-point difference was considered to correspond to a 20% to 30% greater reduction with opioids than with placebo.

In a study examining the efficacy and safety of potent opioids used in the treatment of severe chronic noncancer pain, Kalso and colleagues [35] analyzed data from 1145 patients initially randomized in 15 placebo-controlled trials. Four studies tested intravenous opioids in neuropathic pain in a crossover design with 115 of 120 patients completing the protocols. Using either pain-intensity difference or pain relief as the endpoint, all 4 intravenous studies reported average pain relief of 30% to 60% with opioid. Eleven studies (1025 patients) compared oral opioids with placebo for 4 days to 8 weeks. Six of the 15 trials had an open-label follow-up of 6 to 24 months. The mean decrease in pain intensity in most studies was at least 30% with opioids and was comparable in neuropathic and musculoskeletal pain. Approximately 80% of patients noted at least one adverse effect. The most common adverse effects were constipation (41%), nausea (32%), and somnolence (29%). Only 44% of 388 patients on open-label treatments were still on opioids after therapy for between 7 and 24 months. Adverse effects and lack of efficacy were two common reasons for discontinuation.

Watson and colleagues [36] surveyed 102 patients who had PNCP in a neurologic practice and were followed by a neurologist every 3 months for 1 year or more (median 8 years; range 1–22 years). They reported that approximately one third of patients (34 out of 102) had a change in their pain status from either severe to moderate as measured by a 0 to 10 numerical rating scale (mild, 1–3; moderate, 4–7; severe, 8–10) and a category scale (absent, mild, moderate, severe, very severe), and as noted when considering pain with movement. They queried patients as to whether they were satisfied with pain relief despite adverse events. Forty-five patients (44%) answered that they were satisfied and 57 (56%) replied that they were not satisfied. However, of the 86 patients assessed for disability, 47 (54%) had significant improvement in their disability status on opioids. Also, there was some pain improvement on opioids in 78 (91%) of 102 patients, and the patients chose to continue opioid therapy for some analgesia despite adverse effects.

Opioids have been and continue to be a mainstay agent for intraspinal therapy, which is an option for the treatment of intractable persistent pain that is unresponsive to less-invasive approaches. The Polyanalgesic Consensus Conference 2003 was organized to review current literature, revise the algorithm for drug selection developed in 2000, and develop current guidelines, among other goals. The guidelines developed at the Polyanalgesic Consensus Conference 2003 suggest that the first-line intraspinal agent should be an opioid alone, such as morphine sulfate or hydromorphone. The guidelines also recommend switching from one agent to another if the maximum dose is reached or side effects occur [37].

Overall, the use of LTOT for PNCP may provide significant analgesia with minimal side effects for many years. However:

- LTOT may not be optimal for all patients.
- LTOT does not provide good or excellent analgesia in all patients.
- LTOT is not devoid of side effects.
- LTOT should be monitored to assess efficacy, side effects, and aberrant drug behavior.
- LTOT can be successfully withdrawn in selected patients who may do better without opioids.
- Prescribing LTOT for PNCP remains an art that may be used alone or in conjunction with other therapeutic options but typically not as a first-line agent for patients who have not tried previous treatments.

Analgesic tolerance

Definitions

The American Academy of Pain Medicine, the American Pain Society, and the American Society of Addiction Medicine recognize the following consensus definitions:

> Addiction is a primary, chronic, neurobiologic disease with genetic, psychosocial, and environmental factors influencing its development and manifestations. It is characterized by behaviors that include one or more of the following: impaired control over drug use, compulsive use, continued use despite harm, and craving.
>
> Physical dependence is a state of adaptation that is manifested by a drug class specific withdrawal syndrome that can be produced by abrupt cessation, rapid dose reduction, decreasing blood level of the drug, or administration of an antagonist.
>
> Tolerance is a state of adaptation in which exposure to a drug induces changes that result in a diminution of one or more of the drug's effects over time.

Interactions

Perhaps the major impediment to more widespread acceptance of the use of strong opioids in chronic noncancer pain is the real chance of at some point needing to increase the dose of the opioid to achieve the same level of pain relief. Not so long ago, we supposed in cancer pain management that increasing doses were required because the nociceptive stimulus increased with more widespread distribution of tumor as time progressed. An understanding of the interaction of opioids with various central nervous systems now shows that supposition to be simplistic.

Cholecystokinin

Cholecystokinin is a peptide originally thought to be confined to the gastrointestinal tract, but now known to be co-represented in the central nervous system as well. Cholecystokinin acts as an antiopioid peptide in that when it is administered along with an opioid analgesic in various animal pain models, the antinociceptive effect of the opioid is obtunded. When a cholecystokinin antagonist is administered, the antinociceptive effect of the opioid is enhanced. Repeated administration of opioid increases the release of cholecystokinin and mirrors the decreasing effect of that repeatedly administered opioid. When established antinociceptive tolerance is found, it can be reversed by the administration of a cholecystokinin antagonist. When the cholecystokinin antagonist is administered from commencement of the opioid, antinociceptive tolerance is prevented [38,39].

Calcium/calmodulin-dependent protein kinase II

When mice are treated with morphine, tolerance develops as quickly as 2 to 6 hours. If the calcium/calmodulin-dependent protein kinase II inhibitor KN93 is administered to mice that have become tolerant to morphine, their sensitivity to morphine returns, suggesting that calcium/calmodulin-dependent protein kinase II has a direct effect on the development of opioid antinociceptive tolerance [40].

N-methyl-d-Aspartate

It is thought that the nucleus accumbens, part of the amygdala, plays an important part in drug abuse and dependence. When morphine is chronically administered to rats, the levels of the NR1 and NR2B subunits of the N-methyl-d-aspartate (NMDA) receptors in this region are significantly increased [41]. Not only do changes in NMDA receptor function occur in the brain, but also in the spinal dorsal horn. Chronic morphine exposure is associated with an enhanced NMDA receptor function, as measured electrophysiologically, and this again may be implicated in antinociceptive tolerance [42].

Glutamate

When morphine-tolerant mice are examined, they have significantly elevated levels of the vesicular glutamate transporter 1 and the synaptic vesicle-specific small G-protein Rab3A. These elevated levels are associated with enhances spinal cord excitatory synaptic transmission, which in turn suppresses morphine-induced antinociception [43].

Calcium channel currents

In mice treated repeatedly with morphine and made tolerant to its effects, the effectiveness of mu opioid agonists to inhibit the normal calcium channel current in mu opioid receptors on sensory neurons is lost. This loss of effectiveness in inhibiting normal calcium channel current has been postulated to have at least some part to play in opioid antinociceptive tolerance [44].

Gamma amino butyric acid

Gamma amino butyric acid (GABA) A receptor–mediated synaptic transmission is important in nociceptive processing and is a major target when opioids are administered. In the nucleus raphe magnus, a critical site for opioid analgesia, the GABA A receptor–mediated inhibitory postsynaptic current is significantly increased in morphine-tolerant animals. Protein kinase A inhibitors reverse this chronic morphine-induced synaptic adaptation of GABA-mediated inhibitory postsynaptic currents, suggesting that chronic morphine exposure increases GABA synaptic activity [45].

Enkephalins

Mice that have genetic absence of preproenkephalin display blunted morphine antinociceptive tolerance but have normal conditioned place preference [46].

These examples of work recently published on analgesic tolerance with opioids make it clear that analgesic tolerance with opioid use is multifactorial. Thus, it may be naive to think that any one pharmacologic intervention could ever have a chance of preventing the onset of this troublesome side effect of opioid use.

Opioid side effects

Opioid-induced hyperalgesia

Although it is accepted that opioids are a most important treatment for pain, and in particular severe pain, there may be occasions in which it can induce hyperalgesia rather than pain relief [47,48]. This is most easily seen in humans when ultra–short-acting opioids are used. For example, Angst and colleagues [49] have shown that the area of skin with induced mechanical hyperalgesia is significantly increased after discontinuation of a remifentanil infusion. They go on to show that, while hyperalgesic skin enlargement occurs when remifentanil is used alone, no such enlargement takes place following coadministration of the NMDA receptor antagonist S-ketamine with remifentanil. Similarly, Hood and colleagues [50] induced hyperalgesia by applying capsaicin to skin. Remifentanil infusions were commenced and run for 60 to 100 minutes. This remifentanil reduced the area of hyperalgesia. When the remifentanil was discontinued, areas of hyperalgesia and allodynia increased above pretreatment levels by approximately 180%.

Endocrine consequences of long-term administration of opioids

Abs and colleagues [51] have examined the endocrine consequences of long-term intrathecal opioid administration. Their subjects had a mean duration of opioid therapy of 27 months. Decreased libido and impotence were present in 23 of the 24 male subjects studied. Serum testosterone and free androgen were markedly lowered in treated as compared with control male subjects. Decreased libido was found in 22 of 32 women on long-term opioid therapy. All 21 premenopausal females developed either amenorrhea or an irregular menstrual cycle with ovulation in only 1 subject. Serum leuteinizing hormone, estradiol, and progesterone levels were all significantly lower in the opioid treatment subjects. When all subjects were considered together, the urinary-free cortisol excretion over 24 hours was significantly lower than in control subjects. Therefore, the large majority of men and women treated with long-term intrathecal opioid therapy developed hypogonadotrophic hypogonadism.

One option to address this problem in men is the use of a testosterone patch. Daniell and colleagues [52] report an open-label trial of the use of this patch in men who have opioid-induced androgen deficiency and found that use of a testosterone patch normalized hormone levels and seemed to improve several quality-of-life parameters, including sexual function.

Opioids and the immune system

It is becoming increasingly clear that opioid treatment can have effects on immune function. Morphine can decrease the effectiveness of several functions of both natural and adaptive immunity and significantly reduces cellular immunity. In contrast, buprenorphine does not affect cellular immune responses [53].

Constipation

Constipation is a predictable but troubling effect associated with opioid use. Ackerman and colleagues [54] have examined the rate of constipation in patients who have chronic pain and are receiving transdermal fentanyl and controlled-release oxycodone. They included in their analysis 877 patients using transdermal fentanyl and 1218 patients using controlled-release oxycodone for at least 3 consecutive months. Of these patients, 75 had constipation (28 transdermal fentanyl, 47 controlled-release oxycodone). In patients over the age of 65, those taking oxycodone were 7.33 times more likely to be constipated than those using transdermal fentanyl.

Aspects of the use of individual opioids

Transdermal buprenorphine

Buprenorphine is increasingly being used in the management of pain, both related and unrelated to cancer. It seems to have marked antihyperalgesic effects, which increase its utility in the treatment of neuropathic pain. Sittl [55] suggests that the conventional conversion ratio of morphine to transdermal buprenorphine of 75:1 is questionable and should be changed to 100:1.

Transdermal fentanyl

Fentanyl is a synthetic phenylpiperidine mu opioid receptor agonist. It is approximately 80 times more potent than morphine, is highly lipophilic, and binds avidly to plasma proteins. After intramuscular administration of fentanyl citrate, the analgesic onset time is approximately 7 to 15 minutes; the time to peak analgesia may be extremely variable but could be approximately 15 to 45 minutes, the analgesic duration is approximately 1 to 2 hours; and the elimination half-life is approximately 2 to 4 hours [56]. Fentanyl is largely metabolized by piperidine N-dealkylation to norfentanyl by way of hepatic microsomal CYP3A4 [56]. Amide hydrolysis to desproprionyl fentanyl and alkyl hydroxylation to hydroxyfentanyl are minor pathways [56]. Hydroxynorfentanyl is a minor secondary metabolite arising from N-dealkylation of hydroxyfentanyl [56].

Use of NSAIDs or weak opioids is the norm in the treatment of osteoarthritis pain. Even with such treatment, some patients continue to suffer pain. Langford and colleagues [57] report their study of 596 patients with defined osteoarthritis of the hip or knee who were randomized to receive either transdermal fentanyl or placebo. If they were taking NSAIDs before inclusion, they were permitted to continue. Acetaminophen was offered as a rescue analgesic. Only 50% of patients completed the study. Transdermal fentanyl, compared to placebo, was shown to have a statistically significant pain-reducing effect. That said, reduction of visual analog scores (0–100) were 20 in the transdermal fentanyl group as opposed to 14.6 in the placebo group, giving a greater reduction with transdermal fentanyl of only 5.4 on this visual analog scale measurement. They also report that nausea, vomiting, and somnolence were more frequently encountered in the transdermal fentanyl group.

Oral transmucosal fentanyl citrate is a candied matrix formulation administered orally as a palatable lozenge on a stick. It is applied against the buccal mucosa and, as it dissolves in saliva, a portion of the drug diffuses across the oral mucosa with the rest being swallowed and partially absorbed in the stomach and intestine. The bioavailability is approximately 50%. Oral transmucosal fentanyl citrate seems to be particularly well suited for breakthrough pain (which is present in approximately two thirds of patients who have cancer with pain) because of its rapid onset. Meaningful analgesia may occur between 5 and 10 minutes after initiating use of oral transmucosal fentanyl citrate. Peak plasma concentrations are achieved at 20 minutes and the duration of analgesia is approximately 2 hours [58]. The US Food and Drug Administration (FDA) issued an approval letter for a fentanyl buccal tablet in June 2006. Fentanyl effervescent buccal tablets enhance buccal delivery of fentanyl using a proprietary drug absorption system [59,60].

Oxycodone

In vitro experiments suggest that circulating metabolites of oxycodone are opioid receptor agonists. In a study of oxycodone in healthy human volunteers, Lalovic and colleagues [61] showed that urinary metabolites of oxycodone derived from N-demethylation, noroxycodone, noroxymorphone, and alpha- and beta-noroxycodone account for approximately 45% of the total, whereas those products of O-demethylation, oxymorphone, and alpha- and beta-oxymorphol, and those of 6-keto-reduction, alpha- and beta-oxycodol account for 11% and 8%, respectively. Noroxycodone and noroxymorphone are the major metabolites in the circulation with elimination half-lives longer than that of oxycodone, but the uptake into the rat brain is significantly lower when compared with oxycodone. They conclude that the opioid effects of oxycodone are related to the parent drug and not to its metabolites.

One major question that continues to be of major relevance is whether individual opioids have distinct advantages over other members of this class. Staahl and colleagues [62] compared the effects of morphine and oxycodone in healthy human volunteers. They used a crossover study design in which each subject received morphine and an equianalgesic dose of oxycodone. They showed that both oxycodone and morphine are equipotent in pain modulation of induced skin and muscle pain. In contrast, when used for mechanically and thermally induced visceral pain of the esophagus, oxycodone produced significantly superior analgesia.

Marshall and colleagues [63] assessed the cost of producing pain relief in patients who have osteoarthritis of the hip or knee when controlled-release oxycodone or a combination of acetaminophen and oxycodone are used. They found that 62% of patients using controlled-release oxycodone alone had pain relief as compared with 46% taking the combination of that drug and acetaminophen. Consequently, from an economic perspective, use of controlled-release oxycodone alone was more cost-effective than use of the combination product.

Morphine

Codeine is to an extent metabolically converted to hydrocodone, but to date it has not been accepted that morphine is converted to hydromorphone. Cone and colleagues [64] studied 13 pain patients taking morphine at a high dose on a long-term basis and known not to be taking hydromorphone.

Urine was collected and analysis revealed the presence of hydromorphone at low levels in 10 of the 13 subjects. This finding is important for interpreting urinary screening of patients taking morphine to determine if they are abusing other opioids at the same time. If hydromorphone is found at low levels, its presence may be due to metabolism of morphine and may not be an indication of concomitant hydromorphone use. If, however, the hydromorphone is found at high levels, its presence is unlikely due solely to metabolism of morphine.

Codeine

Opioids are not used exclusively for the treatment of pain. Codeine, for example, has long been used as an antitussive. Smith and colleagues [65] reported on 21 patients who had chronic obstructive pulmonary disease and complained of cough. These patients were given both codeine and placebo at different times. The investigators found that codeine was no more effective than placebo at reducing cough in patients who had long-standing pulmonary disease.

Remifentanil

The multifactorial nature of opioid analgesic tolerance has already been alluded to. Although antinociceptive tolerance to the effects of opioids is a well-defined entity in animal experimentation, its relevance to human clinical practice is still open to debate. Crawford and colleagues [66], in describing their study of pediatric patients undergoing scoliosis surgery, offer insight into analgesic tolerance with remifentanil, an esterase-metabolized 4-anilidopiperidine ultra–short-acting mu opioid receptor agonist with a half-life of approximately 3 to 10 minutes. Patients received either a continuous intraoperative remifentanil infusion or intermittent bolus dosing with morphine. All patients received morphine as a postoperative analgesic using a patient-controlled analgesia device. Cumulative postoperative morphine consumption was significantly higher in the remifentanil group by a margin of 30%, suggesting that intravenous infusion of remifentanil was associated with the onset of acute analgesic tolerance.

Oxymorphone

Oxymorphone, a 3-0-demethylation metabolite of oxycodone, is a potent opioid that has a three to five times higher mu opioid receptor affinity than morphine [67]. Oxymorphone has been studied for postsurgical pain in an oral immediate-release formulation and seems to be effective [68]. Studied as an oral extended-release formulation, oxymorphone may be effective for moderate to severe pain secondary to osteoarthritis [69]. In June 2006, the FDA approved oxymorphone hydrochloride tablets (5 mg, 10 mg), and oxymorphone hydrochloride extended-release tablets (5 mg, 10 mg,

20 mg, 40 mg). Also, oxymorphone extended-release may be equianalgesic to oxycodone controlled-release at half the milligram daily dosage (with comparable safety) [70,71] and may be more potent than morphine at equianalgesic doses [72]. Oxymorphone extended-release uses the TIMERx (Penwest Pharmaceuticals Co., Danbury, Connecticut) delivery system [73] to provide pharmacokinetic characteristics consistent with 12-hour dosing [74]. Major metabolites of oxymorphone include 6-OH-oxymorphone-3-glucuronide. Oxymorphone extended-release does not seem to affect CYP2C9 or CYP3A4 metabolic pathways [75]. Noroxymorphone demonstrated a 3- and 10-fold higher affinity for the mu opioid receptor than oxycodone and noroxycodone, respectively [76].

Summary

Opioids, both weak (referred to as opioids for mild to moderate pain) and strong (referred to as opioids for moderately severe to severe pain), have a well-deserved place in the management of pain, regardless of its type or duration. Evidence recently published confirms the utility of this class of drug in pain management. That said, extensive clinical experience with the use of opioids along with further recently published evidence confirms that opioids are drugs with a definite risk of adverse events. Therefore, careful consideration must be given before prescribing opioids to be certain that the intended benefit of a particular opioid merits its use despite the potential side effects and to determine if the co-prescription of other pharmacologic agents could reduce the risk of adverse events. In acute and cancer pain management, the decisions are easy. Opioids are justifiably prescribed widely. The major issue is their use as a long-term therapy for chronic pain. In the past, there were many exaggerated fears about the use of strong opioids in the management of chronic pain. Opioids are now better understood. Even so, it could be argued that we have reached a stage where too little thought is given to the use of strong opioids in chronic pain treatment. If they were the only agents available, then it would be reasonable for them to be used extensively. However, in many chronic pain conditions, we have useful additions to our therapeutic armamentarium and so the need to select a strong opioid should be reduced. For example, there is a weight of evidence that strong opioids can reduce human neuropathic pain. We now have an increasing array of drugs with proven efficacy in this condition. Some of these have specific indications (eg, pregabalin, lidocaine patch, and duloxetine); others do not, and yet a body of evidence supports their use and they may have a reduced propensity to cause side effects (eg, 5-hydroxytryptamine 3 antagonists, cholecystokinin antagonists, various antiepileptic agents). It could therefore be argued that we should not use strong opioids as an "automatic" first-line treatment option for the management of chronic pain, but reserve them for those patients who fail to respond to other lower-risk options and in whom a proper consideration is given to the long-term consequences of strong opioid use. However, they also should certainly not be withheld as a "last-ditch effort."

Furthermore, it is conceivable that agents potentially on the horizon may hold promise as coanalgesics in combination with opioids that may improve opioid analgesic efficacy. Ibudilast (AV-411) is a nonselective phosphodiesterase inhibitor that is also known to suppress glial cell activation [74]. Preclinical data in multiple rat models of neuropathic pain suggest that ibudilast crosses the blood–brain barrier, is well tolerated, is active after oral administration, reduces glial activation, and alleviates pain, while also enhancing morphine analgesia and attenuating morphine tolerance and withdrawal [74].

The other remarkable feature of the recently published evidence is that we are still amassing insight into how opioids achieve their pain-relieving effects. This deeper understanding shows that the opioids are medications with complex and diverse central and peripheral nervous system effects. To a certain extent, this gives scientific validity for their use. On the other hand, such complex interactions must be associated with a propensity to cause a multitude of effects other than just analgesia (eg, tolerance, addiction, paradoxical pain). Also, prospective long-term well-designed studies of various opioids should be undertaken to elucidate certain adverse effects (eg, opioid effects on sleep and sleep-disordered breathing [sleep apnea]). The opioids therefore represent a well-validated treatment for both acute and chronic pain, but the problems associated with their use dictate that we still need to look for more efficacious and safer drugs. It could be argued that clinicians should no longer weigh just two options for those with chronic pain—either strong opioids for everyone or no strong opioids for anyone. The problem is too complex, and the solution should be tailored to each patient. Strong opioids should be used only after appropriate consideration of their use is made and only after thought is given to possible alternatives.

References

[1] Olsen Y, Daumit GL, Ford DE. Opioid prescriptions by US primary care physicians from 1992 to 2001. J Pain 2006;7:225–35.
[2] Won A, Lapane KL, Vallow S, et al. Long-term effects of analgesics in a population of elderly nursing home residents with persistent non-malignant pain. J Gerontol A Biol Sci Med Sci 2006;61:165–9.
[3] Vestergaard P, Rejnmark L, Mosekilde L. Fracture risk associated with the use of morphine and opiates. J Intern Med 2006;260:76–87.
[4] Kim KS, Lee KW, Lee KW, et al. Adenylyl cyclase type 5 (AC5) is an essential mediator of morphine action. Proc Natl Acad Sci USA 2006;103:3908–13.
[5] Berger B, Rothmaier AK, Wedekind F, et al. Presynaptic opioid receptors on noradrenergic and serotonergic neurons in the human as compared to the rat neocortex. Br J Pharmacol 2006;148:795–80.
[6] Wang JY, Zhao M, Yuan YK, et al. The roles of different subtypes of opioid receptors in mediating the nucleus submedius opioid-evoked antiallodynia in a neuropathic pain model in rats. Neuroscience 2006;138:1319–27.

[7] McNichol E, Strassels SA, Goudas L, et al. NSAIDs or paracetamol, alone or combined with opioids, for cancer pain. Cochrane Database Syst Rev 2005;1:CD005180.

[8] McNichol E, Strassels S, Goudas L, et al. Nonsteroidal anti-inflammatory drugs, alone or combined with opioids, for cancer pain: a systematic review. J Clin Oncol 2004;22: 1975–92.

[9] Reid CM, Martin RM, Sterne JA, et al. Oxycodone for cancer-related pain: meta-analysis of randomized controlled trials. Arch Intern Med 2006;166:837–43.

[10] Zeppetella G, Ribeiro MD. Opioids for the management of breakthrough (episodic) pain in cancer patients. Cochrane Database Syst Rev 2006;1:CD004311.

[11] Ballantyne JC, Carwood CM. Comparative efficacy of epidural, subarachnoid, and intracerebroventricular opioids in patients with pain due to cancer. Cochrane Database Syst Rev 2005;1:CD005178.

[12] Chou R, Clark E, Helfand M. Comparative efficacy and safety of long-acting oral opioids for chronic non-cancer pain: a systematic review. J Pain Symptom Manage 2004;28: 194–5.

[13] Furlan AD, Sandoval JA, Mailis-Gagnon A, et al. Opioids for chronic noncancer pain: a meta-analysis of effectiveness and side effects. CMAJ 2006;174:1589–94.

[14] Duhmke RM, Cornblath DD, Hollingshead JR. Tramadol for neuropathic pain. Cochrane Database Syst Rev 2004;2:CD003726.

[15] Hempenstall K, Nurmikko TJ, Johnson RW, et al. Analgesic therapy in postherpetic neuralgia: a quantitative systematic review. PLoS Med 2005;2:164.

[16] Eisenberg E, McNichol ED, Carr DB. Efficacy of mu-opioid agonists in the treatment of evoked neuropathic pain: systematic review of randomized controlled trials. Eur J Pain 2006;10:667–76.

[17] Holdgate A, Pollock T. Systematic review of the relative efficacy of non-steroidal anti-inflammatory drugs and opioids in the treatment of acute renal colic. BMJ 2004;328:1401.

[18] Rosseland LA. No evidence for analgesic effect of intra-articular morphine after knee arthroscopy: a qualitative systematic review. Reg Anesth Pain Med 2005;30:83–98.

[19] Mercadante S, Bruera E. Opioid switching: a systematic and critical review. Cancer Treat Rev 2006;32:304–15.

[20] Moore RA, McQuay HJ. Prevalence of opioid adverse events in chronic non-malignant pain: systematic review of randomised trials of oral opioids. Arthritis Res Ther 2005;7:1046–51.

[21] Ledeboer A, Hutchinson MR, Watkins LR, et al. Ibudilast (AV-411). A new class therapeutic candidate for neuropathic pain and opioid withdrawal syndromes. Expert Opin Invetig Drugs 2007;16:935–50.

[22] Chou R, Clark E, Helfan M, et al. Comparative efficacy and safety of long-acting oral opioids for chronic non-cancer pain: a systematic review. J Pain Symptom Manage 2003;26: 1026–48.

[23] Portenoy RK. Appropriate use of opioids for persistent non-cancer pain. Lancet 2004;364: 739–40.

[24] A consensus statement prepared on behalf of the Pain Society, the Royal College of Aneasthetists, the Royal College of General Practitioners, and the Royal College of Psychiatrists. Recommendations for the appropriate use of opioids for persistent non-cancer pain, the Pain Society, London (March 2004). Available at: http://www.painsociety.org/pdf/opioids_doc_2004.pdf. Accessed August 9, 2004.

[25] Kalso E, Allan L, Dellemijn PL, et al. Recommendations for using opioids in chronic non-cancer pain. Eur J Pain 2003;7:381–6.

[26] Trescot AM, Boswell MV, Atluri SL, et al. Opioid guidelines in the management of chronic non-cancer pain. Pain Physician 2006;9:1–39.

[27] A joint statement from 21 health organizations and the Drug Enforcement Administration. Promoting pain relief and preventing abuse of pain medications: a critical balancing act. Available at: http://www.medsch.wisc.edu/painpolicy/Consensus2.pdf. Accessed August 4, 2004.

[28] World ·Health Organization. Achieving balance in national opioids control policy: guidelines for assessment. Available at: http://who.int/medicines.docs/pagespublications/ qualitysafetypub.html. Accessed 2005.

[29] Zacny J, Bigelow G, Compton P, et al. College on problems of drug dependence task force on prescription opioid non-medical use and abuse: position statement. Drug Alcohol Depend 2003;69:215–32.

[30] Smith HS. Goal-directed therapy agreements. Journal of Cancer Pain and Symptom Palliation 2005;1:11–3.

[31] Wasan AD, Davar G, Jamison R. The association between negative effect and opioid analgesia in patients with discogenic low back pain. Pain 2005;177:450–61.

[32] Butler SF, Budman SH, Fernandez K, et al. Validation of a screener and opioid assessment measure for patients with chronic pain. Pain 2004;112:65–75.

[33] Webster LR, Webster RM. Predicting aberrant behaviors in opioid-treated patients: preliminary validation of the Opioid Risk Tool. Pain Med 2005;6:432–42.

[34] Eisenberg E, McNicol ED, Carr DB. Efficacy and safety of opioid agonists in the treatment of neuropathic pain of nonmalignant origin: systematic review and meta-analysis trials. JAMA 2005;293:3043–52.

[35] Kalso E, Edwards JE, Moore RA, et al. Opioids in chronic non-cancer pain: a systematic review of efficacy and safety. Pain 2004;112:372–80.

[36] Watson CP, Watt-Watson JH, Chipman ML. Chronic noncancer pain and the long term utility of opioids. Pain Res Manag 2004;9:19–24.

[37] Hassenbusch SJ, Portenoy RK, Cousins M, et al. Polyanalgesic Consensus Conference 2003: an update on the management of pain by intrapsinal drug delivery—report of an expert panel. J Pain Symptom Manage 2004;27:540–63.

[38] McCleane GJ. The role of cholecystokinin antagonists in human pain management: a review. J Neuropathic Pain Symptom Palliation 2005;2:37–44.

[39] McCleane GJ. Cholecystokinin antagonists: can they augment opioid-derived analgesia? J Opioid Manag 2005;1:273–9.

[40] Tang L, Shukla PK, Wang LX, et al. Reversal of morphine antinociceptive tolerance and dependence by the acute supraspinal inhibition of Ca (2 +)/calmodulin-dependent protein kinase II. J Pharmacol Exp Ther 2006;317:901–9.

[41] Bajo M, Crawford EF, Roberto M, et al. Chronic morphine treatment alters expression of N-methyl-D-aspartate receptor subunits in the extended amygdala. J Neurosci Res 2006; 83:532–7.

[42] Zhao M, Joo DT. Subpopulation of dorsal horn neurons displays enhanced N-methyl-D-aspartate receptor function after chronic morphine exposure. Anesthesiology 2006;104: 815–25.

[43] Suzuki M, Narita M, Narita M, et al. Chronic morphine treatment increases the expression of vesicular glutamate transporter 1 in the mouse spinal cord. Eur J Pharmacol 2006;535: 166–8.

[44] Johnson EE, Chieng B, Napier I, et al. Decreased mu-opioid receptor signaling and a reduction in calcium current density in sensory neurons from chronically morphine-treated mice. Br J Pharmacol 2006;148:947–55.

[45] Ma J, Pan ZZ. Contribution of brainstem GABA (A) synaptic transmission to morphine analgesic tolerance. Pain 2006;122:163–73.

[46] Marquez P, Baliram R, Gajawada N, et al. Differential involvement of enkephalins in analgesic tolerance, locomotor sensitization, and conditioned place preference induced by morphine. Behav Neurosci 2006;120:10–5.

[47] Mao J. Opioid-induced abnormal pain sensitivity. Curr Pain Headache Rep 2006;10:67–70.

[48] Angst MS, Clarke JD. Opioid-induced hyperalgesia: a qualitative systematic review. Anesthesiology 2006;104:570–87.

[49] Angst MS, Koppert W, Pahl I, et al. Short-term infusion of the mu-opioid agonist remifentanil in humans causes hyperalgesia during withdrawal. Pain 2003;106:49–57.

[50] Hood DD, Curry R, Eisenach JC. Intravenous remifentanil produces withdrawal hyperalgesia in volunteers with capsaicin-induced hyperalgesia. Anesth Analg 2003;97:810–5.

[51] Abs R, Verhelst J, Maeyaert J, et al. Endocrine consequences of long-term intrathecal administration of opioids. J Clin Endocrinol Metab 2000;85:2215–22.

[52] Daniell HW, Lentz R, Mazer NA. Open-label pilot study of testosterone patch therapy in men with opioid-induced androgen deficiency. J Pain 2006;7:200–10.

[53] Sacerdote P. Opioids and the immune system. Palliat Med 2006;20S:S9–15.

[54] Ackerman SJ, Knight T, Schein J, et al. Risk of constipation in patients prescribed fentanyl transdermal system or oxycodone hydrochloride controlled-release in a California Medicaid population. Consult Pharm 2004;19:118–32.

[55] Sittl R. Transdermal buprenorphine in cancer pain and palliative care. Palliat Med 2006;20S: S25–30.

[56] Janicki PK, Parris WC. Clinical pharmacology of opioids. In: Smith HS, editor. Drugs for pain. Philadelphia: Hanley and Belfus; 2003. p. 97–118.

[57] Langford R, McKenna F, Ratcliffe S, et al. Transdermal fentanyl for improvement of pain and functioning in osteoarthritis: a randomized, placebo-controlled trial. Arthritis Rheum 2006;54:1829–37.

[58] Lichtor JL, Sevarino FB, Joshi GP, et al. The relative potency of oral transmucosal fentanyl citrate compared with intravenous morphine in the treatment of moderate to severe postoperative pain. Anesth Analg 1999;89:732–8.

[59] Pather SI, Siebert JM, Hontz J, et al. Enhanced buccal delivery of fantanyl using the OraVescent drug delivery system. Drug Deliv Tech 2001;1:54–7.

[60] Durfee S, Messina J, Khankari R. Fentanyl effervescent buccal tablets: enhanced buccal absorption. Am J Drug Deliv 2006;4:1–5.

[61] Lalovic B, Kharasch E, Hoffer C, et al. Pharmacokinetics and pharmacodynamics of oral oxycodone in healthy human subjects: role of circulating active metabolites. Clin Pharmacol Ther 2006;79:461–79.

[62] Staahl C, Christrup LL, Andersen SD, et al. A comparative study of oxycodone and morphine in a multi-modal, tissue-differentiated experimental pain model. Pain 2006;123:28–36.

[63] Marshall DA, Strauss ME, Pericak D, et al. Economic evaluation of controlled-release oxycodone vs oxycodone-acetaminophen for osteoarthritis pain of the hip or knee. Am J Manag Care 2006;12:205–14.

[64] Cone EJ, Heit HA, Caplan YH, et al. Evidence of morphine metabolism to hydromorphone in pain patients chronically treated with morphine. J Anal Toxicol 2006;30:1–5.

[65] Smith J, Owen E, Earis J, et al. Effect of codeine on objective measurement of cough in chronic obstructive pulmonary disease. J Allergy Clin Immunol 2006;117:831–5.

[66] Crawford MW, Hickey C, Zaarour C, et al. Development of acute opioid tolerance during infusion of remifentanil for pediatric scoliosis surgery. Anesth Analg 2006;102:1662–7.

[67] Childers SR, Creese I, Snowman AM, et al. Opiate receptor binding affected differentially by opiates and opioid peptides. Eur J Pharmacol 1979;55:11–8.

[68] Gimbel J, Ahdieh H. The efficacy and safety of oral immediate release oxymorphone for postsurgical pain. Anesth Analg 2004;99:1472–7.

[69] Matsumoto AK, Babul N, Ahdieh H. Oxymorphone extended-release tablets relieve moderate to severe pain and improve physical function in osteoarthritis: results of a randomized double-blind, placebo—and active—controlled phase III trial. Pain Med 2005;6:357–66.

[70] Gabrail NY, Dvergsten C, Ahdieh H. Establishing the dosage equivalency of oxymorphone extended release and oxycodone controlled release in patients with moderate to severe cancer pain. Curr Med Res Opin 2004;20:911–8.

[71] Hale ME, Dvergsten C, Gimbel. Efficacy and safety of oxymorphone extended release in chronic low back pain: results of a randomized, double-blind, placebo—and active-controlled phase III study. J Pain 2005;6:21–8.

[72] Sloan P, Slatkin N, Ahdieh H. Effectiveness and safety of oral extended-release oxymorphone for the treatment of cancer pain: a pilot study. Support Care Cancer 2005;13:57–65.

[73] Pharmaceuticals P. TIMERx control release delivery systems. Available at: http://www. penwest.com/timerx.html. Accessed January 10, 2005.

[74] Adams MP, Ahdieh H. Pharmacokinetics and dose-proportionality of oxymorphone extended release and its metabolites: results of a randomized crossover study. Pharmacotherapy 2004;24:468–76.

[75] Adams MP, Ahdieh H. Single- and multiple-dose pharmacokinetic and dose-proportionality study of oxymorphone immediate-release tablets. Drugs R D 2005;6:91–9.

[76] Lalovic B, Phillips B, Risler LL, et al. Quantitative contribution of CYP2D6 and CYP3A to oxycodone metabolism in human liver and intestinal microsomes. Drug Metab Dispos 2004; 32:447–54.

ANESTHESIOLOGY
CLINICS

Anesthesiology Clin
25 (2007) 809–823

Documentation and Potential Tools in Long-Term Opioid Therapy for Pain

Howard S. Smith, MD, FACP[a],*,
Kenneth L. Kirsh, PhD[b]

[a]Albany Medical College, Department of Anesthesiology, 47 New Scotland Avenue,
MC-131 Albany, New York 12208, USA
[b]Pharmacy Practice and Science, University of Kentucky, 725 Rose Street, 401C,
Lexington, KY 40536-0082, USA

Tremendous progress has been made in the study and treatment of pain in the past 2 decades [1,2]. Efforts have been undertaken to make pain assessment and treatment a priority of medical care and to use all of the weapons in our arsenal to bring relief to the millions of people with chronic pain [3,4]. However, this progress has been somewhat tempered by the souring of the regulatory climate and the growth of prescription drug abuse. Because of this, there has been a trend for clinicians to shy away from using high opioid doses or even using this modality at all in the treatment of chronic pain [5–7].

Despite these setbacks, the use of long-term opioid therapy (LTOT) to treat chronic noncancer pain is growing, based in part on evidence from clinical trials and a growing consensus among pain specialists [8–12]. The appropriate use of these drugs requires skills in opioid prescribing, knowledge of addiction medicine principles, and a commitment to perform and document a comprehensive assessment repeatedly over time. Inadequate assessment can lead to undertreatment, compromise the effectiveness of therapy when implemented, and prevent an appropriate response when problematic drug-related behaviors occur [13–15].

Fortunately, there is a growing interest in the development of tools that can be useful for screening patients up front to determine relative risk for patients having problems with prescription drug abuse or misuse. Regarding

A version of this article originally appeared in the 91:2 issue of Medical Clinics of North America.
* Corresponding author.
E-mail address: SmithH@mail.amc.edu (H.S. Smith).

doi:10.1016/j.anclin.2007.07.005

brief screening instruments, a number have arisen, including the Screening Tool for Addiction Risk (STAR) [16], Drug Abuse Screening Test (DAST) [17], Screener and Opioid Assessment for Patients with Pain (SOAPP) [18], and the Opioid Risk Tool (ORT) [19] among others. The choice in tools for more thorough ongoing assessment, however, has been somewhat more limited up until now and will be the focus of our discussion.

Regulatory agencies, state medical boards, and various peer-review groups among others not only expect appropriate medical care but also require proper documentation. In cases of LTOT for chronic pain, aside from the usual "SOAP" (ie, subjective/objective/assessment/plan)-style medical progress notes, various other issues may deserve documentation. Although there are no explicit requirements spelled out as to what and how to document issues related to LTOT, it is felt by some that the use of specific tools/instruments in the chart on some or all visits may boost adherence to documentation expectations as well as consistency of such documentation. Assessment tools may also be helpful in the analysis of persistent pain [20].

It must be cautioned that physicians who adequately assess patients before and during opioid therapy may still encounter problems as a result of poor documentation. In a chart review of 300 patients with chronic pain, 61% had no documentation of a treatment plan [21]. Similarly, a review of the initial consultation notes of 513 patients with acute musculoskeletal pain revealed that only 43% of historical findings and 28% of physical examination findings were documented [22]. In a review of 520 randomly selected visits at an outpatient oncology practice, quantitative assessment of pain scores occurred in less than 1% of cases and qualitative assessment of pain occurred in only 60% of cases [23]. Finally, a review of medical records of 111 randomly selected patients who underwent urine toxicology screens in a cancer center found that documentation was infrequent: 37.8% of physicians failed to list a reason for the test, and 89% of the charts did not include the results of the test [24].

Areas of interest for documentation

Clearly, strategies are needed to translate these recommendations for patient assessment during long-term opioid therapy to frontline practice. This effort would certainly benefit from the availability of a consistent method of documentation. As one potential framework, it is important to consider four main domains in assessing pain outcomes and to better protect your practice for those patients you maintain on an opioid regimen: (1) pain relief, (2) functional outcomes, (3) side effects, and (4) drug-related behaviors. These domains have been labeled the "Four A's" (Analgesia, Activities of daily living, Adverse effects, and Aberrant drug-related behaviors) for teaching purposes [25]. There are, of course, many different ways to think about these domains, and multiple attempts to capture them will be discussed in this article.

The Pain Assessment and Documentation Tool

The Pain Assessment and Documentation Tool (PADT) is a simple charting device based on the 4 A's concept that is designed to focus on key outcomes and provide a consistent way to document progress in pain management therapy over time. Twenty-seven clinicians completed the preliminary version of the PADT for 388 opioid-treated patients [26,27]. Nineteen clinicians (17 physicians, 1 nurse, and 1 psychologist) participated in a debriefing phase. Twelve of the 19 clinicians had participated in the field trial before the debriefing. The debriefing interview for these clinicians used the same standard questions to evaluate both the original and revised PADT.

The result of this work is a brief, two-sided chart note that can be readily included in the patient's medical record. It was designed to be intuitive, pragmatic, and adaptable to clinical situations. In the field trial, it took clinicians between 10 and 20 minutes to complete the tool. The revised PADT is substantially shorter and should require a few minutes to complete. By addressing the need for documentation, the PADT can assist clinicians in meeting their obligations for ongoing assessment and documentation. Although the PADT is not intended to replace a progress note, it is well suited to complement existing documentation with a focused evaluation of outcomes that are clinically relevant and address the need for evidence of appropriate monitoring.

The decision to assess the four domains subsumed under the shorthand designation, the "Four A's," was based on clinical experience, the positive comments received by the investigators during educational programs on opioid pharmacotherapy for noncancer pain, and an evolving national movement that recognizes the need to approach opioid therapy with a "balanced" response. This response recognizes both the legitimate need to provide optimal therapy to appropriate patients and the need to acknowledge the potential for abuse, diversion, and addiction [25]. The value of assessing pain relief, side effects, and aspects of functioning has been emphasized repeatedly in the literature [21,28–31]. Documentation of drug-related behaviors is a relatively new concept that is being explored for the first time in the PADT.

Assessing opioid therapy adverse effects

Documentation of adverse effects in a majority of charts from many pain clinics tend to be addressed (or in many cases not addressed) in their charts by a brief note of the presence or absence of one or more adverse effects (eg, nausea, constipation, itching), noted by busy clinicians. Similar to the goal of the PADT, having a standardized form that is used at every visit and filled out by the patients before being seen by health care providers may provide certain advantages.

Patients with persistent pain on oral opioid therapy have asked to "come off" the opioids because of adverse effects, even if they perceived that opioids were providing reasonable analgesic effects [32]. The distress that may be caused by opioid adverse effects may also be seen with acute postoperative pain patients, who may occasionally ask to stop their opioids despite that they are perceived as effective analgesics, because of the significant distress and suffering that they perceive they are experiencing from an opioid adverse effect.

It therefore appears crucial to assess opioid adverse effects. Ideally, this should be done in a manner as to be able to follow trends as well as compare the patients' perceived intensity of the adverse effects versus the intensity of pain or other symptoms or adverse effects.

One available tool for the quantification of adverse effects is the Numerical Opioid Side Effect (NOSE) assessment tool (see Fig. 1) [33]. The NOSE instrument is self-administered, can be completed by the patient in minutes, and can be entered into electronic databases or inserted into a hard-copy chart on each patient visit. The NOSE assessment tool is easy to administer as well as easy to interpret and may provide clinicians with important

	Not Present									As Bad As You Can Imagine	
	0	1	2	3	4	5	6	7	8	9	10
1. Nausea, vomiting, and/or lack of appetite	O	O	O	O	O	O	O	O	O	O	O
2. Fatigue, sleepiness, trouble concentrating, hallucinations, and/or drowsiness/somnolence	O	O	O	O	O	O	O	O	O	O	O
3. Constipation	O	O	O	O	O	O	O	O	O	O	O
4. Itching	O	O	O	O	O	O	O	O	O	O	O
5. Decreased sexual desire/function and/or diminished libido	O	O	O	O	O	O	O	O	O	O	O
6. Dry Mouth	O	O	O	O	O	O	O	O	O	O	O
7. Abdominal pain or discomfort/cramping or bloating	O	O	O	O	O	O	O	O	O	O	O
8. Sweating	O	O	O	O	O	O	O	O	O	O	O
9. Headache and/or dizziness	O	O	O	O	O	O	O	O	O	O	O
10. Urinary retention	O	O	O	O	O	O	O	O	O	O	O

Fig. 1. Numerical Opioid Side Effect (NOSE) assessment tool.

clinical information that could potentially impact various therapeutic decisions. Although most clinicians probably routinely assess adverse effects of treatments, it is sometimes difficult to find legible, clear, and concise documentation of such information in outpatient records. Furthermore, the documentation that does exist may not always attempt to "quantify" the intensity of treatment-related adverse effects or lend itself to looking at trends.

Assessing LTOT efficacy

The Initiative on Methods, Measurements, and Pain Assessment in Clinical Trials (IMMPACT) recommended that six core outcome domains ([1] pain, [2] physical functions, [3] emotion, [4] participant rating of improvement and satisfaction with treatment, [5] symptoms and adverse events, and [6] participant disposition) should be considered when designing chronic pain clinical trials [34]. The authors believe that the use of a unidimensional tool such as the numerical rating scale-11 (NRS-11) provides a suboptimal assessment of chronic pain as well as LTOT efficacy. Clinicians should attempt to assess multiple domains (preferably with multidimensional tools) in efforts to achieve a global picture of the patient's baseline status as well as the patient's response to LTOT in various domains.

It has been proposed that the use of a collection of various tools may provide adjunct information and help clinicians to create a more complete picture regarding longitudinal trends of overall progress/functioning for their patients with chronic pain on LTOT [35]. Assessing individual outcomes during outpatient multidisciplinary chronic pain treatment is often an extremely challenging task. There are many tools and instruments currently available, but the Treatment Outcomes in Pain Survey tool (TOPS) has been specifically designed to assess and follow outcomes in the chronic pain population and has been described as an augmented SF-36 [36,37]. The Medical Outcomes Study (MOS) Short Form 36-item questionnaire (SF-36) compares the health status of large populations without a preponderance of one single medical condition [38]. The SF-36 assesses eight domains, but it has not been found to be especially useful for following the changes in function and pain in chronic pain populations.

The eight domains of the SF-36 are bodily pain (BP), general health (GH), mental health (MH), physical functioning (PF), role emotional (RE), social functioning (SF), role physical (RP), and vitality (VT). The TOPS scale initially had nine domains, but one (satisfaction with outcomes) was modified in subsequent versions. The nine domains of TOPS are Pain Symptom, Family/Social Disability, Functional Limitations, Total Pain Experience, Objective Work Disability, Life Control, Solicitous Responses, Passive Coping, and Satisfaction with Outcomes. This enhanced SF-36 (TOPS scale) was constructed by obtaining patient data from the SF-36 with 12 additional role-functioning questions. These additional questions were taken in part from the 61-item Multidimensional Pain Inventory (MPI) [39] and the 10-item Oswestry Disability Questionnaire [40], with four additional pain-related questions that are similar to those found in the MOS pain-related sections [41], the Brief Pain Inventory [28], and a six-item coping scale from the MOS [41].

The section adapted from the Oswestry Disability Questionnaire (designed for back pain patients) includes questions that relate to impairment (pain), physical functioning (how long the patient can sit or stand), and disability (ability to travel or have sexual relations) [40]. The patient-generated index is an instrument that attempts to individualize a patient's perception of his or her quality of life [42].

Although the TOPS instrument is an extremely useful tool, it is time-consuming, is based entirely on the patient's subjective responses, and requires that the clinician has access, whether by a special computer program or by sending forms away, for scoring. As a result, it may not be an ideal instrument to use in every pain clinic and may not provide the clinician with an answer immediately of how the patient is doing relative to previous visits (although it may have that potential with adequate time, scanning equipment, and computer software).

Translational analgesia

A concept that may possess potential utility for clinicians is translational analgesia. Translational analgesia refers to improvements in physical, social, or emotional function that are realized by the patient as a result of improved analgesia, or essentially what did the pain relief experienced by the patient "translate" into in terms of perceived improved quality of life [43]. In most cases, a sustained and significant improvement in pain perception that is deemed worthwhile to the patient should "translate" into improvement in quality of life or improved social, emotional, or physical function. Improvements in social, emotional, or physical domains are often spontaneously reported by patients, but in most cases should be able to be ascertained or elicited via "focused" interview techniques with the patient, significant others, and family; "focused" physical exam; or a combination of any of these. Improvements may be subtle and could include a range of daily function activities or other signs (eg, going out more with friends, doing laundry, showing improved mood/relations with family members). It is important to note that this issue is certainly not exclusive to opioid therapy and is thought to apply to other treatments.

The authors do not deem it inappropriate or inhumane to taper relatively "high-dose" opioid therapy in a patient with chronic pain who notes that his or her NRS-11 "pain score" has dropped from 9/10 to 8/10 after escalating to over a gram of long-acting morphine preparation per day but in whom the patient as well as the patient's family or significant other cannot describe (and the clinician cannot elicit) any significant "translational analgesia."

A patient with chronic pain who demonstrates a failure to "get off the couch," despite equivocal or minimally improved analgesia, should not be considered as a therapeutic success. But, should this viewpoint be seen as cruel or as a punishment for these patients? Rome and colleagues [44] demonstrated that at least a subpopulation of patients seems to do better after tapering off opioids. Furthermore, more evidence regarding the hyperalgesic actions of opioids in certain circumstances is mounting [45,46].

The periodic assessment of the patient with chronic pain should be performed in multiple domains (eg, social domain, analgesia domain, functional domain, emotional domain). The authors believe the relatively common practice of evaluating patients with chronic pain by obtaining an NRS-11 pain score at each assessment and basing opioid analgesic treatment solely on this score to be suboptimal. Although tools exist that assess multiple domains used in research, there is no simple, convenient, and universally acceptable instrument that is used in busy clinical pain practices.

To address this issue, a recent tool has been developed. The SAFE score (see section titled "The SAFE score") is a multidomain assessment tool that may have potential utility for rapid dynamic assessment in the busy clinic setting [47,48]. The SAFE score is a clinician-generated tool and may best be used in conjunction with the translational analgesic score (TAS) (a patient-generated tool) as an adjunct. These are discussed, in turn, in the following two sections.

The translational analgesic score

The translational analgesic score (TAS) is a patient-generated tool that attempts to quantify the degree of "translational analgesia" (see Fig. 2) [48]. It is simple, rapid, user-friendly, and suitable for use in busy pain clinics. The patient can be handed the TAS sheet with questions to fill out at each visit while in the waiting room and the responses are averaged for an overall score that is recorded in the chart. The authors encourage clinicians to have all patients write down specific examples of things that they can now do or do frequently that they couldn't do or did rarely when their pain was less controlled. Alternatively, the patients' responses can be entered into a computerized record (with graphs of trends) if the pain clinic's medical records are electronic.

In the sample provided, the patient answered all 10 questions with responses, hence, the average is the sum of all responses (26) divided by 10. Therefore, the TAS is 2.6. A patient, who at each visit consistently has a TAS of 10.0, clearly represents a therapeutic success on their current treatment. Conversely, a patient who at each visit consistently has a TAS of 0.0 would represent a suboptimal therapeutic result (by TAS criteria). Clinicians are encouraged to document at least one or two specific examples of translational analgesia (eg, perhaps various activities that the patient can

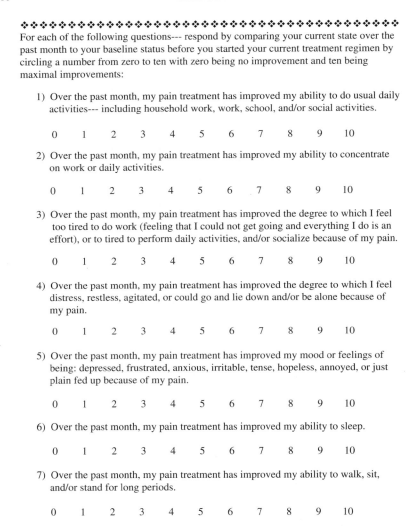

❖❖❖

For each of the following questions--- respond by comparing your current state over the past month to your baseline status before you started your current treatment regimen by circling a number from zero to ten with zero being no improvement and ten being maximal improvements:

1) Over the past month, my pain treatment has improved my ability to do usual daily activities--- including household work, work, school, and/or social activities.

   0   1   2   3   4   5   6   7   8   9   10

2) Over the past month, my pain treatment has improved my ability to concentrate on work or daily activities.

   0   1   2   3   4   5   6   7   8   9   10

3) Over the past month, my pain treatment has improved the degree to which I feel too tired to do work (feeling that I could not get going and everything I do is an effort), or to tired to perform daily activities, and/or socialize because of my pain.

   0   1   2   3   4   5   6   7   8   9   10

4) Over the past month, my pain treatment has improved the degree to which I feel distress, restless, agitated, or could go and lie down and/or be alone because of my pain.

   0   1   2   3   4   5   6   7   8   9   10

5) Over the past month, my pain treatment has improved my mood or feelings of being: depressed, frustrated, anxious, irritable, tense, hopeless, annoyed, or just plain fed up because of my pain.

   0   1   2   3   4   5   6   7   8   9   10

6) Over the past month, my pain treatment has improved my ability to sleep.

   0   1   2   3   4   5   6   7   8   9   10

7) Over the past month, my pain treatment has improved my ability to walk, sit, and/or stand for long periods.

   0   1   2   3   4   5   6   7   8   9   10

Fig. 2. The Translational Analgesic Score (TAS).

now perform as a result of pain relief or can now perform frequently as a result of pain relief that the patient could not do or only do infrequently before therapy) on the bottom or reverse side of the TAS score sheet. Treatment decisions regarding escalation or tapering of opioids, changing agents, adding agents, obtaining consultations, instituting physical medicine or behavioral medicine techniques, remain the medical judgment of practitioners and should be based on a careful reevaluation of the patient and not based on a number.

8) Over the past month, my pain treatment has improved my ability to go up stairs, and/or move or lift objects.

0   1   2   3   4   5   6   7   8   9   10

9) Over the past month, my pain treatment has improved the extent to which my pain interferes with optimal interpersonal relationships and/or intimacy.

0   1   2   3   4   5   6   7   8   9   10

10) Over the past month, to what degree have you, your significant other, your family, your co-workers, and/or your friends noticed any improvements in your socializing, recreational activities, physical functioning, concentration, mood, interpersonal relationships, activities of daily living, and/or overall quality of life?

0   1   2   3   4   5   6   7   8   9   10

--- Please write below--- specific examples of things you can now do or currently do frequently that you couldn't do or only did rarely when your pain was not controlled as well as it is now.

TAS = _____

❖❖❖

The TAS is expressed as a number between 0 to 10 with a decimal being the average of the responses to the ten questions (or less--- if the patient is paraplegic then they would not answer the questions regarding going up stairs, etc.).

As an example, a patient's response to the TAS tool is shown below:
1) Over the past month, my pain treatment has improved my ability to do usual daily activities--- including household work, work, school, and/or social activities.

0   1   2   3   •   5   6   7   8   9   10

2) Over the past month, my pain treatment has improved my ability to concentrate on work or daily activities.

0   1   2   •   4   5   6   7   8   9   10

3) Over the past month, my pain treatment has improved the degree to which I feel too tired to do work (feeling that I could not get going and everything I do is an effort), or to tired to perform daily activities, and/or socialize because of my pain.

0   1   2   •   4   5   6   7   8   9   10

Fig. 2 (*continued*).

The concept of translational analgesia is not meant to imply that opioids should be tapered, weaned, or discontinued. If a patient has a TAS that is very low and essentially unchanged over time (especially in conjunction with a SAFE score in the "red zone"), then this should prompt the clinician to reevaluate the patient and consider a change in therapy. This could mean pursuing various therapeutic options including perhaps increasing the dose

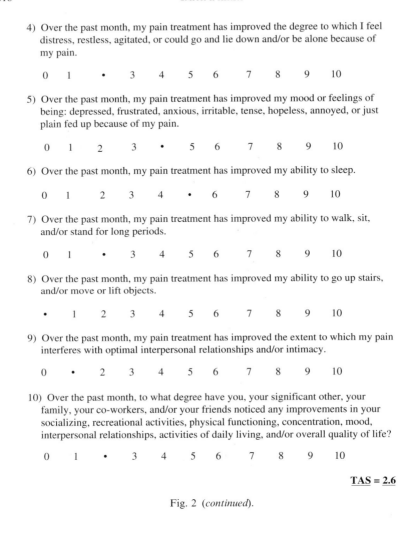

4) Over the past month, my pain treatment has improved the degree to which I feel distress, restless, agitated, or could go and lie down and/or be alone because of my pain.

0   1   •   3   4   5   6   7   8   9   10

5) Over the past month, my pain treatment has improved my mood or feelings of being: depressed, frustrated, anxious, irritable, tense, hopeless, annoyed, or just plain fed up because of my pain.

0   1   2   3   •   5   6   7   8   9   10

6) Over the past month, my pain treatment has improved my ability to sleep.

0   1   2   3   4   •   6   7   8   9   10

7) Over the past month, my pain treatment has improved my ability to walk, sit, and/or stand for long periods.

0   1   •   3   4   5   6   7   8   9   10

8) Over the past month, my pain treatment has improved my ability to go up stairs, and/or move or lift objects.

•   1   2   3   4   5   6   7   8   9   10

9) Over the past month, my pain treatment has improved the extent to which my pain interferes with optimal interpersonal relationships and/or intimacy.

0   •   2   3   4   5   6   7   8   9   10

10) Over the past month, to what degree have you, your significant other, your family, your co-workers, and/or your friends noticed any improvements in your socializing, recreational activities, physical functioning, concentration, mood, interpersonal relationships, activities of daily living, and/or overall quality of life?

0   1   •   3   4   5   6   7   8   9   10

TAS = 2.6

Fig. 2 (*continued*).

of opioids. However, if a patient has a high TAS and a SAFE score in the green zone, the patient should probably continue LTOT.

The SAFE score

Another tool that has been advocated to help with this purpose is called the SAFE score [47,48]. Although it has not yet been rigorously validated, it is simple and practical and may possess clinical utility. It is a score generated by the health care provider that is meant to reflect a multidimensional assessment of outcome to opioid therapy. It is not meant to replace more elaborate patient-based assessment tools but could possibly serve as an adjunct and possibly in the future shed some light on the difference between patients' perception of how they are doing on opioid treatment versus the physician-based view of outcome.

At each visit, the clinician rates the patient's functioning and pain relief in four domains. The domains assessed include social functioning (S), analgesia or pain relief (A), physical functioning (F), and emotional functioning (E). Together, the ratings in each of the four domains are combined to yield a "SAFE" score. The "SAFE" score can range from 4 to 20.

The SAFE tool is both practical in its ease and clinically useful (Fig. 3). The goals of the SAFE tool are multifold. Specifically, they include the need to demonstrate that the clinician has routinely evaluated the efficacy of the treatment from multiple perspectives; guide the clinician toward a broader view of treatment options beyond adjusting the medication regimen; and document the clinician's rationale for continuation, modification, or cessation of opioid therapy.

Interpretation of scores

Scores can be broken down into three distinct categories. First, the *green zone* represents a SAFE score of 4 to 12 or decrease of 2 points in total score

	Rating	Criterion				
Social Marital, family, friends, leisure, recreational		1 supportive harmonious socializing engaged	2	3	4	5 conflictual discord isolated bored
Analgesia Intensity, frequency, duration		1 comfortable effective controlled	2	3	4	5 intolerable ineffective uncontrolled
Function Work, ADL's, home management, school, training, physical activity		1 independent active productive energetic	2	3	4	5 dependent unmotivated passive deconditioned
Emotional Cognitive, stress, attitude, mood, behavior, neuro-vegetative signs		1 clear relaxed optimistic upbeat composed	2	3	4	5 confused tense pessimistic depressed distressed
Total Score						

The patient's status in each of the four domains is rated as follows:

1 = Excellent
2 = Good
3 = Fair
4 = Borderline
5 = Poor

Fig. 3. Sample SAFE form.

Example A

Social	3
Analgesia	2
Function	3
Emotional	3
Green Zone "SAFE" score	11

Example B

Social	2
Analgesia	4
Function	3
Emotional	1
Green Zone "SAFE" score	10

Fig. 4. Green zone cases using the SAFE scoring tool.

from baseline. With a score in the green zone, the patient is considered to be doing well and the plan would be to continue with the current medication regimen or consider reducing the total dose of the opioids. Second, the *yellow zone* represents a SAFE score of 13 to 16 or a rating of 5 in any category or an increase of 2 or more from baseline in the total score. With a score in the yellow zone, the patient should be monitored closely and reassessed frequently. Finally, the *red zone* represents a SAFE score greater than or equal to 17. With a score in the red zone, a change in the treatment would be warranted.

Once the color determination is made, a decision can be made regarding treatment options. Treatment options depend on the pattern of scores. If attempts are made to address problems in specific domains and the patient is still not showing an improvement in the SAFE score, then the patient may not be an appropriate candidate for long-term opioid therapy.

Fig. 4 illustrates green zone cases. In example A, there is good analgesic response to opioids, with a fair response in the other domains. No change in treatment would be necessary unless adverse reactions to the medications require an adjustment or discontinuation. In example B, there is borderline analgesic response, but good social and emotional responses and a fair physical functioning response. Some pain specialists may determine that the medication regimen should be optimized. For others, this pattern of ratings may reflect a reasonable improvement in quality of life for the patient. Therefore, continuing the present medication regimen would be a reasonable option.

Fig. 5 illustrates how the SAFE tool can be used to track changes in the status of the same patient on two consecutive visits. In the change in scores

Example C

Social	5
Analgesia	3
Function	5
Emotional	5
Red Zone "SAFE" score	18

Example D

Social	3
Analgesia	4
Function	3
Emotional	3
Green Zone "SAFE" score	13

Fig. 5. Tracking an overall positive change in status using the SAFE scoring tool.

Example E

Social	3
Analgesia	2
Function	3
Emotional	3
Green Zone "SAFE" score	11

Example F

Social	3
Analgesia	2
Function	4
Emotional	4
Yellow Zone "SAFE" score	13

Fig. 6. Tracking an overall negative change in status using the SAFE scoring tool.

from example C to example D, although analgesia deteriorates from fair to borderline, there is significant improvement in the other domains. The clinician may feel this is satisfactory for this particular patient and continue with the current medication regimen. Once again, too narrow a focus on analgesic response may lead to unnecessary dose escalation. This case also illustrates the situation in which even though the total score at visit D is greater than 12 and would be a *yellow zone*, it is assigned as a *green zone* because there was a decrease of more than 2 in the total score. Alternately, the clinician may determine that a borderline analgesic response is not optimal. The choices for intervention may include rotating to another opioid agent, increasing the current opioid dose, adding adjuvant medications, referring for nonpharmacological treatment, or discontinuing high-dose opioids.

Fig. 6 illustrates again a single patient on two consecutive visits. Here, analgesia has remained good over time, but there has been a negative impact on the domains of function and emotion. Pain specialists who are focused on the pain scores of such a patient may be comfortable with continuing the established treatment plan. However, using SAFE, an expanded view of the patient's overall status will alert the clinician to monitor the patient's physical and emotional functioning in future visits. If the ratings in the psychological and physical domains persist, then the clinician may recommend that the patient pursue psychosocial treatment or physical rehabilitation in addition to maintaining the medication regimen.

Summary

Assessment and documentation are cornerstones for both protecting your practice and obtaining optimal patient outcomes while on opioid therapy. There are a growing number of assessment tools for clinicians to guide the evaluation of a group of important outcomes during opioid therapy and provide a simple means of documenting patient care. They all have the capability to prove helpful in clinical management and offer mechanisms for documenting the types of practice standards that those in the regulatory and law enforcement communities seek to ensure.

References

[1] Berry PH, Dahl JL. The new JCAHO pain standards: implications for pain management nurses. Pain Manag Nurs 2000;1(1):3–12.

[2] SUPPORT Study Principal Investigators. A controlled trial to improve care for seriously ill hospitalized patients: a study to understand prognoses and preferences for outcomes and risks of treatment (SUPPORT). JAMA 1995;274:1591.

[3] Osterweis M, Kleinman A, Mechanic D, editors. Pain and disability: clinical, behavioral, and public policy perspectives. [Report of the Committee on Pain, Disability, and Chronic Illness Behavior, Institute of Medicine, National Academy of Sciences.]. Washington, DC: National Academy Press; 1987.

[4] Verhaak PFM, Kerssens JJ, Dekker J, et al. Prevalence of chronic benign pain disorder among adults: a review of the literature. Pain 1998;77:231–9.

[5] Cicero TJ, Inciardi JA, Munoz A. Trends in abuse of Oxycontin and other opioid analgesics in the United States: 2002–2004. J Pain 2005;6(10):662–72.

[6] Lipman AG. Does the DEA truly seek balance in pain medicine? J Pain Palliat Care Pharmacother 2005;19(1):7–9.

[7] Passik SD, Kirsh KL. Fear and loathing in the pain clinic. Pain Med 2006;7(4):363–4.

[8] Collett BJ. Opioid tolerance: the clinical perspective. Br J Anaesth 1998;81:58–68.

[9] Portenoy RK. Opioid therapy for chronic nonmalignant pain: a review of critical issues. J Pain Symptom Manage 1996;11:203–17.

[10] Portenoy RK. Opioid therapy for chronic nonmalignant pain. Pain Res Manage 1996;1:17–28.

[11] Urban BJ, France RD, Steinberger EK, et al. Long-term use of narcotic/antidepressant medication in the management of phantom limb pain. Pain 1986;24:191–6.

[12] Zenz M, Strumpf M, Tryba M. Long-term oral opioid therapy in patients with chronic nonmalignant pain. J Pain Symptom Manage 1992;7:69–77.

[13] Joint Commission on the Accreditation of Healthcare Organizations. Patient rights and organization ethics. Referenced from the comprehensive accreditation manual for hospitals, update 3, 1999. Available at: http://www.jointcommission.org. Accessed September 2006.

[14] Max MB, Payne R, Edwards WT, et al. Principles of analgesic use in the treatment of acute pain and cancer pain. 4th ed. Glenview, IL: American Pain Society; 1999.

[15] Katz N. The impact of pain management on quality of life. J Pain Symptom Manage 2002; 24(suppl 1):S38–47.

[16] Friedman R, Li V, Mehrotra D. Treating pain patients at risk: evaluation of a screening tool in opioid-treated pain patients with and without addiction. Pain Med 2003;4(2):182–5.

[17] Gavin DR, Ross HE, Skinner HA. Diagnostic validity of the drug abuse screening test in the assessment of DSM-III drug disorders. Br J Addict 1989;84(3):301–7.

[18] Butler SF, Budman SH, Fernandez K, et al. Validation of a screener and opioid assessment measure for patients with chronic pain. Pain 2004;112(1–2):65–75.

[19] Webster LR, Webster RM. Predicting aberrant behaviors in opioid-treated patients: preliminary validation of the Opioid Risk Tool. Pain Med 2005;6(6):432–42.

[20] Wincent A, Linden Y, Arner S. Pain questionnaires in the analysis of long lasting (chronic) pain conditions. Eur J Pain 2003;7:311–21.

[21] Clark JD. Chronic pain prevalence and analgesic prescribing in a general medical population. J Pain Symptom Manage 2002;23:131–7.

[22] Solomon DH, Schaffer JL, Katz JN, et al. Can history and physical examination be used as markers of quality? An analysis of the initial visit note in musculoskeletal care. Med Care 2000;38:383–91.

[23] Rhodes DJ, Koshy RC, Waterfield WC, et al. Feasibility of quantitative pain assessment in outpatient oncology practice. J Clin Oncol 2001;19:501–8.

[24] Passik SD, Schreiber J, Kirsh KL, et al. A chart review of the ordering and documentation of urine toxicology screens in a cancer center: do they influence patient management? J Pain Symptom Manage 2000;19:40–4.

[25] Passik SD, Weinreb HJ. Managing chronic nonmalignant pain: overcoming obstacles to the use of opioids. Adv Ther 2000;17:70–83.
[26] Passik SD, Kirsh KL, Whitcomb LA, et al. A new tool to assess and document pain outcomes in chronic pain patients receiving opioid therapy. Clin Ther 2004;26(4):552–61.
[27] Passik SD, Kirsh KL, Whitcomb LA, et al. Monitoring outcomes during long-term opioid therapy for non-cancer pain: results with the pain assessment and documentation tool. Journal of Opioid Management 2005;1(5):257–66.
[28] Daut R, Cleeland C, Flannery R. Development of the Wisconsin Brief Pain Questionnaire to assess pain in cancer and other diseases. Pain 1983;17:197–210.
[29] Cleeland CS, Ryan KM. Pain assessment: global use of the Brief Pain Inventory. Ann Acad Med Singapore 1994;23:129–38.
[30] Melzack R. The McGill Pain Questionnaire: major properties and scoring methods. Pain 1975;1:277–99.
[31] McCarberg BH, Barkin RL. Long-acting opioids for chronic pain: pharmacotherapeutic opportunities to enhance compliance, quality of life, and analgesia. Am J Ther 2001;8:181–6.
[32] Kalso E, Edwards JE, Moore RA, et al. Opioids in chronic non-cancer pain: systematic review of efficacy and safety. Pain 2004;112:372–80.
[33] Smith HS. The Numerical Opioid Side Effect (NOSE). Assessment tool. Journal of Cancer Pain and Symptom Palliation 2005;1:3–6.
[34] Turk DC, Dworkin RH, Allen RR, et al. Core outcome domains for chronic pain clinical trials: IMMPACT recommendations. Pain 2003;106:337–45.
[35] Smith HS. Translational analgesia and the translational analgesic score. Journal of Cancer Pain and Symptom Palliation 2005;1:15–9.
[36] Rogers WH, Wittink H, Wagner A, et al. Assessing individual outcomes during outpatient multidisciplinary chronic pain treatment by means of an augmented SF-36. Pain Med 2000; 1:44–54.
[37] Rogers WH, Wittink H, Ashburn MA, et al. Using the "TOPS," an outcome instrument for multidisciplinary outpatient pain treatment. Pain Med 2000;1:55–67.
[38] Ware JE Jr, Sherbourne CD, The MOS. 36-item short-form health survey (SF-36). I. Conceptual Framework and Item Selection. Med Care 1992;30:473–83.
[39] Kerns R, Turk D, Rudy T. The West Haven-Yale Multidimensional Pain Inventory (WHYMPI). Pain 1985;23:345–6.
[40] Fairbanks J, Couper J, Davies J, et al. The Oswestry low back pain disability questionnaire. Physiotherapy 1980;66:271–3.
[41] Tarlor A, Ware J Jr, Greenfield S, et al. The Medical Outcomes Study: an application of methods for monitoring the results of medical care. JAMA 1989;262:925–30.
[42] Ruta DA, Garratt AM, Leng M, et al. A new approach to quality of life: the patient-generated index. Med Care 1994;32:1109–26.
[43] Smith HS. Perspectives in persistent noncancer pain. Journal of Cancer Pain and Symptom Palliation 2005;1:31–2.
[44] Rome JD, Townsend CP, Bruce BK, et al. Chronic noncancer pain rehabilitation with opioid withdrawal: comparison of treatment outcomes based on opioid use status at admission. Mayo Clin Proc 2004;79:759–68.
[45] Holtman JR, Wala EP. Characterization of morphine-induced hyperalgesia in male and female rats. Pain 2005;114:62–70.
[46] Ruscheweyh R, Sand Kuhler J. Opioids and central sensitization: II. Induction and reversal of hyperalgesia. Eur J Pain 2005;9:149–52.
[47] Smith H, Audette J, Witkower A. Assessing analgesic therapeutic outcomes. In: Smith H, editor. Drugs for pain. Philadelphia (PA): H. Hanley and Belfus; 2003. p. 499–508.
[48] Smith HS, Audette J, Witkower A. Playing It "SAFE". Journal of Cancer Pain and Symptom Palliation 2005;1:3–10.

ELSEVIER
SAUNDERS

Anesthesiology Clin
25 (2007) 825–839

ANESTHESIOLOGY
CLINICS

Topical Analgesics

Gary McCleane, MD, FFARCSI

Rampark Pain Centre, 2 Rampark Dromore Road, Lurgan BT66 7JH, Northern Ireland, UK

Among the drugs with well-known peripheral effects are nonsteroidal anti-inflammatory drugs (NSAIDs), local anesthetics, and capsaicin. Less well appreciated is the fact that nitrates, tricyclic antidepressants (TCAs), glutamate receptor antagonists, α-adrenoerecptor antagonists, and cannabinoids may have an analgesic effect when applied topically. The rational for the analgesic effects of these compounds, when applied topically, is discussed in this article.

To patients, it makes sense to apply pain relief directly to where they feel pain. They "know" that oral medication can produce side effects, whereas topical agents are less likely to do so. Knowledgeable physicians, however, understand that pain is influenced by peripheral and central factors. They understand that significant opportunity exists to augment inhibitory or to lessen facilitatory influences on the pain stimulus, and therefore, in general, seem to prefer systemically active agents. Increasing evidence, however, backed up by clinical use, now suggests that topically applied medication can be at least as effective as that administered by the oral route and, in general, has a more favorable side effect profile than orally active agents. In this article, the author looks at medications that have a tradition of topical use and at newer additions to this range of drugs. Although a rich variety of potential pharmacologic targets exists peripherally, to date, only some of these are amenable to currently available therapeutic entities; it is on these that concentration is focused.

Not all medication applied to the skin has a local, peripheral action. Drugs such as fentanyl and buprenorphine, which can be applied to the skin, have predominately central effects. This type of administration is known as "transdermal" to distinguish it from the "topical" analgesics— drugs that are applied to skin and have a predominate peripheral effect.

A version of this article originally appeared in the 91:1 issue of Medical Clinics of North America.

E-mail address: gary@mccleane.freeserve.co.uk

Anti-inflammatory agents

Nonsteroidal anti-inflammatory drugs

Among the most widely used topical agents are the NSAIDs. These agents are known to reduce the production of prostaglandins that sensitize nerve endings at the site of injury. This effect occurs due to the inhibition of the cyclooxygenase (COX) enzyme that converts arachidonic acid liberated from the phospholipid membrane by phospholipases to prostanoids such as prostaglandin. At least two forms of COX are thought to be important. COX1 is normally expressed in tissues such as stomach and kidneys and plays a physiologic role in maintaining tissue integrity [1]. A second form, COX2, plays a role in pain and inflammation [1]. The analgesic effects of NSAIDs can be dissociated from anti-inflammatory effects, and this may reflect additional spinal and supraspinal actions of NSAIDs to inhibit various aspects of central pain processing [2]. Recent evidence suggests that a third COX, COX3, which is predominately centrally distributed, may also be involved in NSAID or acetaminophen action [3]; however, its role remains uncertain.

When NSAIDs are applied topically, bioavailability and plasma concentrations are 5% to 15% of those achieved by systemic delivery [4]. In human experimental pain models, topically applied NSAIDs produce analgesia in models of cutaneous pain [5–8] and muscle pain [9]. In terms of clinical use, three major reviews—one examining use in musculoskeletal and soft tissue pain [10], another looking at data accrued in over 10,000 patients in 86 trials [11], and the last looking primarily at chronic rheumatic disease [4]—concluded that there was clear and significant evidence that topical NSAIDs have pain-relieving properties.

When NSAIDs are applied topically, relatively high concentrations occur in the dermis, whereas levels in adjacent muscle are as high as when the NSAID is given systemically [4]. Gastrointestinal side effects occur less frequently than when the drug is given orally but are still more likely in patients who have previously demonstrated such responses to oral medication [10].

Perhaps the greatest danger of topical NSAID use is the risk of polypharmacy. A number of over-the-counter topical and oral NSAIDs are now available, and the risk of overdosing with several different preparations taken at the same time and all containing NSAID is very real.

Nitrates

Conventionally used in the treatment of ischemic heart disease, it now seems that nitrates also have potent analgesic and anti-inflammatory effects. It is known that exogenous nitrates stimulate the release of nitric oxide (NO) [12]. This substance is known to be a potent mediator in a wide variety of different cellular systems such as the endothelium and the central and peripheral nervous system. It is released from the endothelium and from neutrophils and macrophages—all known to be intimately involved in the inflammatory process. It appears that NO exerts its effect by stimulating increases in guanylate cyclase, thereby increasing levels of 3′,5′-cyclic GMP [13]. Cholinergic drugs such as acetylcholine produce analgesia in a similar fashion by releasing NO and increasing NO at the nociceptor level [14].

In addition to this action, NO may activate ATP-sensitive potassium channels and activate peripheral antinociception [15]. Endogenous NO levels may be increased if glutamate levels are increased [16]. Glutamate is known to be an excitatory amino acid, activating N-methyl-D-aspartate (NMDA) receptors, thereby initiating sensitization and protracting the pain process.

Topical nitrate, in the form of glyceryl trinitrate (GTN), has been shown to effectively reduce the pain of osteoarthritis [17], supraspinatus tendonitis [18], and infusion-related thrombophlebitis [19]. In addition, it may reduce the pain and inflammation caused by sclerosant treatment of varicose veins [20] and may even be useful in the treatment of vulvar pain [21]. A number of reports suggest that topical nitrates may enhance the analgesic effectiveness of strong opioids [22–24], but it is likely that this effect is due to systemic absorption of the nitrate and a consequent central action. The predominant side effect associated with topical nitrate use is headache. Currently, patch formulations deliver a relatively large amount of nitrate and, therefore, the incidence of headache is high. Should lower dose patches become available, the utility of this treatment would be increased. GTN is also available in an ointment formulation. Measurement and consistency of dosing are problematic with the ointment formulation, and because there is only a small difference between a potentially analgesic dose and one that causes headache, GTN ointment use is less practical than the use of the patch varieties.

Topical nitrates can therefore be considered when pain is localized and particularly in patients in whom NSAIDs are contraindicated. Nitrates are devoid of the renal, gastrointestinal, and hematologic side effects of NSAIDs.

Local anesthetics

Gels/creams

Several topical local anesthetic preparations are available in gel, cream, and patch form. Amethocaine is available as a gel and lidocaine/prilocaine is presented as a cream. The cream contains a eutectic mixture of lidocaine and prilocaine and its use has become established in the anesthetizing of skin before cannula insertion. It also has demonstrable benefit in reducing the pain of other procedures including lumbar puncture, intramuscular injections, and circumcision [25]. Although lidocaine/prilocaine cream is not

US Food and Drug Administration (FDA) approved for any neuropathic pain condition, several studies have been undertaken in patients who have postherpetic neuralgia (PHN). Two of these studies were uncontrolled and showed a pain-reducing effect [26,27], whereas a randomized controlled study of the same condition failed to show any benefit [28]. Caution should be used with long-term use of this preparation because prilocaine use has been associated with the onset of methemoglobinemia.

Patches

Lidocaine is available in a topically applied patch at a 5% strength. In the United States, this preparation is approved by the FDA for the treatment of PHN. Its efficacy in this pain condition is supported by several trials that also confirm that it is well tolerated [29,30]. Not only can pain levels in patients who have PHN be reduced but measures of quality of life also show improvement [31]. In one study of patients who had PHN, 66% of subjects reported reduced pain intensity when up to three lidocaine 5% patches were used for 12 hours each day [31].

Although lidocaine 5% is indicated for use in PHN, it may also be efficacious in other pain conditions. When used in the treatment of focal neuropathic pain conditions such as mononeuropathies and intercostal and ilioinguinal neuralgia, one controlled study confirmed a pain-reducing effect [32]. In an open-label study of 16 patients who had "refractory" neuropathic pain (including patients who had post-thoracotomy pain, complex regional pain syndrome, postamputation pain, neuroma pain, painful diabetic neuropathy, meralgia parasthetica, and postmastectomy pain), 81% of subjects experienced notable pain relief [33]. In this report, *refractory* was defined as those who had failed to gain pain relief or who experienced unacceptable side effects with opiates, anticonvulsants, antidepressants, or antiarrhythmic agents.

Capsaicin

Capsaicin use has a long history in medical practice. Extract of chili pepper was reported in the midnineteenth century to reduce chilblain pain and toothache [34]. It has now been shown to reduce the pain associated with painful diabetic neuropathy [35–38], PHN [39–41], chronic distal painful polyneuropathy [42], oral neuropathic pain [43], surgical neuropathic pain [44], and the pain associated with Guillain-Barré syndrome [45]. In the treatment of non-neuropathic pain, capsaicin has a role, with evidence of a pain-relieving effect in osteoarthritis [46–51] and neck pain [52].

It appears that capsaicin achieves its pain-relieving effect by reversibly depleting sensory nerve endings of substance P [53,54] and by reducing the density of epidermal nerve fibers, also in a reversible fashion [55].

When used clinically, the major impediment to better compliance is the intense burning sensation associated with capsaicin's use. This sensation generally reduces with repeated administration, although when capsaicin cream is applied outside the normal area of application, discomfort is again apparent. It has been shown that coadministration of GTN can reduce the discomfort associated with application [50,56,57] and enhance the analgesic effect of the capsaicin [50]. Alternatively, preapplication of lidocaine 5% cream can also reduce application-associated discomfort [58].

Some patients experience bouts of sneezing when capsaicin is used, which is normally caused by overapplication and drying of the cream on the skin and then nasal inhalation of the capsaicin dust from the application site. Care must always be used so that capsaicin is not applied to moist areas because this is associated with increased burning sensation.

Tricyclic antidepressants

TCAs, when taken orally, have a long pedigree in pain management. Their use is established in a broad range of pain conditions. Their pain-relieving effect is independent of their antidepressant effect. It is unfortunate that their use is also associated with a significant risk of side effects (eg, dry mouth, sedation, urinary retention, and weight gain), which reduces compliance. In contrast, when TCAs are applied topically, side effects are relatively rare, yet a very real chance of pain relief exists. Any relief obtained by topical TCA use can be rationalized by their possible peripheral actions.

Adenosine receptors

At peripheral nerve terminals in rodents, adenosine A_1 receptor activation produces antinociception by decreasing cyclic AMP levels in the sensory nerve terminals, whereas adenosine A_2 receptor activation produces pronociception by increasing cyclic AMP levels in the sensory nerve terminals. Adenosine A_3 receptor activation produces pain behaviors due to the release of histamine and serotonin from mast cells and subsequent actions in the sensory nerve terminal [59]. Caffeine acts as a nonspecific adenosine receptor antagonist. When systemic caffeine is administered with systemic amitriptyline, the normal effect on thermal hyperalgesia is blocked. When amitriptyline is administered into a rodent paw that has neuropathic pain, an antihyperalgesic effect is recorded (but not when it is given into the contralateral paw). This antihyperalgesic effect is blocked by caffeine [60], suggesting that at least part of the effect of peripherally applied amitriptyline is mediated through peripheral adenosine receptors.

Sodium channels

Sudoh and colleagues [61] injected various TCAs by a single injection into rat sciatic notches. These investigators measured the duration of complete sciatic nerve blockade and compared these values with that of bupivacaine. They found that amitriptyline, doxepin, and imipramine produced a longer complete sciatic nerve block than bupivacaine, whereas trimipramine and desipramine produced a shorter block. Nortriptyline and maprotiline failed to produce any block. When the effect of topical application of amitriptyline is compared with that of lidocaine, amitriptyline is seen to produce longer cutaneous analgesia [62].

These studies suggest, therefore, that from a mode-of-action perspective, TCAs could have an analgesic effect when applied peripherally.

Animal evidence of an antinociceptive effect of peripherally applied tricyclic antidepressants

Neuropathic pain

When amitriptyline is applied to rodent paws made neuropathic by a chronic nerve constriction injury, an antinociceptive effect is observed. When the amitriptyline is applied to the contralateral paw, no antinociceptive effect is observed in the paw on the injured side [63,64]. When desipramine and the selective serotonin reuptake inhibitor fluoxetine are considered, desipramine has a similar antinociceptive effect when applied topically, whereas fluoxetine does not [65].

Formalin test

It seems that when amitriptyline [66–68] and desipramine [65] are coadministered peripherally with formalin, the first- and second-phase responses are reduced.

When amitriptyline is administered peripherally along with formalin, Fos immunoreactivity in the dorsal region of the spinal cord is significantly lower than in animals in which formalin is administered alone [68].

Visceral pain

Using a noxious colorectal distension model in the rat, Su and Gebhart [69] showed that the antidepressants imipramine, desipramine, and clomipramine reduce the response to noxious colorectal distension by 20%, 22%, and 46%, respectively, compared with control-treated animals.

Thermal injury

Thermal hyperalgesia is produced by exposing a rodent hindpaw to 52°C for 45 seconds. Locally applied amitriptyline at the time of thermal injury may produce antihyperalgesic and analgesic effects, depending on the concentration used. When the amitriptyline is applied after the injury, the analgesic effect, but not the antihyperalgesic effect, is retained [70].

Human pain

Human evidence of an analgesic effect with the topical application of TCAs is limited. A small randomized, placebo-controlled trial of 40 subjects who had neuropathic pain of mixed etiology produced a reduction of 1.18 on a 0-to-10 linear visual analog score relative to placebo use with the application of a doxepin 5% cream. Minor side effects were seen in only 3 subjects [71]. A larger randomized controlled trial involving 200 subjects, again with neuropathic pain of mixed etiology, suggested that doxepin 5% cream reduced the linear visual analog score by about 1 relative to placebo and that time to effect was about 2 weeks. Again, side effects were minor and infrequent [72]. A pilot study examining the effect of topical amitriptyline application failed to produce any pain relief, but the maximum therapy duration was 7 days [73]; the study may have been terminated before the time to maximal effect had been reached.

Case reports have been made of a useful reduction in pain when doxepin 5% cream was applied topically in subjects who had complex regional pain syndrome type I [74] and when doxepin was used as an oral rinse in patients who had oral pain as a result of cancer or cancer therapy [75].

Although the human evidence of an analgesic effect with topical doxepin is interesting, more study is needed to verify its effects and the effects of other TCAs when used by this route of administration. Evidence suggests that the effect of topically applied doxepin is a local effect and that the consequences of systemic administration and, hence, systemic side effects can be substantially reduced. Doxepin in a 5% cream formulation is currently available and is indicated in the treatment of itch associated with eczema.

Glutamate receptor antagonist

It has recently become apparent that glutamate receptors are expressed on peripheral nerve terminals and that these may contribute to peripheral nociceptive signaling. Ionotropic and metabotropic glutamate receptors are present on membranes of unmyelinated peripheral axons and axon terminals in the skin [76,77], and peripheral inflammation increases the proportions of unmyelinated and myelinated nerves expressing ionotropic glutamate receptors [78]. Local injections of NMDA and non-NMDA glutamate receptor agonists to the rat hindpaw [79,80] or knee joint [81] enhance pain behaviors generating hyperalgesia and allodynia. Injections of metabotropic glutamate receptor agonists produce similar actions [76,82]. Local application of glutamate receptor antagonists inhibits pain behavior following formalin application [81].

In humans, ketamine, a noncompetitive NMDA receptor antagonist, enhances the local anesthetic and analgesic effects of bupivicaine in acute postoperative pain by a peripheral mechanism [83]. When a thermal injury was inflicted in volunteers, one study suggested that subcutaneous injection of ketamine produces long-lasting reduction in hyperalgesia [84], whereas another study failed to confirm this result [85]. That said, not only may any analgesic effect produced by peripheral ketamine application be due to its glutamate receptor activity but ketamine may also block voltage-sensitive

calcium channels, alter cholinergic and monoaminergic actions, and interfere with opioid receptors [86–88].

Isolated case reports suggest that topical ketamine can reduce sympathetically maintained pain [89] and pain of malignant origin [90], again suggesting that perhaps glutamate receptor antagonists may have some analgesic
effect when applied topically.

α-Adrenoreceptor antagonists

Clonidine, an α_2-adrenoreceptor agonist can be obtained in cream and
patch formulations. It can have peripheral and central action when applied
topically. Clonidine patches have been reported to reduce the hyperalgesia
associated with sympathetically maintained pain but not the hyperalgesia
in patients who have sympathetically independent pain [91]. Clonidine
cream may also have some pain-relieving effect in orofacial neuralgia-like
pain [92]. The effect of clonidine in sympathetically maintained pain may
be related to its effect of reducing presynaptic norepinephrine release from
sympathetic nerves. In patients who have sympathetically maintained
pain, localized norepinephrine injection worsens the mechanical and thermal
hyperalgesia in some [93,94] and in those who have peripheral nerve injury
[95] and PHN [96].

When clonidine is injected into the knee joint after arthroscopy, pain relief is observed [97,98]; when injected along with bupivicain [99,100] and
morphine [101], the analgesic effect of these drugs is enhanced.

Cannabinoids

Cannabinoids (CBs) can act at peripheral sites to produce analgesia by
virtue of their effect on CB_1 and CB_2 receptors. In animal models, peripheral
administration of agents selective for CB_1 receptors produces local analgesia
in the formalin test [102], the carrageenan hyperalgesia model [103], and the
nerve injury model [104]. This effect may be obtained because of the effects
of these agents on the sensory nerve terminal to inhibit release of calcitonin
gene–related peptide [103] or by inhibiting effects of nerve growth factor
[105]. CB_2 receptor mechanisms may play a prominent role in inflammatory
pain [105].

Opioids

The analgesic effects of systemic opioids are well established and beyond
question. Recently, transdermal formulations of fentanyl and buprenorphine have been introduced. Although they are applied to skin, it is likely
that their predominant effect is central.

It is now apparent that opioid receptors are not exclusively located in the central nervous system. It appears that opioid receptors are synthesized in dorsal root ganglia and transported into peripheral terminals of primary afferent neurons [106,107]. Both mu and delta opioid receptors can be identified in fine cutaneous nerves in opioid-naïve animals [108]. When a ligature is placed on the rat sciatic nerve, β-endorphin binding sites accumulate proximally and distally to the ligature site [109]. When inflammation is induced, the number of β-endorphin binding sites on both sides of the ligature massively increases [109].

From the human clinical perspective, a number of reports suggest that the knowledge of a peripheral representation of opioid receptors may have practical application. Topical morphine, provided as an oral rinse, has been shown to reduce mucositis-related pain in patients undergoing chemotherapy for head and neck carcinomas [110,111], whereas other case reports suggest that topical opioids may reduce pain from skin ulcer [112,113]. In patients undergoing dental extractions, mixed results have been obtained, with some reporting enhanced relief when morphine is applied locally after dental extraction [114,115] and others reporting no such effect [116]. It has also been suggested that intravesical, strong opioids can reduce painful bladder spasms [117,118].

Despite these suggestions from the literature, two systematic reviews failed to find any evidence of a pain-relieving effect when morphine was used by peripheral application [119,120].

Summary

Our knowledge and understanding of the pathophysiology and treatment of pain is increasing; however, we should not lose sight of the simple opportunities that exist for intercepting pain at peripheral targets. Although systemic medication often has peripheral and central modes of action, the appeal for provision of medication close to where these peripheral targets exist should be high. If these sites can be attacked with relatively high concentrations of active drug while keeping systemic levels of that drug below the level at which systemic side effects become apparent, then this should lead to desirable outcomes. Even though the number of true topical agents with an indication for this use is small, a number of other topical agents are available that evidence suggests have the possibility of being effective. Given the increased understanding of pain, the likelihood of further topical agents becoming available is high.

References

[1] Vane JR, Bakhle YS, Botting J. Cyclo-oxygenase 1 and 2. Annu Rev Pharmacol Toxicol 1998;38:97–120.

[2] Yaksh TL, Dirig DM, Malmberg AB. Mechanisms of action of nonsteroidal anti-inflammatory drugs. Cancer Investig 1998;16:509–27.

[3] Chandrasekharan NV, Dai H, Roos KL, et al. Cox-3, a cyclo-oxygenase-1 variant inhibited by acetaminophen and other analgesic/antipyretic drugs. Cloning, structure and expression. Proc Natl Acad Sci U S A 2002;99:13926–31.

[4] Heyneman CA, Lawless-Liday C, Wall GC. Oral versus topical NSAIDs in rheumatic diseases. A comparison. Drugs 2000;60:555–74.

[5] Kress M, Reeh PW. Chemical excitation and sensitization in nociceptors. In: Cavero F, Belmonte C, editors. Neurobiology and nociceptors. Oxford (UK): Oxford University Press; 1996. p. 258–97.

[6] Steen KH, Reeh PW, Kreysel HW. Topical acetylsalicylic, salicylic acid and indomethacin suppresses pain from experimental tissue acidosis in human skin. Pain 1995;62:339–47.

[7] Steen KH, Reeh PW, Kreysel HW. Dose-dependent competitive block by topical acetylsalicylic acid and salicylic acid of low pH-induced cutaneous pain. Pain 2001;64:71–82.

[8] Schmelz M, Kress M. Topical acetylsalicylate attenuates capsaicin induced pain, flare and allodynia but not thermal hyperalgesia. Neurosci Lett 1996;214:72–4.

[9] Steen KH, Wegner H, Meller ST. Analgesic profile of peroral and topical ketoprofen upon low pH-induced muscle pain. Pain 2001;93:23–33.

[10] Vaile JH, Davis P. Topical NSAIDs for musculoskeletal conditions. A review of the literature. Drugs 1998;56:783–99.

[11] Moore RA, Tramer MR, Carrol D, et al. Quantitative systematic review of topically applied non-steroidal anti-inflammatory drugs. BMJ 1998;316:333–8.

[12] Feelisch M, Noack EA. Correlation between nitric oxide formation during degradation of organic nitrates and activation of guanylate cyclase. Eur J Pharmacol 1987;139:19–30.

[13] Knowles RG, Palacios M, Palmer RM, et al. Formation of nitric oxide from L-arginine in the central nervous system: a transduction mechanism for stimulation of soluble guanylate cyclase. Proc Natl Acad Sci U S A 1989;86:5159–62.

[14] Duarte ID, Lorenzetti BB, Ferreira SH. Acetylcholine induces peripheral analgesia by the release of nitric oxide. In: Moncada S, Higgs A, editors. Nitric oxide from L-arginine. A bioregulatory system. Amsterdam: Elsevier; 1990. p. 165–70.

[15] Soares A, Leite R, Patsuo M, et al. Activation of ATP sensitive K channels: mechanisms of peripheral antinociceptive action of the nitric oxide donor, sodium nitroprusside. Eur J Pharmacol 2000;14:67–71.

[16] Okuda K, Sakurada C, Takahashi M, et al. Characterization of nociceptive responses and spinal release of nitric oxide metabolites and glutamate evoked by different concentrations of formalin in rats. Pain 2001;92:107–15.

[17] McCleane GJ. The addition of piroxicam to topically applied glyceryl trinitrate enhances its analgesic effect in musculoskeletal pain: a randomised, double-blind, placebo-controlled study. Pain Clin 2000;12:113–6.

[18] Berrazueta JR, Losada A, Poveda J, et al. Successful treatment of shoulder pain syndrome due to supraspinatus tendonitis with transdermal nitroglycerin. A double blind study. Pain 1996;66:63–7.

[19] Berrazeuta JR, Poveda JJ, Ochoteco JA, et al. The anti-inflammatory and analgesic action of transdermal glyceryl trinitrate in the treatment of infusion related thrombophlebitis. Postgrad Med J 1993;69:37–40.

[20] Berrazueta JR, Fleitas M, Salas E, et al. Local transdermal glyceryl trinitrate has an anti-inflammatory action on thrombophlebitis induced by sclerosis of leg varicose veins. Angiology 1994;45:347–51.

[21] Walsh KE, Berman JR, Berman LA, et al. Safety and efficacy of topical nitroglycerin for treatment of vulvar pain in women with vulvodynia: a pilot study. J Gend Specif Med 2002;5:21–7.

[22] Lauretti GR, de Oliveira R, Reis MP, et al. Transdermal nitroglycerine enhances spinal sufentanil postoperative analgesia following orthopaedic surgery. Anesthesiology 1999;90: 734–9.

[23] Lauretti GR, Lima IC, Reis MP. Oral ketamine and transdermal nitroglycerin as analgesic adjuvants to oral morphine therapy for cancer pain management. Anesthesiology 1999;90: 1528–33.

[24] Lauretti GR, Perez MV, Reis MP, et al. Double-blind evaluation of transdermal nitroglycerine as an adjuvant to oral morphine for cancer pain management. J Clin Anesth 2002;14: 83–6.

[25] Galer BS. Topical medications. In: Loeser JD, editor. Bonica's management of pain. Philadelphia: Lippincott-Williams & Wilkins; 2001. p. 1736–41.

[26] Attal N, Brasseur L, Chauvin M. Effects of single and repeated applications of a eutectic mixture of local anesthetics (EMLA®) cream on spontaneous and evoked pain in post-herpetic neuralgia. Pain 1999;81:203–9.

[27] Litman SJ, Vitkun SA, Poppers PJ. Use of EMLA® cream in the treatment of post-herpetic neuralgia. J Clin Anesth 1996;8:54–7.

[28] Lycka BA, Watson CP, Nevin K, et al. EMLA® cream for the treatment of pain caused by post-herpetic neuralgia: a double-blind, placebo controlled study. Proceedings of the Annual Meeting of the American Pain Society. Glenview (IL): American Pain Society; 1996. A111 (abstract).

[29] Rowbotham MC, Davies PS, Verkempinck C, et al. Lidocaine patch: double-blind controlled study of a new treatment method for post-herpetic neuralgia. Pain 1996;65:39–44.

[30] Galer BS, Rowbotham MC, Perander J, et al. Topical lidocaine patch relieves post-herpetic neuralgia more effectively than vehicle patch: results of an enriched enrolment study. Pain 1999;80:533–8.

[31] Katz NP, Davis MW, Dworkin RH. Topical lidocaine patch produces a significant improvement in mean pain scores and pain relief in treated PHN patients: results of a multicenter open-label trial. J Pain 2001;2:9–18.

[32] Meier T, Wasner G, Faust M, et al. Efficacy of lidocaine 5% patch in treatment of focal peripheral neuropathic pain syndromes: a randomized, double-blind, placebo-controlled study. Pain 2003;106:151–8.

[33] Devers A, Galer BS. Topical lidocaine patch relieves a variety of neuropathic pain conditions: an open-label study. Clin J Pain 2000;16:205–8.

[34] Capsaicin Study Group. Treatment of painful diabetic neuropathy with topical capsaicin. Arch Intern Med 1991;151:2225–9.

[35] Tandan R, Lewis GA, Krusinski PB, et al. Topical capsaicin in painful diabetic neuropathy. Diabetes Care 1992;15:8–13.

[36] Capsaicin Study Group. Effect of treatment with capsaicin on daily activities of patients with painful diabetic neuropathy. Diabetes Care 1992;15:159–65.

[37] Chad DA, Aronin N, Lundstorm R, et al. Does capsaicin relieve the pain of diabetic neuropathy? Pain 1990;42:387–8.

[38] Bernstein JE, Korman NJ, Bickers DR, et al. Topical capsaicin treatment of chronic postherpetic neuralgia. J Am Acad Dermatol 1989;21:265–70.

[39] Watson CP, Tyler KL, Bickers DR, et al. A randomized vehicle controlled trial of topical capsaicin in the treatment of postherpetic neuralgia. Clin Ther 1993;15:510–26.

[40] Watson CP, Evans R, Watt VR. Post herpetic neuralgia and topical capsaicin. Pain 1988; 33:333–40.

[41] Low PA, Opfer-Gehrking TL, Dyck PJ, et al. Double blind, placebo controlled study of the application of capsaicin cream in chronic distal painful polyneuropathy. Pain 1995;45: 163–8.

[42] Epstein JB, Marcoe JH. Topical application of capsaicin for treatment of oral neuropathic pain and trigeminal neuralgia. Oral Surg Oral Med Oral Pathol 1994;77:135–40.

[43] Ellison N, Loprinzi CL, Kugler J, et al. Phase III placebo controlled trial of capsaicin cream in the management of surgical neuropathic pain in cancer patients. J Clin Oncol 1997;15: 2974–80.

[44] Morgenlander JC, Hurwitz BJ, Massey EW. Capsaicin for the treatment of pain in Guillain-Barré syndrome. Ann Neurol 1990;12:199.

[45] Turnbull A. Tincture of capsicum as a remedy for chilblains and toothache. Dublin (Ireland): Dublin Medical Press; 1850. p. 95–6.

[46] Altman RD, Aven A, Holmburg CE, et al. Capsaicin cream 0.025% as monotherapy for osteoarthritis: a double blind study. Sem Arth Rheum 1994;23S:25–33.

[47] Deal CL. The use of topical capsaicin in managing arthritis pain: a clinician's perspective. Sem Arth Rheum 1994;23S:48–52.

[48] Deal CL, Schnitzer TJ, Lipstein E, et al. Treatment of arthritis with topical capsaicin: a double blind trial. Clin Ther 1991;13:383–95.

[49] McCarthy GM, McCarty DJ. Effect of topical capsaicin in the therapy of painful osteoarthritis of the hands. J Rheumatol 1992;19:604–7.

[50] McCleane GJ. The analgesic efficacy of topical capsaicin in enhanced by glyceryl trinitrate in painful osteoarthritis: a randomized, double-blind, placebo controlled study. Eur J Pain 2000;4:355–60.

[51] Schnitzer T, Morton C, Coker S. Topical capsaicin therapy for osteoarthritis pain: achieving a maintenance regimen. Sem Arth Rheum 1994;23S:34–40.

[52] Mathias BJ, Dillingham TR, Zeigler DN, et al. Topical capsaicin for chronic neck pain. Am J Phys Med Rehabil 1995;74:39–44.

[53] Fitzgerald M. Capsaicin and sensory neurones. Pain 1983;15:109–30.

[54] Rains C, Bryson HM. Topical capsaicin. A review of its pharmacological properties and therapeutic potential in post herpetic neuralgia, diabetic neuropathy and osteoarthritis. Drugs Aging 1995;7:317–28.

[55] Nolano M, Simone DA, Wendelschafer-Crabb G, et al. Topical capsaicin in humans: parallel loss of epidermal nerve fibers and pain sensation. Pain 1999;81:135–41.

[56] Walker RA, McCleane GJ. The addition of glyceryl trinitrate to capsaicin cream reduces the thermal allodynia associated with the use of capsaicin in humans. Neurosci Lett 2002;323:78–80.

[57] McCleane GJ, McLaughlin M. The addition of GTN to capsaicin cream reduces the discomfort associated with application of capsaicin alone. A volunteer study. Pain 1998;78: 149–51.

[58] Yosipovitch G, Mailback HI, Rowbotham MC. Effect of EMLA pre-treatment on capsaicin-induced burning and hyperalgesia. Acta Derm Venereol 1999;79:118–21.

[59] Sawynok J. Adenosine receptor activation and nociception. Eur J Pharmacol 1998;317: 1–11.

[60] Esser MJ, Sawynok MJ. Caffeine blockade of the thermal antihyperalgesic effect of acute amitriptyline in a rat model of neuropathic pain. Eur J Pharmacol 2000;399:131–9.

[61] Sudoh Y, Cahoon EE, Gerner P, et al. Tricyclic antidepressant as long acting local anesthetics. Pain 2003;103:49–55.

[62] Haderer A, Gerner P, Kao G, et al. Cutaneous analgesia after transdermal application of amitriptyline versus lidocaine in rats. Anesth Analg 2003;96:1707–10.

[63] Esser MJ, Sawynok J. Acute amitriptyline in a rat model of neuropathic pain: differential symptom and route effects. Pain 1999;80:643–53.

[64] Esser MJ, Chase T, Allen GV, et al. Chronic administration of amitriptyline and caffeine in a rat model of neuropathic pain: multiple interactions. Eur J Pharmacol 2001;430: 211–8.

[65] Sawynok J, Esser MJ, Reid AR. Peripheral antinociceptive actions of desipramine and fluoxetine in an inflammatory and neuropathic pain test in the rat. Pain 1999;82:149–58.

[66] Sawynok J, Reid AR, Esser MJ. Peripheral antinociceptive action of amitriptyline in the rat formalin test: involvement of adenosine. Pain 1999;80:45–55.

[67] Sawynok J, Reid A. Peripheral interactions between dextromethorphan, ketamine and amitriptyline on formalin-evoked behaviours and paw edema in rats. Pain 2003;102:179–86.

[68] Heughan CE, Allen GV, Chase TD, et al. Peripheral amitriptyline suppresses formalin-induced Fos expression in the rat spinal cord. Anesth Analg 2002;94:427–31.

[69] Su X, Gebhart GF. Effects of tricyclic antidepressants on mechanosensitive pelvic nerve afferent fibers innervating the rat colon. Pain 1998;76:105–14.

[70] Oatway M, Reid A, Sawynok J. Peripheral antihyperalgesic and analgesic actions of ketamine and amitriptyline in a model of mild thermal injury in the rat. Anesth Analg 2003;97:168–73.

[71] McCleane GJ. Topical doxepin hydrochloride reduces neuropathic pain: a randomized, double-blind, placebo controlled study. Pain Clin 1999;12:47–50.

[72] McCleane GJ. Topical application of doxepin hydrochloride, capsaicin and a combination of both produces analgesia in chronic human neuropathic pain: a randomized, double-blind, placebo-controlled study. Br J Clin Pharmacol 2000;49:574–9.

[73] Lynch ME, Clarke AJ, Sawynok J. A pilot study examining topical amitriptyline, ketamine, and a combination of both in the treatment of neuropathic pain. Clin J Pain 2003;19:323–8.

[74] McCleane GJ. Topical application of doxepin hydrochloride can reduce the symptoms of complex regional pain syndrome: a case report. Injury 2002;33:88–9.

[75] Epstein JB, Truelove EL, Oien H, et al. Oral topical doxepin rinse: analgesic effect in patients with oral mucosal pain due to cancer or cancer therapy. Oral Oncol 2001;37:632–7.

[76] Zhou S, Komak S, Du J, et al. Metabotropic glutamate 1α receptors on peripheral primary afferent fibers: their role in nociception. Brain Res 2001;913:18–26.

[77] Carlton SM, Hargett GL, Coggeshall RE. Localization and activation of glutamate receptors in unmyelinated axons of rat glabrous skin. Neurosci Lett 1995;197:25–8.

[78] Carlton SM, Coggeshall RE. Inflammation-induced changes in peripheral glutamate receptor populations. Brain Res 1999;820:63–70.

[79] Zhou S, Bonasera L, Carlton SM. Peripheral administration of NMDA, AMPA or KA results in pain behaviour in rats. Neuroreport 1996;7:895–900.

[80] Jackson DL, Graff CB, Richardson JD. Glutamate participates in the peripheral modulation of thermal hyperalgesia in rats. Eur J Pharmacol 1995;284:321–5.

[81] Lawland NB, Willis WD, Westlund KN. Excitatory amino acid receptor involvement in peripheral nociceptive transmission in rats. Eur J Pharmacol 1997;324:169–77.

[82] Walker K, Reeve A, Bowes M, et al. mGlu5 receptors and nociceptive function II. mGlu5 receptors functionally expressed on peripheral sensory neurones mediate inflammatory hyperalgesia. Neuropharmacology 2001;40:10–9.

[83] Tverskoy M, Oren M, Vaskovich M, et al. Ketamine enhances local anesthetic and analgesic effects of bupivicaine by a peripheral mechanism: a study in postoperative patients. Neurosci Lett 1996;215:5–8.

[84] Warncke T, JØrum E, Stubhaug A. Local treatment with the N-methyl-D-aspartate receptor antagonist ketamine, inhibits development of secondary hyperalgesia in man by a peripheral action. Neurosci Lett 1997;227:1–4.

[85] Pedersen JL, Galle TS, Kehlet H. Peripheral analgesic effects of ketamine in acute inflammatory pain. Anesthesiology 1998;89:58–66.

[86] Hirota K, Lambert DG. Ketamine: its mechanism(s) of action and unusual clinical uses. Br J Anaesth 1996;77:441–4.

[87] Meller ST. Ketamine: relief from chronic pain through actions at the NMDA receptor? Pain 1996;68:435–6.

[88] Sawynok J, Reid AR. Modulation of formalin-induced behaviours and edema by local and systemic administration of dextromethorphan, memantine and ketamine. Eur J Pharmacol 2002;450:115–21.

[89] Crowley KL, Flores JA, Hughes CN, et al. Clinical application of ketamine ointment in the treatment of sympathetically maintained pain. Int J Pharmaceutical Compounding 1998;2:122–7.

[90] Wood RM. Ketamine for pain in hospice patients. Int J Pharmaceutical Compounding 2000;4:253–4.

[91] Davis CL, Treede RD, Raja SN, et al. Topical application of clonidine relieves hyperalgesia in patients with sympathetically maintained pain. Pain 1991;47:309–17.

[92] Epstein JB, Grushka M, Le N. Topical clonidine for orofacial pain: a pilot study. J Orofac Pain 1997;11:346–52.

[93] Torebjörk E, Wahren L, Wallin G, et al. Noradrenaline-evoked pain in neuralgia. Pain 1995;63:11–20.

[94] Ali Z, Raja SN, Wesselmann U, et al. Intradermal injection of norepinephrine evokes pain in patients with sympathetically maintained pain. Pain 2000;88:161–8.

[95] Chabal C, Jacobson L, Mariano A, et al. The use of oral mexiletine for the treatment of pain after peripheral nerve injury. Anesthesiology 1992;76:513–7.

[96] Choi B, Rowbotham MC. Effect of adrenergic receptor activation on post-herpetic neuralgia pain and sensory disturbances. Pain 1997;69:55–63.

[97] Gentili M, Houssel P, Osman H, et al. Intra-articular morphine and clonidine produce comparable analgesia but the combination is not more effective. Br J Anaesth 1997;79:660–1.

[98] Gentili M, Juhel A, Bonnet F. Peripheral analgesic effect of intra-articular clonidine. Pain 1996;64:593–6.

[99] Reuben SS, Connelly NR. Postoperative analgesia for outpatient arthroscopic knee surgery with intraarticular clonidine. Anesth Analg 1999;88:729–33.

[100] Joshi M, Reuben SS, Kilaru PR, et al. Postoperative analgesia for outpatient arthroscopic knee surgery with intraarticular clonidine and/or morphine. Anesth Analg 2000;90:1102–6.

[101] Buerkle H, Huge V, Wolfgart M, et al. Intra-articular clonidine analgesia after knee arthroscopy. Eur J Anaesthesiol 2000;17:295–9.

[102] Calignano A, La Ranna G, Giuffrida A, et al. Control of pain initiation by endogenous cannabinoids. Nature 1998;394:277–81.

[103] Richardson JD, Kilo S, Hargreaves KM. Cannabinoids reduce hyperalgesia and inflammation via interaction with peripheral CB1 receptors. Pain 1998;75:111–9.

[104] Fox A, Kesingland A, Gentry C, et al. The role of central and peripheral cannabinoid$_1$ receptors in the antihyperalgesic activity of cannabinoids in a model of neuropathic pain. Pain 2001;92:91–100.

[105] Rice AS, Farquhar-Smith WP, Nagy I. Endocannabinoids and pain: spinal and peripheral analgesia in inflammation and neuropathy. Prostaglandins Leukot Essent Fatty Acids 2002;66:243–56.

[106] Zhou L, Zhang Q, Stein C, et al. Contribution of opioid receptors on primary afferent versus sympathetic neurons to peripheral opioid analgesia. J Pharmacol Exp Ther 1998;286: 1000–6.

[107] Stein C, Schafer H, Hassan AH. Peripheral opioid receptors. Ann Med 1995;27:219–21.

[108] Coggeshall RE, Zhou S, Carlton SM. Opioid receptors on peripheral sensory axons. Brain Res 1997;764:126–32.

[109] Hassan AH, Ableitner A, Stein C, et al. Inflammation of the rat paw enhances axonal transport of opioid receptors in the sciatic nerve and increases their density in the inflamed tissue. Neuroscience 1993;55:185–95.

[110] Cerchietti LC, Navigante AH, Bonomi MR, et al. Effect of topical morphine for mucositis-associated pain following concomitant chemoradiotherapy for head and neck carcinoma. Cancer 2002;95:2230–6.

[111] Cerchietti LC, Navigante AH, Körte MW, et al. Potential utility of the peripheral analgesic properties of morphine in stomatitis-related pain: a pilot study. Pain 2003;105:265–73.

[112] Krajnik M, Zylicz Z, Finlay I, et al. Potential uses of topical opioids in palliative care— report of 6 cases. Pain 1999;80:121–5.

[113] Twillman RK, Long TD, Cathers TA, et al. Treatment of painful skin ulcers with topical opioids. J Pain Symptom Manage 1999;17:288–92.

[114] Likar R, Sittl R, Gragger K, et al. Peripheral morphine analgesia in dental surgery. Pain 1998;76:145–50.

[115] Likar R, Koppert W, Blatnig H, et al. Efficacy of peripheral morphine analgesia in inflamed, non-inflamed perineural tissue of dental surgery patients. J Pain Symptom Manage 2001;21:330–7.

[116] Moore RJ, Seymour RA, Gilro J, et al. The efficacy of locally applied morphine in postoperative pain after bilateral third molar surgery. Br J Clin Pharmacol 1994;37:227–30.

[117] Duckett JW, Cangiano T, Cubina M, et al. Intravesical morphine analgesia after bladder surgery. J Urol 1997;157:1407–9.

[118] McCoubrie R, Jeffrey D. Intravesical diamorphine for bladder spasm. J Pain Symptom Manage 2003;25:1–2.

[119] Picard PR, Tramer MR, McQuay HJ, et al. Analgesic efficacy of peripheral opioids (all except intra-articular): a qualitative systematic review of randomised controlled trials. Pain 1997;72:309–18.

[120] Gupta A, Bodin L, Holmstrom B, et al. A systematic review of the peripheral analgesic effects of intraarticular morphine. Anesth Analg 2001;93:761–70.

ANESTHESIOLOGY
CLINICS

Anesthesiology Clin
25 (2007) 841–851

Myofascial Trigger Points

Elizabeth Demers Lavelle, MD[a], William Lavelle, MD[b],*, Howard S. Smith, MD, FACP[a]

[a]*Department of Anesthesiology, Albany Medical Center,
43 New Scotland Avenue, Albany, NY 12208, USA*
[b]*Department of Orthopaedic Surgery, 1367 Washington Avenue,
Albany Medical Center, Albany, NY 12206, USA*

A myofascial trigger point is a hyperirritable point in skeletal muscle that is associated with a hypersensitive palpable nodule [1]. Approximately 23 million Americans have chronic disorders of the musculoskeletal system [2]. Painful conditions of the musculoskeletal system, including myofascial pain syndrome, constitute some of the most important chronic problems that are encountered in a clinical practice.

Definitions

Myofascial pain syndrome is defined as sensory, motor, and autonomic symptoms that are caused by myofascial trigger points. The sensory disturbances that are produced are dysesthesias, hyperalgesia, and referred pain. Coryza, lacrimation, salivation, changes in skin temperature, sweating, piloerection, proprioceptive disturbances, and erythema of the overlying skin are autonomic manifestations of myofascial pain.

Travell and Simons [1] defined the myofascial trigger point as "a hyperirritable spot, usually within a taut band of skeletal muscle or in the muscle fascia which is painful on compression and can give rise to characteristic referred pain, motor dysfunction, and autonomic phenomena" [1]. When the trigger point is pressed, pain is caused and produces effects at a target, the zone of reference, or referral zone [3,4]. This area of referred pain is the feature that differentiates myofascial pain syndrome from fibromyalgia. This pain is reproduced reliably on palpation of the trigger point, despite the

---

A version of this article originally appeared in the 91:2 issue of Medical Clinics of North America.

* Corresponding author.
E-mail address: lavellwf@yahoo.com (W. Lavelle).

doi:10.1016/j.anclin.2007.07.003   *anesthesiology.theclinics.com*

fact that it is remote from its source of origin. This referred pain rarely co-incides with dermatologic or neuronal distributions, but follows a consistent pattern [5].

Etiology

Trigger points may develop after an initial injury to muscle fibers. This injury may include a noticeable traumatic event or repetitive microtrauma to the muscles. The trigger point causes pain and stress in the muscle or muscle fiber. As the stress increases, the muscles become fatigued and more susceptible to activation of additional trigger points. When predisposing factors combine with a triggering stress event, activation of a trigger point occurs. This theory is known as the "injury pool theory" [1].

Pathophysiology

There is no pathologic or laboratory test for identifying trigger points. Therefore, much of the pathophysiologic research on trigger points has been directed toward verifying common theories of their formation. Fig. 1 provides an example of the theory behind the formation of myofascial trigger points.

The local twitch response (LTR) has been described as a characteristic response of myofascial trigger points. LTR is a brisk contraction of the muscle fibers in and around the taut band elicited by snapping palpation or rapid

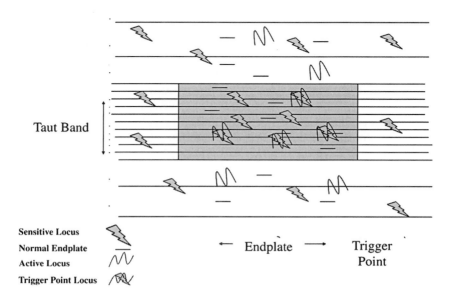

Fig. 1. Myofascial trigger point loci.

insertion of a needle into the myofascial trigger point [6]. The sensitive site where an LTR is found has been termed the "sensitive locus." Based on observations during successful trigger point injections, a model with multiple sensitive loci in a trigger point region was proposed [6]. In a recent histologic study, the sensitive loci correlated with sensory receptors [7,8].

In a study by Hubbard and Berkoff, spontaneous electrical activity was demonstrated at sites in a trigger point region, whereas similar activity was not found at adjacent nontender sites [6]. The site where the spontaneous electrical activity is recorded is termed the "active locus." To elicit and record spontaneous electrical activity, high-sensitivity recording and a gentle insertion technique into the trigger point must be used [6]. The waveforms of the spontaneous electrical activity correspond closely to previously published reports of motor endplate noise [9,10]. Therefore, the spontaneous electrical activity likely is one type of endplate potential, and the active loci probably are related closely to motor endplates.

It was hypothesized that a myofascial trigger point locus is formed when a sensitive locus, the nociceptor, and an active locus—the motor endplate—coincide. It is possible that sensitive loci are distributed widely throughout the entire muscle, but are concentrated in the trigger point region. This explains the finding of elicitation of referred pain when "normal" muscle tissue is needled or high pressure is applied (Fig. 2).

Diagnosis

The diagnosis of myofascial pain is best made through a careful analysis of the history of pain along with a consistent physical examination [11]. The diagnosis of myofascial pain syndrome, as defined by Simons and colleagues [12], relies on eight clinical characteristics (Box 1). Identification of the pain distribution is one of the most critical elements in identifying and treating myofascial pain. The physician should ask the patient to identify the most intense area of pain using a single finger. There also is an associated consistent and characteristic referred pain pattern on palpation of this trigger point. Often, this referred pain is not located in the immediate vicinity of the trigger point, but is found commonly in predictable patterns. These patterns are described clearly in *Travell and Simon's Myofascial Pain and Dysfunction: The Trigger Point Manual* [12]. Pain can be projected in a peripheral referral pattern, a central referral pattern, or a local pain pattern (Fig. 3). When a hyperintense area of pain is identified, its area of referred pain should be identified [4].

The palpable band is considered critical in the identification of the trigger point. Three methods have been identified for trigger point palpation: flat palpation, pincer palpation, and deep palpation. Flat palpation refers to sliding a fingertip across the muscle fibers of the affected muscle group. The skin is pushed to one side, and the finger is drawn across the muscle

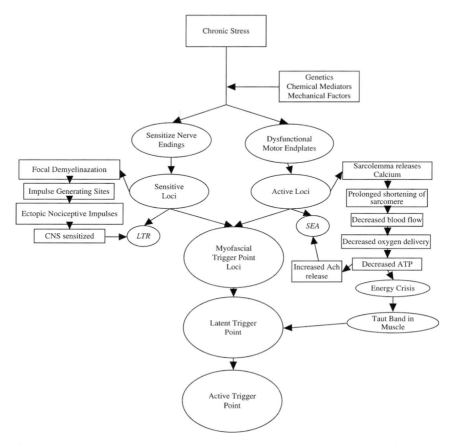

Fig. 2. Pathophysiology of myofascial trigger points. Ach, acetylcholine; CNS, central nervous system; LTR, local twitch response; SEA, spontaneous electrical activity.

fibers. This process is repeated with the skin pushed to the other side. A taut band may be felt passing under the physician's finger. Snapping palpation, like plucking of a violin, is used to identify the specific trigger point. Pincer palpation is a method that involves firmly grasping the muscle between the thumb and forefinger. The fibers are pressed between the fingers in a rolling manner while attempting to locate a taut band. Deep palpation may be used to find a trigger point that is obscured by superficial tissue. The fingertip is placed over the muscle attachment of the area suspected of housing the trigger point. When the patient's symptoms are reproduced by pressing in one specific direction, a trigger point may be presumed to be located [2].

    Several devices have been developed to assist in the location of a myofascial trigger point. Fisher [13] developed a pressure threshold measuring gauge to assist in the diagnosis and location of the myofascial trigger point. It is a hand-held device calibrated in kg/cm^2. Pressure is increased gradually

---

Box 1. Clinical characteristics of myofascial pain syndrome

Onset description and immediate cause of the pain

Pain distribution pattern

Restricted range of motion with increased sensitivity to
stretching

Weakened muscle due to pain with no muscular atrophy

Compression causing pain similar to the patient's chief complaint

A palpable taut band of muscle correlating with the patient's
trigger point

LTR elicited by snapping palpation or rapid insertion of a needle

Reproduction of the referred pain with mechanical stimulation of
the trigger point

---

and evenly until the patient reports discomfort. The pressure measurement is then recorded. Contralateral pressure measurements are taken to establish relative sensitivity of the point in question; a difference of 2 kg/cm^2 is considered an abnormal reading [14]. An electromyogram (EMG) also may assist in the diagnosis of the trigger point [15,16]. When the active locus is entered, the peak amplitudes often are off the scale of the EMG monitor. Although this method may seem to be useful scientifically, significant clinical results have not been found.

Noninvasive techniques for management

Spray (freeze) and stretch

Travell and Simons [1] advocated passive stretching of the affected muscle after application of sprayed vapocoolant to be the "single most effective

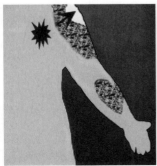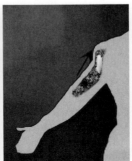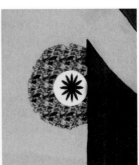

Peripheral Projection of Pain   Central Projection of Pain   Local Pain

Fig. 3. Trigger points and their reference zones.

treatment" for trigger point pain. The proper technique depends on patient education, cooperation, compliance, and preparation. The patient should be positioned comfortably, ensuring that the trigger point area is well supported and under minimal tension. Position should place one end of the muscle with the trigger point zone securely anchored. The patient should be marked after careful diagnosis of the trigger point region, and the reference zone should be noted. The skin overlying the trigger point should be anesthetized with a vapocoolant spray (ethyl chloride or dichlorodifluoromethane-trichloromonofluoromethane) over the entire length of the muscle [12]. This spray should be applied from the trigger point toward the reference zone until the entire length of the muscle has been covered. The vapocoolant should be directed at a 30° angle to the skin. Immediately after the first vapocoolant spray pass, passive pressure should be applied to the other end of the muscle, resulting in a stretch. Multiple slow passes of spray over the entire width of the muscle should be performed while maintaining the passive muscle stretch. This procedure is repeated until full range of motion of the muscle group is reached, with a maximum of three repetitions before rewarming the area with moist heat. Care must be taken to avoid prolonged exposure to the vapocoolant spray, assuring that each spray pass lasts less than 6 seconds. Patients must be warned not to overstretch muscles after a therapy session.

Physical therapy

Some of the best measures to relieve cyclic myofascial pain involve the identification of perpetuating factors. Physical therapists assist patients in the determination of predisposing activities. With routine follow-up, they are often able to correct elements of poor posture and body mechanics [1].

Transcutaneous electrical stimulation

Transcutaneous electrical stimulation (TENS) is used commonly as adjuvant therapy in chronic and acute pain management. Placement of the TENS electrode is an empiric process and may involve placement at trigger point sites or along zones of referred pain [17].

Ultrasound

Ultrasound may be used as an adjunctive means of treatment. Ultrasound transmits vibration energy at the molecular level; approximately 50% reaches a depth of 5 mm.

Massage

Massage was advocated by Simons and colleagues [12]. Their technique was described as a "deep stroking" or "stripping" massage. The patient is positioned comfortably to allow the muscle group being treated to be lengthened and relaxed as much as possible.

Ischemic compression therapy

The term "ischemic compression therapy" refers to the belief that the application of pressure to a trigger point produces ischemia that ablates the trigger point. Pressure is applied to the point with increasing resistance and maintained until the physician feels a relief of tension. The patient may feel mild discomfort, but should not experience profound pain. The process is repeated for each band of taut muscle encountered [12].

Invasive techniques for management

Trigger point injection remains the treatment with the most scientific evidence and investigation for support. Typically, it is advocated for trigger points that have failed noninvasive means for treatment. Injections are highly dependent of the clinician's skill to localize the active trigger point with a small needle.

Various injected substances have been investigated. These include local anesthetics, botulism toxin, sterile water, sterile saline, and dry needling. One common finding with these techniques is that, at least anecdotally, the duration of pain relief following the procedure outlasts the duration of action of the injected medication.

The universal technique for injection

The patient should be positioned in a recumbent position for the prevention of syncope, assistance in patient relaxation, and decreased muscle tension. The trigger point must then be identified correctly. The palpable band is considered critical in the identification of the trigger point. This can be done with any of the three methods described above. The trigger point should be marked clearly. Then, the skin is prepared in a sterile fashion. Various physicians use different skin preparations for their local procedures. One common skin preparation technique is to cleanse the skin with a topical alcohol solution followed by preparation with povidone-iodine [12]. A 22-gauge 1.5-inch needle is recommended for most superficial trigger points. Deeper muscles may be reached using a 21-gauge 2-inch or 2.5-inch needle. The needle should never be inserted to the hub because this is the weakest point on the needle [18].

Once the skin is prepared and the trigger point is identified, the overlying skin is grasped between the thumb and index finger or between the index and middle finger. The needle is inserted approximately 1 to 1.5 cm away from the trigger point to facilitate the advancement of the needle into the trigger point at a 30° angle. The grasping fingers isolate the taut band and prevent it from rolling out of the trajectory of the needle. A "fast-in, fast-out" technique should be used to elicit an LTR. This local twitch was shown to predict the effectiveness of the trigger point injection [19]. After entering the trigger point, the needle should be aspirated to ensure that the lumen of a local blood vessel has not been violated. If the physician chooses to inject an agent, a small volume should be injected at this time. The needle may be withdrawn to the level of the skin without exiting, and it should be redirected to the trigger point repeating the process. The process of entering the trigger point and eliciting LTRs should proceed, attempting to contact as many sensitive loci as possible (Fig. 4).

An integral part of trigger point therapy is postprocedural stretching. After trigger point injection, the muscle group that was injected should undergo a full active stretch.

Complications of trigger point injections

As with the introduction of any foreign body through the skin, the risk for skin or soft tissue infection is a possibility. Injection over an area of infected skin is contraindicated. The physician should never aim the needle at an intercostal space to avoid the complication of a pneumothorax. Hematoma formation following a trigger point injection can be minimized with proper injection technique and holding pressure over the surrounding soft tissue after withdrawal of the needle [12,20].

Medications for injection

Local anesthetics

Local anesthetics are the substances that have been investigated most frequently for the treatment of myofascial trigger points. Local anesthetic

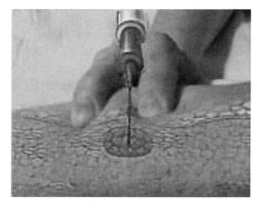

Fig. 4. Injection technique. The trigger point is positioned between two fingers to prevent the sliding of the trigger point during injection. The fingers are pressed downward and apart to maintain pressure and ensure hemostasis.

injections were shown to improve measures on a pain scale, range of motion, and algometry pressure thresholds. The volume of local anesthetic injected also has been investigated, and small volumes are considered the most effective. Typically, less than 1 mL of local agent should be injected in a highly controlled manner. The primary use for a local anesthetic is to prevent local soreness. Procaine is selected often because it is selective for small, unmyelinated fibers that control pain perception rather than motor control. Lidocaine is a common substitute for procaine, but no experimental comparisons are available in the literature [12,21].

Corticosteroids

Local steroid injections offer the potential advantage of control of local inflammatory response; however, the theory that a trigger point is due to a local energy crisis does not support their clinical use. Steroids are used commonly by the orthopedic surgeon and rheumatologist to treat local conditions, such as trigger finger and tennis elbow. They carry the added dangers of local myotoxicity, subcutaneous tissue damage, and skin discoloration [12].

Botulinum toxin

Localized injection of a small amount of commercially prepared botulism toxin A relaxes an overactive muscle by blocking the release of acetylcholine. This essentially denervates the muscle until new synaptic contacts can be established. When injecting botulism toxin, the physician should remember that the toxin does not discriminate between trigger points and normal motor endplates. The physician should be careful to localize the trigger point before injection [22,23].

Dry needling

Dry needling involves multiple advances of a needle into the muscle at the region of the trigger point. Much like any injection technique, the physician should aim to elicit an LTR, reproduction of the patient's symptomatology, and relief of muscle tension [7,24].

Summary

Myofascial pain syndromes are a widely recognized phenomenon among physicians and represent a common pain disorder in the American population. A myofascial trigger point is "a hyperirritable spot, usually within a taut band of skeletal muscle or in the muscle fascia. The spot is painful on compression and can give rise to characteristic referred pain, motor dysfunction, and autonomic phenomena" [1]. Many treatment strategies, both invasive and noninvasive, have been recognized for myofascial trigger points.

References

[1] Travell JG, Simons DG. Myofascial pain and dysfunction: the trigger point manual. Baltimore (MD): Williams and Wilkins; 1983.

[2] Imamura ST, Fischer AA, Imamura M, et al. Pain management using myofascial approach when other treatment failed. Physical Medicine & Rehabilitation Clinics of North America 1997;8(1):179–96.

[3] Maigne J, Maigne R. Trigger point of the posterior iliac crest: painful iliolumbar ligament insertion or cutaneous dorsal ramus pain? An anatomic study. Arch Phys Med Rehabil 1991;72(9):734–7.

[4] Sola A, Bonica J. Myofascial pain syndromes. In: Bonica J, Loeser J, Chapman S, et al, editors. The management of pain. Baltimore (MD): Lippincott Williams & Wilkins; 1996. p. 352–67.

[5] Long S, Kephart W. Myofascial pain syndrome. In: Ashburn M, Rice L, editors. The management of pain. New York: Churchill Livingstone, Inc.; 1998. p. 299–321.

[6] Simons D. Single-muscle myofascial pain syndromes. In: Tollison CD, Satterthwaite CD, Tollison J, editors. Handbook of pain management. 2nd edition. Baltimore (MD): Williams & Wilkins; 1994. p. 539–55.

[7] Hong C-Z. Trigger point injection: dry needling vs. lidocaine injection. Am J Phys Med Rehabil 1994;73:156–63.

[8] Hong C-Z, Chen J-T, Chen S-M, et al. Histological findings of responsive loci in a myofascial trigger spot of rabbit skeletal muscle fibers from where localized twitch responses could be elicited [abstract]. Arch Phys Med Rehabil 1996;77:962.

[9] Simons DG. Do endplate noise and spikes arise from normal motor endplates? Am J Phys Med Rehabil 2001;80:134–40.

[10] Simons DG, Hong C-Z, Simons LS. Endplate potentials are common to midfiber myofascial trigger points. Am J Phys Med Rehabil 2002;81:212–22.

[11] Graff-Radford S. Myofascial pain: diagnosis and management. Curr Pain Headache Rep 2004;8:463–7.

[12] Simons DG, Travell JG, Simons LS. Travell and Simon's myofascial pain and dysfunction: the trigger point manual. 2nd edition. Baltimore (MD): Williams and Wilkins; 1998.

[13] Fischer AA. Pressure threshold meter: its use for quantification of tender points. Arch Phys Med Rehabil 1986;67:836.

[14] Hong C-Z, Chen Y-N, Twehous D, et al. Pressure threshold for referred pain by compression on the trigger point and adjacent areas. Journal of Musculoskeletal Pain 1996;4: 61–79.

[15] Hubbard D, Berkhoff G. Myofascial trigger points show spontaneous needle EMG activity. Spine 1993;18:1803–7.

[16] Simons DG, Hong C-Z, Simons LS. Prevalence of spontaneous electrical activity at trigger spots and at control sites in rabbit skeletal muscle. Journal of Musculoskeletal Pain 1995;3: 35–48.

[17] Graff-Redford SB, Reeves JL, Baker RL, et al. Effects of transcutaneous electrical nerve stimulation on myofascial pain and trigger point sensitivity. Pain 1989;37:1–5.

[18] Ruane J. Identifying and injecting myofascial trigger points. Phys Sportsmed 2001;29(12): 49–53.

[19] Hong C-Z, Simons DG. Response to standard treatment for pectoralis minor myofascial pain syndrome after whiplash. Journal of Musculoskeletal Pain 1993;1:89–131.

[20] Hong C-Z, Simons D. Pathophysiologic and electrophysiologic mechanisms of myofascial trigger points. Arch Phys Med Rehabil 1998;79:863–72.

[21] Hubbard D. Chronic and recurrent muscle pain: pathophysiology and treatment, and review of pharmacologic studies. Journal of Musculoskeletal Pain 1996;4:123–43.
[22] Acquandro MA, Borodic GE. Treatment of myofascial pain with botulism toxin A. Anesthesiology 1994;80:705–6.
[23] Cheshire WP, Abashian SW, Mann JD. Botulism toxin in the treatment of myofascial pain syndrome. Pain 1994;59:65–9.
[24] Chen J, Chung K, Hou C, et al. Inhibitory effect of dry needling on the spontaneous electrical activity recorded from myofascial trigger points of rabbit skeletal muscle. Am J Phys Med Rehabil 2001;80:729–35.

ELSEVIER
SAUNDERS

Anesthesiology Clin
25 (2007) 853–862

ANESTHESIOLOGY
CLINICS

Intra-Articular Injections

William Lavelle, MD[a],*,
Elizabeth Demers Lavelle, MD[b], Lori Lavelle, DO[c]

[a]Department of Orthopaedic Surgery, Albany Medical Center, 1367 Washington Avenue,
Albany, NY 12206, USA
[b]Department of Anesthesiology, Albany Medical Center, 43 New Scotland Avenue, Albany,
NY 12208, USA
[c]Department of Rheumatology, Altoona Arthritis and Osteoporosis Center,
1125 Old Route 220N, Duncansville, PA 16635, USA

Intra-articular injections are one method that physicians may use to treat joint pain. Corticosteroids were the first substances to be injected commonly into the intra-articular space. In the 1950s, corticosteroids were found to lower indicators of the inflammatory response, including the interarticular leukocyte count [1,2]. The indications and effectiveness of intra-articular steroid injections have been debated since their introduction. More recently, viscosupplementation has gained popularity. Local anesthetics also have become common additions to intra-articular injections. Anesthesiologists and orthopedic surgeons have started to explore the use of intra-articular opiates for postoperative analgesia.

Injections for chronic joint pain

Steroid injections

Joint aspiration was described as early as the 1930s. The first intra-articular injectates, which yielded little benefit, were formalin and glycerin, lipodol, lactic acid, and petroleum jelly [3,4]. Hollander [5,6] attempted joint injections with hydrocortisone acetate and found that his patients had a much better clinical response in a series of more than 100,000 injections

A version of this article originally appeared in the 91:2 issue of Medical Clinics of North America.
* Corresponding author.
E-mail address: lavellwf@yahoo.com (W. Lavelle).

in 4000 patients. From the 1950s to the present, physicians have used corticosteroid injections routinely to treat joint pain.

Clinical efficacy has been shown for intra-articular injections of steroids in the treatment of rheumatoid arthritis. In a randomized study, patients who were treated with intra-articular injections demonstrated significantly better pain control and range of motion than did those who were treated with mini-pulse systemic steroids. Patient evaluation of disease activity, tender joint count, blood pressure, side effects, calls to the physician, and hospital visits were significantly better ($P < .05$) for those who were treated with intra-articular steroids [7].

Mechanism of action of intra-articular steroid injections

Steroids possess anti-inflammatory properties. On the cellular level, steroids are highly lipophilic and are believed to bind to the cell's nucleus. It is believed that steroids act by altering transcription. Intra-articular steroids seem to reduce the number of lymphocytes, macrophages, and mast cells [8,9]; this, in turn, reduces phagocytosis, lysosomal enzyme release, and the release of inflammatory mediators [1]. Inflammation is reduced, particularly through reductions in the release of interleukin-1, leukotrienes, and prostaglandins [10,11]. With the reduction of these inflammatory mediators, pain symptoms often are improved.

Because they are injected locally, intra-articular steroids avoid most of the systemic effects of oral steroids, including muscle weakness, skin thinning resulting in easy bruising, peptic ulceration, and aggravation of diabetes.

Skin preparation

Skin preparation is as individualized as that seen for surgical site preparation. In a survey of orthopedists and rheumatologists, approximately half used alcohol swabs and the other half used chlorhexidine or povidine-iodine. Less than 20% used sterile towels to isolate the injection site, and only 32.5% of respondents used sterile gloves [12]. The authors recommend preparation with alcohol followed by preparation with Betadine and the use of sterile gloves.

Choice of steroid

Based strictly on chemical structure, the duration of effect should be inversely proportional to the solubility of the steroid (Table 1). There have been conflicting studies on the duration of action of various steroids. Little data exist touting the true efficacy of one agent over another. In most cases, the choice of steroid is related to the personal preference of the physician rather than true science. In a survey performed on members of the 1994 American College of Rheumatology, approximately one third favored

Table 1
Steroid solubility

Steroid	Solubility (% wt/vol)
Hydrocortisone acetate	0.002
Methylprednisolone acetate	0.001
Prednisolone tebutate	0.001
Triamcinolone acetate	0.004
Triamcinolone hexacetonide	0.0002

methylprednisolone, one third favored triamcinolone hexacetonide, and one fifth favored triamcinolone acetonide [9,13].

Use of local anesthetic

At times, local anesthetics (eg, lidocaine) are combined with the steroid. Some physicians contend that the local agent dilutes the steroid crystals, but it is unclear whether this process has any impact on the effect of the steroid. Lidocaine may have a transient anti-inflammatory effect in and of itself [14,15].

Adverse reactions

The most obvious concern about intra-articular injections is infection; however, few orthopedists and rheumatologists have encountered a case of poststeroid septic arthritis [12]. Avoidance of this complication depends on strict adherence to sterile technique. Suspicion of an intra-articular infection or an overlying soft tissue infection contraindicates the injection of a joint with corticosteroid. Other contraindications include a local fracture of total joint. Recent reports found infection rates of between 1 in 3000 and 1 in 50,000 [12]. *Staphylococcus aureus* is the most common infecting organism [12,16].

Mild local reactions do occur after injection. Postinjection flares occurred in about 2% to 6% of patients and were believed to result from chemical synovitis in response to the injected crystals [17]. Facial flushing may be seen in up to 15% of patients, mostly in women [8]. Skin or fat atrophy may be observed at the actual site of needle entry [17]. There is some concern regarding the use of intra-articular steroid injections in the diabetic population. Transient increases in blood glucose may be seen in patients receiving corticosteroid injections; however, in a study of diabetic patients who received soft tissue injections of methylprednisolone acetate, there was no detectable effect on blood glucose levels in the 14 days after injection [18]. Intra-articular steroids also transiently affect the hypothalamic–pituitary– adrenal axis. These changes, which include a 21.5% reduction in serum cortisol levels, typically normalize within 3 days, although an episode of Cushing's syndrome was reported [19,20].

Joint destruction after repetitive injections is a common concern. Animal studies have been suggestive of damage to articular cartilage because of intra-articular steroid injections; however, there are no human data to corroborate this claim [10]. Because of fear of possible joint destruction, many physicians recommend 3 months between injections of the same joint [13,21].

Clinical trials

One of the largest clinical trials of intra-articular steroid injections was done in the 1950s by Hollander [5,6]. Hydrocortisone injections of 1034 knees with osteoarthritis revealed an 80% success rate. Since that time, a multitude of studies proved the excellent short-term pain relief (1–4 weeks) gained from injected corticosteroids [21]. Longer-term results were not proved in consecutive studies; however, the short-term pain relief may allow the patient to return to baseline function and improve one's ability to perform physical therapy [22,23].

An adjunct to the success of steroid treatment in the patient who has an effusion may be the aspiration of that effusion. Eighty-four patients who had osteoarthritis were randomized to receive triamcinolone hexacetonide or placebo. Patients who received the steroid reported a statistically significant improvement in pain, distance walked in 1 minute, and Health Assessment Questionnaire score. Among patients who were treated with steroids, those who had an effusion that was aspirated at the time of injection showed greater improvement ($P < .05$) [24]. Joint lavage similarly improved pain and function if performed at the time of steroid injection [25].

Hyaluronic acid

Intra-articular steroids are not the only materials that are injected intra-articularly in the treatment of osteoarthritis. A randomized, placebo-controlled study compared more than 100 patients who received hyaluronic acid, corticosteroid (methylprednisolone acetate), or isotonic saline. These injections were placed with the aid of ultrasound. Injections were administered at 14-day intervals, with each patient receiving three injections. Significant improvement was seen at 3 months in the population that was treated with corticosteroid compared with patients who were treated with saline ($P = .006$ at 14 days, $P = .006$ at 28 days, and $P = .58$ at 3 months), whereas improvement in the group that was treated with hyaluronic acid failed to reach statistical significance ($P = .069$ at 14 days, $P = .14$ at 28 days, and $P = .57$ at 3 months). Statistically, there was no significant difference between hyaluronic acid and corticosteroid at any time point ($P > .21$) [26].

Postoperative intra-articular analgesia

The analgesic effects of intra-articular agents in the postoperative period are controversial; however, their use is becoming more common in the outpatient orthopedic setting [27]. The use of peripheral blocks for extremity surgery requires greater skill in placement and has a potential for significant complications [27]. Arthroscopy has been described as a method for orthopedic improvement with decreased morbidity, but not one of decreased pain [28,29]. Poor pain control may prevent a procedure from being acceptable in an outpatient setting, therefore, postoperative analgesia becomes an important consideration for outpatient surgery centers. Intra-articular analgesia techniques are used most commonly for knee and shoulder surgery. With some debate, intra-articular administration of local agents has proven effective for knee arthroscopy [30–38]; however, pain control for the shoulder has proven a greater task. Severe pain scores have been reported for even the most minor shoulder procedures [39].

Local agents

Most anesthesiologists and orthopedic surgeons select bupivacaine because of its long duration of action. This does not preclude the use of other local agents. The literature on the use of intra-articular local anesthetics includes numerous studies, but it is difficult to interpret because of the use of confounding agents, such as intra-articular opiates, clonidine, and nonsteroidals. A large number of these studies also is flawed with regard to study design, data collection, and reporting. A systematic review of double-blind, randomized, controlled trials that compared intra-articular local with placebo or no intervention and found a statistically significant improved pain after intra-articular local in pain scores. Pain scores were significantly lower in the treatment group and the amount of supplemental analgesics requested was reduced by 10% to 50%. The presence of hemarthrosis, which can increase the level of pain and decrease the concentration of local agents, is another factor that may alter the activity of intra-articular local analgesia [37]. Although the data from this review seem to indicate that intra-articular local analgesia is only mildly effective, its use in the outpatient orthopedic setting is a popular and safe adjuvant [40].

A continuous infusion of intra-articular analgesia was examined. In a prospective randomized trial of 50 subjects who underwent acromioplasty and rotator cuff repair and received a multiorifice catheter placed in the subacromial space, no statistically significant difference in pain scores or patient-controlled analgesic use was detected [41].

Opiates

Opioid receptors have been discovered in the peripheral nervous system. Mu, delta, and kappa receptors were found on peripheral nerves [37,42]. The effectiveness of opiates in inflamed tissues has been explained by a disruption in the perineurium, allowing for easier access of opioids to neuronal receptors. This also may be associated with an unmasking or up-regulation of inactive opiate receptors [37,43]. It was proposed that the effects of intra-articular morphine might simply be due to systemic absorption; however, the plasma concentration achieved from an intra-articular injection would be far too low for a systemic effect to be observed [37]. Within the joint itself, the relative concentration is high.

Kalso and colleagues [44] reviewed 36 randomized controlled trials. Four of the six studies that compared opiates with placebo found greater efficacy for intra-articular morphine. Four of the six studies that compared intra-articular morphine with intravenous or intramuscular morphine showed greater efficacy for intra-articular morphine. Several dosages were used with varying effects in the literature reviewed. Specifically, the minimum dose tested (0.5 mg) did not show efficacy, but a dose of 1 mg did. No greater effect was found when a dose of 1 mg was compared with 2 mg [44,45].

In a review by Gupta and colleagues [46], a meta-analysis was completed on the pooled data of 19 prospective, placebo-controlled, randomized studies in which intra-articular morphine was used. Within these studies, visual analog scores were collected at the early phase (0–2 hours), the intermediate phase (2–6 hours), and the late phase (6–24 hours). This analysis concluded that although no clear dose-response effect was seen, a definite, but mild, analgesic effect was present.

Another recent review is a bit more skeptical. Rosseland and colleagues reviewed randomized controlled trials that involved the use of intra-articular morphine [29]. In the 43 publications included, some of which were included in the reviews by Kalso and colleagues [44] and Gupta and colleagues [46], 23 were believed to be of low scientific quality with poor randomization and blinding or unsound statistics. Thirteen were believed to have usable information; however, four of the positive outcomes were believed to be due to the uneven distribution of patients whose natural course was low postoperative pain. The only randomized control trial that Rosseland believed was adequate was negative [47].

Clonidine

Intra-articular clonidine also has been investigated. Clonidine is an α-agonist that was shown to prolong the duration of local anesthetics. In a controlled study, 40 patients who underwent knee arthroscopy were randomized to receive intra-articular clonidine in combination with 1 mg of morphine. Patients who received clonidine had significantly longer analgesia durations [37].

Many physicians who participate in outpatient orthopedic surgery recommend a multimodal approach consisting of intra-articular agents, including local analgesia, an opiate, and an adjunct (eg, clonidine) [37]. The specifics of the injectate are left to the individual. Local analgesia seems to be helpful early in the postoperative period (2-4 hours) to prevent a deleterious physiologic pain response. Intra-articular morphine may be more

Subacromial Space   Glenohumeral Space   Acromialclavicular Space

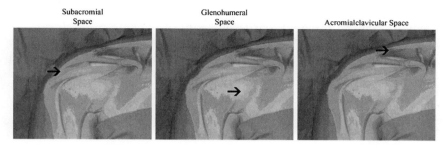

Fig. 1. Spaces in the shoulder that may be treated by an intra-articular injection.

helpful in the hours afterward. In general, the use of pre-emptive and multimodal analgesia is important to abate postoperative pain, with an emphasis on minimizing systemic narcotic analgesia, which has the deleterious effects of respiratory depression, sedation, nausea, puritis, and delayed discharge [37].

Techniques to improve placement

Figs. 1 and 2 illustrate the anatomic locations for injections into the shoulder and knee. It is truly with repetition that the physician becomes facile with most intra-articular injections. Image guidance with the aid of ultrasound or fluoroscopy is a valuable tool to help access difficult joints, such as the hip. Fluoroscopy and a radiopaque tracer allow for documented delivery of an agent into a joint. Aspiration of synovial fluid before injection of a steroid is one method that may allow for improved accuracy.

Lateral Para patella Portal   Medial Para patella Portal   Superior Lateral Portal

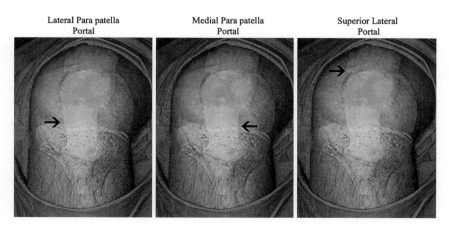

Fig. 2. Different approaches used to access the knee for an intra-articular injection.

One study examined this question. A recent article assessed the accuracy of needle placement in the intra-articular space of the knee using three common knee joint portals. The investigators documented the location of the injected fluid by fluoroscopic imaging. They found far more success with a lateral midpatellar injection than with either of the other injection portals [47].

Summary

Intra-articular injections provide physicians with one modality to treat chronic or acute joint pain. Whatever method is chosen, careful attention to the anatomic landmarks and experience are critical to the successful placement of an intra-articular injection. Intra-articular steroid injections have been used for management of inflammatory joint diseases, such as arthritis. Occasionally, local anesthetics are injected in combination with the steroids. New studies found that intra-articular injections may be helpful for the management of postoperative pain, particularly with the use of opiates.

References

[1] Snibbe JC, Gambardella RA. Use of injections for osteoarthritis in joints and sports activity. Clin Sports Med 2005;24(1):83–91.

[2] Hollander JL, Brown EM Jr, Jessar RA, et al. Hydrocortisone and cortisone injected into arthritic joints; comparative effects of and use of hydrocortisone as a local antiarthritic agent. JAMA 1951;147(17):1629–35.

[3] Pemberton R. Arthritis and rheumatoid conditions. Their nature and treatment. Philadelphia: Lea and Febiger; 1935.

[4] Ropes MW, Bauer W. Synovial fluid changes in joint disease. Cambridge (MA): Harvard University Press; 1953.

[5] Hollander JL. Hydrocortisone and cortisone injected into arthritic joints. Comparative effects of and use of hydrocortisone as a local antiarthritic agent. JAMA 1951;147:1629.

[6] Hollander JL. Intrasynovial corticosteroid therapy: a decade of use. Bull Rheum Dis 1961; 11:239.

[7] Furtado RN, Oliveira LM, Natour J. Polyarticular corticosteroid injection versus systemic administration in treatment of rheumatoid arthritis patients: a randomized controlled study. J Rheumatol 2005;32(9):1691–8.

[8] Cole BJ, Schumacher HR Jr. Injectable corticosteroids in modern practice. J Am Acad Orthop Surg 2005;13(1):37–46.

[9] Centeno LM, Moore ME. Preferred intraarticular corticosteroids and associated practice: a survey of members of the American College of Rheumatology. Arthritis Care Res 1994; 7(3):151–5.

[10] Uthman I, Raynauld JP, Haraoui B. Intra-articular therapy in osteoarthritis. Postgrad Med J 2003;79(934):449–53.

[11] Wilder RL. Corticosteroids. In: Klippel JH, Cornelia WM, Wortmann RL, editors. Primer on rheumatic diseases. Atlanta (GA): Arthritis Foundation; 1997. p. 427–31.

[12] Charalambous CP, Tryfonidis M, Sadiq S, et al. Septic arthritis following intra-articular steroid injection of the knee–a survey of current practice regarding antiseptic technique used during intra-articular steroid injection of the knee. Clin Rheumatol 2003;22(6):386–90.

[13] Rozental TD, Sculco TP. Intra-articular corticosteroids: an updated overview. Am J Orthop 2000;29(1):18–23.

[14] Schumacher HR Jr. Aspiration and injection therapies for joints. Arthritis Rheum 2003; 49(3):413–20.

[15] Paul H, Clayburne G, Schumacher HR. Lidocaine inhibits leukocyte migration and phagocytosis in monosodium urate crystal-induced synovitis in dogs. J Rheumatol 1983;10(3): 434–9.

[16] von Essen R, Savolainen HA. Bacterial infection following intra-articular injection. A brief review. Scand J Rheumatol 1989;18(1):7–12.

[17] Kumar N, Newman RJ. Complications of intra- and peri-articular steroid injections. Br J Gen Pract 1999;49(443):465–6.

[18] Slotkoff A, Clauw D, Nashel D. Effect of soft tissue corticosteroid injection on glucose control in diabetics. Arthritis Rheum 1994;37(Suppl 9):S347.

[19] Emkey RD, Lindsay R, Lyssy J, et al. The systemic effect of intraarticular administration of corticosteroid on markers of bone formation and bone resorption in patients with rheumatoid arthritis. Arthritis Rheum 1996;39(2):277–82.

[20] Roberts WN, Babcock EA, Breitbach SA, et al. Corticosteroid injection in rheumatoid arthritis does not increase rate of total joint arthroplasty. J Rheumatol 1996;23(6):1001–4.

[21] Chumacher HR, Chen LX. Injectable corticosteroids in treatment of arthritis of the knee. Am J Med 2005;118(11):1208–14.

[22] Godwin M, Dawes M. Intra-articular steroid injections for painful knees. Systematic review with meta-analysis. Can Fam Physician 2004;50:241–8.

[23] Arroll B, Goodyear-Smith F. Corticosteroid injections for painful shoulder: a meta-analysis. Br J Gen Pract 2005;55(512):224–8.

[24] Gaffney K, Ledingham J, Perry JD. Intra-articular triamcinolone hexacetonide in knee osteoarthritis: factors influencing the clinical response. Ann Rheum Dis 1995;54(5):379–81.

[25] Ravaud P, Moulinier L, Giraudeau B, et al. Effects of joint lavage and steroid injection in patients with osteoarthritis of the knee: results of a multicenter, randomized, controlled trial. Arthritis Rheum 1999;42(3):475–82.

[26] Qvistgaard E, Christensen R, Torp-Pedersen S, et al. Intra-articular treatment of hip osteoarthritis: a randomized trial of hyaluronic acid, corticosteroid, and isotonic saline. Osteoarthritis Cartilage 2006;14(2):163–70.

[27] Savoie FH, Field LD, Jenkins RN, et al. The pain control infusion pump for postoperative pain control in shoulder surgery. Arthroscopy 2000;16(4):339–42.

[28] Rawal N. Incisional and intra-articular infusions. Best Pract Res Clin Anaesthesiol 2002; 16(2):321–43.

[29] Rosseland LA, Helgesen KG, Breivik H, et al. Moderate-to-severe pain after knee arthroscopy is relieved by intraarticular saline: a randomized controlled trial. Anesth Analg 2004; 98(6):1546–51.

[30] Geutjens G, Hambidge JE. Analgesic effects of intraarticular bupivacaine after day-case arthroscopy. Arthroscopy 1994;10(3):299–300.

[31] Morrow BC, Milligan KR, Murthy BV. Analgesia following day-case knee arthroscopy–the effect of piroxicam with or without bupivacaine infiltration. Anaesthesia 1995;50(5):461–3.

[32] Vranken JH, Vissers K, de Jongh R, et al. Intraarticular sufentanil administration facilitates recovery after day-case knee arthroscopy. Anesth Analg 2001;92:625–8.

[33] Henderson RC, Campion ER, DeMasi RA, et al. Postarthroscopy analgesia with bupivacaine. A prospective, randomized, blinded evaluation. Am J Sports Med 1990;18(6):614–7.

[34] Osborne D, Keene G. Pain relief after arthroscopic surgery of the knee: a prospective, randomized, and blinded assessment of bupivacaine and bupivacaine with adrenaline. Arthroscopy 1993;9(2):177–80.

[35] Aasbo V, Raeder JC, Grogaard B, et al. No additional analgesic effect of intra-articular morphine or bupivacaine compared with placebo after elective knee arthroscopy. Acta Anaesthesiol Scand 1996;40(5):585–8.

[36] Highgenboten CL, Jackson AW, Meske NB. Arthroscopy of the knee. Ten-day pain profiles and corticosteroids. Am J Sports Med 1993;21(4):503–6.

[37] Reuben SS, Sklar J. Pain management in patients who undergo outpatient arthroscopic surgery of the knee. J Bone Joint Surg Am 2000;82-A(12):1754–66.

[38] Dye SF, Vaupel GL, Dye CC. Conscious neurosensory mapping of the internal structures of the human knee without intraarticular anesthesia. Am J Sports Med 1998;26(6):773–7.

[39] Ritchie ED, Tong D, Chung F, et al. Suprascapular nerve block for postoperative pain relief in arthroscopic shoulder surgery: a new modality? Anesth Analg 1997;84(6):1306–12.

[40] Meinig RP, Holtgrewe JL, Wiedel JD, et al. Plasma bupivacaine levels following single dose intraarticular instillation for arthroscopy. Am J Sports Med 1988;16(3):295–300.

[41] Boss AP, Maurer T, Seiler S, et al. Continuous subacromial bupivacaine infusion for postoperative analgesia after open acromioplasty and rotator cuff repair: preliminary results. J Shoulder Elbow Surg 2004;13(6):630–4.

[42] Stein C, Millan MJ, Shippenberg TS, et al. Peripheral opioid receptors mediating antinociception in inflammation. Evidence for involvement of mu, delta and kappa receptors. J Pharmacol Exp Ther 1989;248(3):1269–75.

[43] Stein C, Yassouridis A. Peripheral morphine analgesia. Pain 1997;71(2):119–21.

[44] Kalso E, Tramer MR, Carroll D, et al. Pain relief from intra-articular morphine after knee surgery: a qualitative systematic review. Pain 1997;71(2):127–34.

[45] Allen GC, St Amand MA, Lui AC, et al. Postarthroscopy analgesia with intraarticular bupivacaine/morphine. A randomized clinical trial. Anesthesiology 1993;79(3):475–80.

[46] Gupta A, Bodin L, Holmstrom B, et al. A systematic review of the peripheral analgesic effects of intraarticular morphine. Anesth Analg 2001;93(3):761–70.

[47] Jackson DW, Evans NA, Thomas BM. Accuracy of needle placement into the intra-articular space of the knee. J Bone Joint Surg Am 2002;84-A(9):1522–7.

ELSEVIER
SAUNDERS

Anesthesiology Clin
25 (2007) 863–882

ANESTHESIOLOGY
CLINICS

Intrathecal Analgesia

Steven P. Cohen, MD[a,b,*], Anthony Dragovich, MD[b]

[a]Pain Management Division, Department of Anesthesiology, Johns Hopkins School of
Medicine, 550 North Broadway, Suite 301, Baltimore, MD 21205, USA
[b]Department of Surgery, Walter Reed Army Medical Center, Anesthesia Service,
6900 Georgia Avenue, NW, Washington, DC 20307, USA

The discovery of opioid receptors in neural tissue in the early 1970s [1,2] provided the impetus for the treatment of pain by injecting analgesic medications directly into the spinal canal, first in experimental animals [3], then in cancer patients [4]. In many respects the treatment of cancer pain with intrathecal (IT) opioids is an ideal scenario, given the high incidence of severe pain in terminal patients [5], the likelihood of developing dose-limiting side effects when oral opioids are used to treat pain, and concerns regarding issues of tolerance, dependence, and addiction. Previous reviews have demonstrated excellent outcomes using IT analgesia in patients with malignancies, although for financial reasons some experts recommend tunneled epidural catheters in lieu of implantable infusion devices in patients with life expectancies under 3 months [6].

The main controversy surrounding spinal analgesia is whether it is effective in the long term for nonmalignant pain. Current issues that permeate the ongoing debate on opioid use for noncancer pain include evidence that opioid-induced hyperalgesia accounts for a significant component of narcotic tolerance; literature suggesting that whereas opioids do provide short-term pain relief, their long-term ability to attenuate pain and improve function are less convincing; and higher estimates from better studies on the incidence of addiction in chronic pain patients [7–9].

A version of this article originally appeared in the 91:2 issue of Medical Clinics of North America.

The opinions or assertions contained herein are the private views of the authors and are not to be construed as official or as reflecting the views of the Department of the Army or the Department of Defense.

Funded in part by the John P. Murtha Neuroscience and Pain Institute, Johnstown, PA, and the U.S. Department of Defense.

* Corresponding author.

E-mail address: scohen40@jhmi.edu (S.P. Cohen).

We believe that implantable IT pumps have a place in the treatment of chronic, nonmalignant pain, albeit with certain caveats. Similar to prescribing oral and parenteral opioids, patients should be screened for signs of abuse, aberrant behavior, and psychological conditions that might predispose patients to failure before embarking on an IT trial. Although IT pumps are less prone to abuse than systemic opioids and carry almost no risk of diversion, the dependent relationship established by the implantation of an IT infusion device makes risk stratification just as essential [10]. A recent report by Kittelberger and colleagues [11] described a patient with failed back surgery syndrome (FBSS) who self-extracted hydromorphone from his pump.

Consideration should also be given to the likelihood of treatment success. Patients who have not acquiesced to trials with less invasive treatments are probably poor candidates for IT therapy. Certain medical conditions are more amenable to IT therapy than others. For example, IT baclofen is well-documented to be an effective treatment for spasticity-related pain, and zicontide was demonstrated in a recent multicenter randomized, controlled study to be effective in AIDS [12]. For opioid therapy, there are studies that support treatment in herpes zoster, but little evidence for their use in fibromyalgia.

Finally, in patients who otherwise meet criteria for consideration of IT therapy, a trial with either IT or epidural medications is of paramount importance. This holds true irrespective of the intended analgesic medication(s). But short-term trials are not without drawbacks. Some limitations of IT trials include the lack of standardization regarding the types (combinations) and doses of medications administered, limited outcome measures, and the fact that while short-term trials may predict short- and intermediate-term pain relief, their ability to prognosticate long-term outcomes is less established. For long-term therapy, the main factors limiting success are the development of tolerance and side effects, neither of which can be accurately predicted with a short-term trial (Box 1).

Opioids

Opioid receptors are characterized into three subtypes: mu, delta, and kappa, all of which are G-protein complexes [13]. The analgesic and nonanalgesic effects of opioids are mediated pre- and postsynaptically. Opioid binding to presynaptic terminals results in inhibition of substance P and calcitonin gene-related peptide release through suppression of voltage-gated calcium channels [14]. Postsynaptically, opioids cause inhibition of adenyl cyclase and activation of inwardly rectifying potassium currents resulting in neuronal hyperpolarization [15].

The effects of opioids are determined by their affinity for endogenous receptors and their ability to reach those receptors. In general, there is

---

Box 1. Selection criteria for intrathecal pump placement

- Stable medical condition amenable to surgery
- Clear organic pain generator
- No psychological or sociological contraindication
- No familial contraindication such as severe codependent behavior
- Documented responsible behavior and stable social situation
- Good pain relief with oral or parenteral opioids
- Intolerable side effects from systemic opioid therapy
- Baseline neurological exam and psychological evaluation
- Failure of more conservative therapy including trials with nonopioid medications and nerve blocks
- Constant or almost constant pain requiring around-the-clock opioid therapy
- High degree of tolerance to opioids may limit effectiveness of intrathecal therapy
- No tumor encroachment of thecal sac in cancer patients
- Life expectancy > 3 months
- No practical issues that might interfere with device placement, maintenance, or assessment (eg, morbid obesity, severe cognitive impairment)
- Positive response to an intrathecal trial

---

a positive correlation between the degree of water solubility and both the spread of analgesia and side effects. Highly water-soluble opioids like morphine exhibit a greater degree of rostral spread when injected intrathecally, which may improve analgesia in conditions requiring higher spinal levels or more extensive coverage. Conversely, many of the most common (pruritis and vomiting) and feared (delayed respiratory depression) adverse effects of spinal opioids are a result of interactions with opioid receptors in the brain, and thus are more frequently encountered with hydrophilic drugs like morphine (Table 1).

There is increasing evidence that IT opioids are superior to oral delivery in malignant pain, especially when narcotic dosage is limited by side effects.

Table 1
Conversion ratios between commonly used opioid agonists

Opioid	Oral	Parenteral	Epidural	Intrathecal	Hydrophilicity
Morphine	300	200	10	1	High
Hydromorphone	60	20	2	0.2	Intermediate
Meperidine	3000	1000	100	10	Low
Fentanyl	—	1	0.1	0.01	Low
Sufentanil	—	0.1	0.01	0.001	Low

In a multicenter, randomized trial, Smith and colleagues [16] compared IT drug delivery to comprehensive medical management (CMM) in 200 cancer patients. The mean visual analogue scale (VAS) pain score in the IT group fell 52%, which favorably compared with the 39% decrease in the CMM group. Toxicity scores in the CMM group fell 17% versus 50% in pump patients. Although not considered a primary outcome measure, 6-month survival in the IT drug delivery group was 54% compared with 37% in CMM patients. Whereas the large majority of studies assessing IT opioids in cancer pain have demonstrated reduced pain and improved function and quality of life, not all have been uniformly positive. In a multicenter, prospective, open-label study, Rauck and colleagues [17] evaluated a patient-activated IT morphine delivery system in 119 cancer patients with either refractory pain or uncontrollable side effects. One-month postimplant, the mean numerical pain score decreased from 6.1 to 4.2 (31%), a difference that persisted for 13 months. A statistically significant reduction was also noted for toxicity and oral opioid requirements. However at the final 16-month follow-up, the difference between baseline and current pain scores was no longer significant.

The evidence supporting IT opioids in nonmalignant pain is less robust than for cancer pain. To some extent, this may be because of different pain mechanisms characterizing the two conditions. In cancer, between 75% and 90% of pain is either nociceptive or mixed nociceptive-neuropathic in origin [18,19]. In nonmalignant pain, the etiology is more variable. For the chronic nonmalignant conditions most amenable to spinal analgesia such as FBSS, neuropathic pain tends to play a significant role. Numerous preclinical [20] and clinical [21] studies have shown neuropathic pain to be less responsive to opioids than nociceptive pain.

Thimineur and colleagues [22] conducted a prospective study comparing outcomes for chronic nonmalignant pain in patients who received IT opioid therapy (n = 38) with patients who either failed their trial or refused pump implant (n = 31), and newly referred patients who were not offered IT therapy (n = 41). During the 3-year study, VAS pain scores, functional capacity, and mood scores improved significantly in the pump recipients, while they either declined or stayed the same in nonpump recipients. However, most IT patients continued to suffer from moderate to severe pain. The authors concluded that while patients with severe, refractory pain will likely improve with IT therapy, their overall pain and symptom severity will remain high. To summarize the existing studies evaluating IT opioids for noncancer pain, most show significant short- to intermediate-term improvement for both neuropathic and nociceptive pain, but rarely is pain completely eradicated, and improvement in other outcome parameters (eg, mood and functional capacity) is less impressive (Table 2).

The most frequent causes of reoperation are catheter-related complications (migration, coiling, obstruction, breakage, and so forth), which range between 20% and 40%. Intrathecal granuloma formation is a serious complication that has the potential to cause spinal cord compression and neurological devastation. The etiology has not been fully elucidated, but the phenomenon appears to be related to concentration (>25 mg/mL), daily dosage (>10 mg/d), and duration of therapy. However in one review, 39% of morphine-related granulomas were associated with concentrations less than 25 mg/mL, 30% occurred despite doses of under 10 mg/d, and some were noted after within 1 month after initiating therapy [41].

Because of decreased dosing, IT therapy is associated with a lower incidence of many side effects than oral or parenteral use. Nevertheless, the route is not devoid of adverse effects. The most frequent side effects of IT opioids are constipation, urinary retention, nausea/vomiting, sweating, and libido disturbances secondary to hypogonadotrophic hypogonadism [42]. With few exceptions (eg, sweating, peripheral edema, constipation) these adverse effects tend to diminish with time [27]. The mechanism(s) of opioid-induced leg edema is not fully known but may involve partial sympathetic blockade. In one study, Aldrete and da Silva [43] found that among the 22% of FBSS patients who developed lower extremity edema necessitating discontinuation or dose reduction, all had evidence of venous stasis before pump insertion (Table 3).

Local anesthetics

The most widely used spinal analgesics are local anesthetics (LA), which are used to provide both surgical anesthesia and pain relief. The mechanism of action by which LA work is via the blockade of sodium channels, the pivotal event in the depolarization of neurons. As such, LA block the transmission of all neurons, not just the A delta and C fibers responsible for pain.

Numerous studies have documented good intermediate to long-term outcomes mixing LA with opioids and other IT analgesics. Two studies by Sjoberg and colleagues [44,45] conducted in more than 100 cancer patients found the combination of IT morphine and bupivacaine resulted in adequate pain relief in almost 100% of subjects. However, the mean follow-up period in these studies was less than 1 month. In a retrospective study by van Dongen and colleagues [46], the authors found that the addition of IT bupivacaine to opioids resulted in adequate analgesia in 10 of 17 cancer patients who failed IT opioid therapy. The mean follow-up in this study was 112 days. In a later, double-blind, randomized trial comparing IT morphine alone to IT morphine and bupivacaine in 20 cancer patients, the same group found the combination group developed less opioid tolerance than the morphine-only group [47]. The authors concluded the combination of IT bupivacaine and morphine provided synergistic analgesic effects.

Similarly beneficial results have been reported with IT LA-opioid combinations in noncancer pain. Krames [6] reported the addition of bupivacaine to IT opioids either decreased opioid side effects or enhanced analgesia in

Table 2
Outcomes with intrathecal opioids for noncancer pain

Study	Study type, no. implanted	Follow-up (mean in years)	Relief of pain, n%*	Condition studied	Comments & complications
Plummer et al [23] 1991	Retrospective, 12	0.5	83	Not mentioned	2 pumps explanted for poor pain relief
Krames and Lanning [24] 1993	Retrospective, 16	2.3	81	NO, NP, Mixed (FBSS)	Used MSO4 or hydromorphone; Bupivacaine added in 13/16 patients
Kanoff [25] 1994	Retrospective, 15	0.2–4.0	73	NP, Mixed (FBSS)	2 terminated therapy; 53% excellent relief
Hassenbusch et al [26] 1995	Prospective comparative, 18	0.8–4.7	61	NP	Used MSO4 or sufentanil; 33% re-operation rate; edema resolved in 3 patients after switch to sufentanil
Winkelmuller and winket maller [27] 1996	Retrospective, 120	0.5–6 (mean 3.4)	77	DA, Mixed (FBSS), NP	92% satisfied; 81% improved quality of life
Paice et al [28] 1996	Retrospective physician survey, 296	1.0	95	Mixed (FBSS), NP, NO, DA	Somatic pain improved more than other types; 21.6% mechanical complication rate
Yoshida et al [29] 1996	Retrospective, 18	2.0	25	Mixed (FBSS)	Performed 1.4 additional procedures per patient
Tutak and Doleys [30] 1996	Retrospective, 26	2.0	77	Not mentioned	11 reoperations

Study	Study type, N		Outcome	Diagnosis	Comments
Angel et al [31] 1998	Prospective observational, 11	0.5–3.0 (mean 2.3)	73	Mixed (FBSS), NP	2 pumps removed for urinary retention
Anderson and Burchiel [32] 1999	Prospective observational, 30	2.0	50% had ≥ 25% pain relief	Mixed (FBSS), NO, DA, NP	20% reoperation rate. Used MSO4 or hydromorphone, with 5 needing bupivacaine
Willis and Odefs [33] 1999	Retrospective study evaluating IT fentanyl after prior opioid failure, 8	2.5	68	Not mentioned	Patients failed IT MSO4 or hydromorphone
Kumar et al [34] 2001	Prospective observational, 16	1–4 (mean 1.5)	NO 57 FBSS 61 DA 75	NO, Mixed (FBSS), DA	3 pumps replaced or explanted; 12 successes
Roberts et al [35] 2001	Retrospective patient survey, 88	3.0	82	Mixed (FBSS), NP, NO	40% of patients required reoperation. 88% satisfaction rate
Anderson et al [36] 2001	Retrospective study evaluating i.t. hydromorphone	0.8	10%; 6 of 16 pts switched to hydromorphone b/c of inadequate analgesia had ≥ 25% pain relief	Mixed (FBSS), NP, NO, DA	All patients failed IT MSO4; Most patients had fewer side effects with hydromorphone
Deer et al [37] 2004	Prospective registry, 136	1.0	62	Mixed (FBSS), NP, NO	21 reoperations to correct mechanical problems; 36 physicians participated
Cherry et al [38] 2003	Case series, 7	2.0–7.0	Angina↓	Angina s/p CABG	Angina improved with IT fentanyl or MSO4

(continued on next page)

Table 2 (*continued*)

Study	Study type, no. implanted	Follow-up (mean in years)	Relief of pain, n%*	Condition studied	Comments & complications
Thimineur et al [22] 2004	Prospective observational with 2 comparative groups, 31	3	27	Not mentioned	Pain, disability, and depression improved in implanted patients while non-pump recipients worsened
Njee et al [39] 2004	Retrospective, 19	0.3–12.0 mean 4.5	NO 64 FBSS 58 NP 25	Mixed (FBSS), NP, NO	10% infection and catheter dislodgement rate; 90% patient satisfaction
Du Pen et al [40] 2006	Retrospective review of IT hydro-morphone, 24	1.0	25 decrease in VAS	Mixed (FBSS), NO, NP	Average dose increase was 600% in 1 year; only 7 patients had 1-year follow-up data

* Relief of pain = the % of patients with either good or excellent relief or ≥ 50% reduction in pain score.
Abbreviations: CABG, coronary artery bypass surgery; DA, deafferentation pain; FBSS. Failed Back Surgery Syndrome; NO, nociceptive pain; NP, Neuropathic pain; FBSS is listed in parenthesis after "mixed" if the most prevalent cause of mixed neuropathic and nociceptive pain was FBSS.

Table 3
Incidence of side effects with long-term intrathecal opioid therapy, %*

Side effect	%
Constipation	57
Sweating	47
Nausea	42
Urinary retention	37
Vomiting	33
Insomnia/nightmares	28
Impotence	21
Confusion	15
Pruritis	14
Edema	7
Disturbance of libido	6
Fatigue	6
Dry mouth	4
Dizziness	4
Loss of appetite	3
Hypothyroidism	2
Amenorrhea	2
Convulsions	1
Provocation of asthma	1

* *Adapted from* Refs. [27,32,34].

77% of 13 patients with nonmalignant pain, with a mean follow-up of al-most 1 year. In a large, retrospective cohort study conducted in 109 patients with FBSS and metastatic cancer of the spine, Deer and colleagues [48] found the combination of opioid and bupivacaine provided superior analge-sia and greater patient satisfaction, and was associated with less medication use than IT opioids alone. The average exposure to bupivacaine was 62 weeks. Excellent results were also reported mixing IT bupivacaine with morphine, clonidine, and midazolam in 26 patients with chronic back and/or leg pain [49] (mean follow-up 27 months).

In clinical practice, effective doses of bupivacaine generally range from 3 to 50 mg/d, although there are some reports of daily doses exceeding 100 mg/d [46,50]. Common side effects of IT LA include numbness, pares-thesias, weakness, and bowel or bladder dysfunction, all of which can be diminished by using combination therapy.

Calcium channel blockers

Voltage-gated calcium channels play an integral role pain transmission. Numerous classes of voltage-sensitive calcium channels have been identified, which are classified as T, L, N, P, Q, and R subtypes. These channels are characterized by biophysical properties such as sensitivity to pharmacolog-ical blocking agents, single-channel conductance kinetics, and voltage-dependence. In animal models of acute pain, there is compelling evidence to support a role for "N-type" calcium channels in nociception, moderate evidence for "L-type" channels, and limited or no evidence for other calcium channels. However, under conditions of persistent nociception induced by chemical, inflammatory, or neuropathic stimuli, all types of calcium channels may play a role in pain maintenance [51,52].

The only calcium channel blocker clinically used to treat chronic pain neuraxially is ziconotide, which blocks N-type calcium channels. Approved by the Food and Drug Administration (FDA) in 2004, ziconotide is a synthetic form of the peptide ω-conotoxin MVIIA isolated from venom produced by the marine snail *Conus magus*. In a multicenter, double-blind, placebo-controlled crossover study evaluating IT ziconotide for the treatment of refractory pain in 111 patients with cancer and AIDS, Staats and colleagues [12] found the treatment group (n = 68) obtained significantly better pain relief than control patients (53.0% versus 17.5%) in all parameters. Thirty-one percent of the ziconotide patients experienced side effects, with the most common being confusion, somnolence, and urinary retention. The observation that there was no loss of efficacy for ziconotide during the 5-day maintenance phase (mean dose 21.8 μg/d) is consistent with animal studies showing a lack of tolerance with calcium channel blockers. In an attempt to reduce side effects, Rauck and colleagues [53] conducted a double-blind, placebo-controlled study using a slower titration schedule and lower maximum dose in 220 patients with chronic, nonmalignant pain (mostly FBSS) refractory to conventional treatment. At the end of the 3-week treatment period, VAS pain scores improved by 15% in the ziconotide group versus 7% in the placebo group. During the treatment period, only 12% of ziconotide patients reported adverse effects.

Although ziconotide is approved only as monotherapy in chronic pain patients who have failed conventional IT therapy, many physicians are using it in combination with opioids and nonopioid analgesics [54]. The major limitations for IT ziconotide are its high cost and the high incidence of side effects, which top 33% in some studies. Adverse effects include psychiatric symptoms, neurological symptoms, cardiovascular events, and gastrointestinal complaints. Currently, IT ziconotide is considered a fourth-line treatment for chronic pain patients [55].

Alpha-2 agonists

Alpha-2 adrenergic receptors play a key role in analgesic effects mediated at peripheral, spinal, and brainstem sites. Several different subtypes of alpha-2 receptors have been identified, although recent studies suggest the alpha-2$_A$ receptor is primarily responsible for analgesia and sedation [56]. Presynaptically, alpha$_2$ agonists bind to receptors on primary afferent neurons, resulting in diminished release of neurotransmitters involved in relaying pain signals. On postsynaptic neurons, they hyperpolarize the cell by increasing potassium conductance through G$_i$ coupled channels. Alpha adrenergic agonists also activate spinal cholinergic neurons, which may potentiate their analgesic effects. In perioperative settings, clonidine has been shown to have synergistic analgesic effects when co-administered with neuraxial LA. However, the evidence that clonidine in combination with opioids is more effective than either agent alone in acute pain settings is weak and inconsistent [57].

The most studied and only FDA-approved alpha-2 agonist for IT use is clonidine. In a prospective, open-label study evaluating combination IT therapy in FBSS, Rainov and colleagues [49] reported good or excellent results at 2-year follow-up in 73% of patients. Sixteen patients received clonidine as part of their IT therapy. Siddall and colleagues [58] conducted a double-blind, placebo-controlled study assessing the efficacy of IT morphine or clonidine, alone or combined, for up to 6 days in 15 patients with central pain secondary to spinal cord injury. The authors found the combination of clonidine and morphine provided significantly better pain relief than saline (37% versus 0% reduction) or either drug alone (20% reduction for morphine, 17% for clonidine). No significant difference was noted in the incidence of side effects.

In addition to prospective studies reporting good outcomes using clonidine in combination with opioids and other analgesics, there are more than 2 dozen reported cases whereby IT clonidine, usually in combination with morphine, provided substantial relief for cancer pain, low back pain (LBP), and even spasticity-related pain in concert with baclofen [59–61]. In 2 retrospective studies, the results are split. Raphael and colleagues [62] reported good outcomes in 74% of patients using combination IT therapy in patients with chronic LBP (clonidine was administered to 27 of 37 patients), with no significant increases in opioid requirements after 2 years of treatment (mean follow-up 4.4 years). However, Ackerman and colleagues [63] reported IT clonidine, with or without opioids, to be of limited value in 15 patients with cancer and chronic nonmalignant pain. The most common side effects of IT clonidine are sedation, hypotension, nausea, and dry mouth. Intrathecal clonidine is recommended in combination with morphine as a second-line therapy for chronic pain [55].

N-methyl-D-aspartate receptor antagonists

Glutamatergic receptors are divided into G-protein coupled (metabotropic) (mGluR) and ion channel (ionotropic) receptors, which include not only N-methyl-D-aspartate (NMDA) receptors, but α-amino-3-hydroxy-5-methylisoxazole-4-propionic acid (AMPA) and kainite receptors. In addition to a binding site for the excitatory neurotransmitter glutamate, the NMDA receptor contains binding sites for the co-agonist glycine, phencyclidine-like compounds, and endogenous protons and polyamines. Following tissue injury, the activation of spinal NMDA receptors induces a state of facilitated processing from repetitive small afferent fiber stimulation, leading to an increased response to high- and low-threshold stimulation, and enhanced receptor field size. This process, known as "wind-up," is responsible for such phenomena such as allodynia and hyperalgesia. In animal studies, selective agonists at the NMDA, AMPA, kainite, and group I mGlu receptors produce spontaneous pain behavior in naïve animals, and allodynia and hyperalgesia in neuropathic and inflammatory models of persistent pain. No AMPA, kainite, or mGluR agonists or antagonists are clinically used in humans.

The most studied NMDA receptor blocker is the noncompetitive antagonist ketamine. In addition to its effects on NMDA receptors, ketamine possesses a plethora of other actions that enhance its analgesic properties. These include blocking non-NMDA glutamate and muscarinic cholinergic receptors, facilitating $GABA_A$ signaling, weakly binding to opioid receptors, and possessing LA and possibly neuroregenerative properties [64].

The results of IT ketamine use in acute and chronic pain have been mixed. In an early study by Bion [65], the administration of hyperbaric ketamine was found to provide adequate anesthesia in 16 patients undergoing lower limb surgery for war injuries. However, more recent studies have reported less-auspicious results. Hawksworth and Serpell [66] found the high incidence of psychomimetic side effects and incomplete anesthesia precluded the use of IT ketamine as a sole anesthetic. Similarly disappointing results were found by Kathirvel and colleagues [67] in 25 women undergoing brachytherapy, and by Togal and colleagues [68] in 40 men undergoing prostate surgery.

For terminal cancer pain, controlled studies and anecdotal experience support the use of IT ketamine in patients refractory to conventional analgesics. Benrath and colleagues [69] reported a patient with metastatic urethral cancer and unremitting neuropathic pain who failed to respond to extremely high doses of IT morphine, bupivacaine, and clonidine. After ketamine was added, a dramatic decrease in pain occurred enabling significant reductions in IT morphine and clonidine, and discontinuation of bupivacaine. Muller and Lemos [70] reported four patients with nociceptive and neuropathic cancer pain who obtained excellent pain relief without tolerance to combination IT therapy with ketamine, morphine, clonidine, and lidocaine. In two of the patients, ketamine was successfully added after tolerance developed to the other three agents. A similar scenario was reported by Vranken and colleagues [71], who described almost complete abolition of neuropathic pain after ketamine was added to the treatment regimen in a cancer patient refractory to IT morphine, bupivacaine, and clonidine. Finally, in a double-blind crossover study comparing the co-administration of low-dose IT ketamine (1 mg) with morphine and IT morphine alone twice daily in 20 patients with terminal cancer, Yang and colleagues [72] found that combination treatment resulted in significantly lower morphine requirements, less rescue medication, and slightly improved pain scores over the 48-hour treatment period. No serious side effects were noted.

The positive reports on the use of IT ketamine for chronic pain remain tempered by questions of neurotoxicity. In the 1990s Karpinski and colleagues [73] reported a terminal cancer patient who received a 3-week IT infusion of racemic ketamine and was found to have subpial vacuolar myelopathy on autopsy. Stotz and colleagues [74] reported a similar finding 2 years later in another cancer patient following a 7-day trial of IT ketamine. These reports led subsequent clinicians to limit IT ketamine administration to preservative-free formulations of the active S(+) enantiomer. However, Vranken and colleagues [75] recently reported severe histopathological abnormalities on postmortem spinal cord examination in a woman with terminal cervical cancer who received excellent pain relief 3 weeks after S(+) ketamine was added to her IT morphine, bupivacaine, and clonidine regimen. Based on the absence of human toxicology studies, mixed reports of animal toxicology studies, and anecdotal reports of neurological injury, IT ketamine should be reserved for terminal patients who fail to derive pain relief from more conventional analgesics.

Gamma-aminobutyric acid agonists

Three subtypes of the GABA receptor have been identified: $GABA_A$, $GABA_B$, and $GABA_C$. When these receptors are activated, an influx of chloride ions enters the cell resulting in hyperpolarization of the cell membrane and decreased neuronal excitability. $GABA_A$ and $GABA_C$ are both ligand-gated chloride channels, and can be differentiated by location and response to antagonists. $GABA_A$, the more clinically relevant of the two, is most prominent in the dorsal horn of the spinal cord.

The $GABA_B$ receptor is a G-protein–linked complex whose activation results in augmentation of potassium channel currents. Like $GABA_A$, $GABA_B$ receptors are found throughout the spinal cord, being located both pre- and postsynaptically. Presynaptic activation results in decreased neurotransmitter release; postsynaptic activation leads to membrane hyperpolarization and decreased opening of voltage-sensitive calcium channels [76].

Although IT midazolam has been shown to have analgesic efficacy in animal models of visceral, inflammatory somatic, and acute nociception [77], there are few clinical studies evaluating its use. In a randomized, double-blind study comparing single-shot epidural steroids with 2 mg of IT midazolam in 25 patients with chronic, mechanical LBP, Serrao and colleagues [78] reported similar improvement in one half to three quarters of patients up to 2-months postinjection. However, the use of rescue medication was less in the midazolam group. Borg and Krijnen [79] treated four patients with chronic benign neurogenic and musculoskeletal pain refractory to conventional analgesics with continuous infusions of up to 6 mg/d of IT midazolam in combination with clonidine or morphine. In all four patients, long-term combination infusion therapy resulted in nearly complete pain relief. Rainov and colleagues [49] published a pilot study evaluating long-term treatment outcomes in 26 patients with chronic low back and leg pain treated with various combinations of IT morphine, bupivacaine, clonidine, and midazolam (n = 10). Although results were not tabulated by individual drug combinations, 73% of patients reported good or excellent outcomes. Similar benefits were noted by Yanez and colleagues [80] who reported excellent pain relief in four patients with cancer and noncancer pain poorly responsive to IT morphine. Based on animal and clinical studies, the use of IT midazolam appears to potentiate the analgesic effects of opioids and clonidine.

Animal studies are mixed regarding the toxicity of IT midazolam, with approximately half reporting neurotoxicity [77,81]. Deleterious effects have been demonstrated across a wide range of species and dosages, using mixtures with and without preservatives. However, these reports are balanced by a plethora of similar studies concluding IT midazolam is no more neurotoxic than saline [82,83]. In a randomized study evaluating the effects of adding 2 mg of midazolam to LA in 1100 patients undergoing spinal anesthesia, Tucker and colleagues [84] found no increase in postoperative neurological symptoms in patients who received combination treatment. The most common side effect of IT midazolam is dose-dependent sedation, with motor weakness occurring only at high doses. Midazolam is currently a fourth-line IT treatment for chronic pain [55].

Preclinical studies with $GABA_B$ agonists in animal models of acute and persistent nociception found that $GABA_B$ agonists such as baclofen produce antinociception and anti-allodynia at doses that do not impair motor function [85]. In a recent review, Slonimski and colleagues [86] eloquently detailed the preclinical evidence demonstrating efficacy for IT baclofen in spasm-induced, neuropathic, sympathetically maintained and acute pain. Intrathecal baclofen has been used to treat spasticity since the mid-1980s, and is FDA-approved for this indication. In a Cochrane review of pharmacological interventions for spinal cord injury (SCI)-induced spasticity, Tarrico and colleagues [87] concluded only IT baclofen has been proven effective. In a similar meta-analysis conducted for spasticity associated with multiple sclerosis (MS), Beard and colleagues [88] found good evidence to support only IT baclofen and botulinum toxin. These findings are consistent with reviews evaluating treatments for spasticity derived from other etiologies.

Clinical studies have also demonstrated IT baclofen to be effective for a wide array of other pain conditions. In a randomized, double-blind cross-over trial, seven women with complex regional pain syndrome (CRPS) were given bolus injections of either baclofen 25, 50, or 75 µg or saline [89]. No difference was found between 25 µg and saline injections. With higher doses, six of seven patients had complete or partial resolution of symptoms and proceeded to pump implantation. Three months postimplant, three women had regained normal hand function and two the ability to walk. Three had marked reductions in pain, four in paresthesias and two in numbness. The beneficial effects of IT baclofen in CRPS is supported by the work of Zuniga and colleagues [90], who reported two cases of refractory CRPS type I successfully treated with baclofen. In both patients, dramatic improvements in autonomic symptoms, and spontaneous and evoked pain were noted.

Intrathecal baclofen is considered the gold standard for spasticity, but anecdotal evidence suggests it may alleviate central pain as well. In a double-blind, placebo-controlled study by Herman and colleagues [91] conducted in patients with MS and SCI, the authors found significant reductions in dysesthetic and spasm-related pain, but no effect on evoked pain. These results are supported by Taira and colleagues [92] who found 9 of 14 patients with central pain secondary to stroke or SCI experienced significant reductions in spontaneous pain, allodynia, and hyperalgesia following an IT baclofen bolus. They are in contrast to the findings of Loubser and Akman, [93] who found that while musculoskeletal pain decreased in a large majority of SCI patients 1 year after initiation of IT baclofen, only 22% experienced a significant decline in neurogenic pain.

In addition to chronic pain associated with spasticity, IT baclofen has been reported to relieve neuropathic pain secondary to FBSS, amputation, and plexopathy [94]. In a recent case series conducted in patients with refractory neuropathic pain, Lind and colleagues [95] treated seven patients with IT baclofen pumps and spinal cord stimulation and four with baclofen

Table 4
Dose range and evidence for efficacy and commonly used intrathecal analgesic agents

Drug	Typical dose range	Clinical evidence for efficacy
Morphine	1–20 mg/d	Strong evidence for cancer pain. Moderate evidence for nonmalignant pain.
Hydromorphone	0.5–10 mg/d	Same as morphine.
Fentanyl	0.02–0.3 mg/d	Same as morphine.
Bupivacaine	4–30 mg/d	Strong evidence for cancer pain. Moderate evidence for nonmalignant pain.
Midazolam	0.2–6 mg/d	Weak evidence for chronic back pain. Anecdotal evidence for neuropathic pain.
Clonidine	0.03–1 mg/d	Weak evidence for cancer pain. Moderate evidence for back pain. Weak evidence for central pain. Moderate evidence for neuropathic pain.
Ketamine	1–50 mg/d	Moderate evidence for cancer pain. Weak evidence for neuropathic pain.
Baclofen	0.05–0.8 mg/d	Strong evidence for muscle spasm–related pain. Weak evidence for central pain. Moderate evidence for neuropathic pain.

alone. Although both groups obtained significant pain relief, a greater reduction in pain scores occurred in the combination group (mean follow-up 35 months).

The most common side effects associated with IT baclofen are drowsiness, cognitive impairment, weakness, gastrointestinal complaints, and sexual dysfunction [96]. Baclofen is currently considered a fourth-line treatment for chronic pain [55] (Table 4).

Summary

Since the advent of implantable IT drug delivery systems over 25 years ago, numerous advances have been made with regard to system technology, pharmacology, and patient selection. Whereas strong evidence exists for the use of IT therapy for cancer pain, the evidence supporting long-term efficacy in noncancer pain is less convincing. However, in carefully selected patients, combination therapy appears to provide the ideal balance between efficacy and side effects, at least for intermediate-term outcomes. Areas most ripe for future investigation include which pain conditions are most amenable to IT therapy, the long-term efficacy of infusion therapy for noncancer pain, particularly in regard to functional improvement, delineating which drug combinations provide the best balance between efficacy and adverse effects, and conducting preclinical and clinical safety studies on promising analgesics such as ketamine and midazolam.

References

[1] Pert CB, Snyder S. Opiate receptor: demonstration in nervous tissue. Science 1973;179(77): 1011–4.

[2] Terenius L. Characteristics of the "receptor" for narcotic analgesics in synaptic plasma membrane fractions from rat brain. Acta Pharmacol Toxicol (Copenh) 1973;33(5):377–84.

[3] Yaksh TL, Rudy TA. Studies on the direct spinal action of narcotics in the production of analgesia in the rat. J Pharmacol Exp Ther 1977;202(2):411–28.

[4] Wang JK, Nauss LA, Thomas JE. Pain relief by intrathecally applied morphine in man. Anesthesiology 1979;50(2):149–51.

[5] Foley KM. Treatment of cancer pain. N Engl J Med 1985;313(2):84–95.

[6] Krames ES. Intrathecal infusional therapies for intractable pain: patient management guidelines. J Pain Symptom Manage 1993;8(1):36–46.

[7] Kalso E, Edwards JE, Moore RA, et al. Opioids in chronic non-cancer pain: systematic review of efficacy and safety. Pain 2004;112(3):372–80.

[8] Ives TJ, Chelminski PR, Hammett-Stabler CA, et al. Predictors of opioid misuse in patients with chronic pain: a prospective cohort study. BMC Health Serv Res 2006;6:46.

[9] Ballantyne JC, Mao J. Opioid therapy for chronic pain. N Engl J Med 2003;349(20):1943–53.

[10] Webster LR, Webster RM. Predicting aberrant behaviors in opioid-treated patients: preliminary validation of the Opioid Risk Tool. Pain Med 2006;6(6):432–42.

[11] Kittelberger KP, Buchheit TE, Rice SF. Self-extraction of intrathecal pump opioid. Anesthesiology 2004;101(3):807.

[12] Staats PS, Yearwood T, Charapata SG, et al. Intrathecal ziconotide in the treatment of refractory pain in patients with cancer or AIDS: a randomized controlled trial. JAMA 2004;291(1):63–70.

[13] Akil H, Watson SJ, Young E, et al. Endogenous opioids: biology and function. Annu Rev Neurosci 1984;7:223–55.

[14] Reisine T. Opiate receptors. Neuropharmacology 1995;34(5):463–72.

[15] Ocana M, Cendan CM, Cobos EJ, et al. Potassium channels and pain: present realities and future opportunities. Eur J Pharmacol 2004;500(1–3):203–19.

[16] Smith TJ, Staats PS, Deer T, et al. Implantable Drug Delivery Systems Study Group. Randomized clinical trial of an implantable drug delivery system compared with comprehensive medical management for refractory cancer pain. Impact on pain, drug-related toxicity, and survival. J Clin Oncol 2002;20(19):4040–9.

[17] Rauck RL, Cherry D, Boyer MF, et al. Long-term intrathecal opioid therapy with a patient-activated, implanted delivery system for the treatment of refractory cancer pain. J Pain 2003; 4(8):441–7.

[18] Zeppetella G, O'Doherty CA, Collins S. Prevalence and characteristics of breakthrough pain in patients with non-malignant terminal disease admitted to a hospice. Palliat Med 2001; 15(3):243–6.

[19] Portenoy RK, Hagen NA. Breakthrough pain: definition, prevalence and characteristics. Pain 1990;41(3):273–81.

[20] Idanpaan-Heikkila JJ, Guilbaud G. Pharmacological studies on a rat model of trigeminal neuropathic pain: baclofen, but not carbamazepine, morphine or tricyclic antidepressants, attenuates the allodynia-like behavior. Pain 1999;79(2–3):281–90.

[21] Hanks GW, Forbes K. Opioid responsiveness. Acta Anaesthesiol Scand 1997;41(1 Pt 2): 154–8.

[22] Thimineur MA, Kravitz E, Vodapally MS. Intrathecal opioid treatment for chronic non-malignant pain: a 3-year prospective study. Pain 2004;109(3):242–9.

[23] Plummer JL, Cherry DA, Cousins MJ, et al. Long-term spinal administration of morphine in cancer and non-cancer pain: a retrospective study. Pain 1991;44(3):215–20.

[24] Krames ES, Lanning RM. Intrathecal infusional analgesia for nonmalignant pain: analgesic efficacy of intrathecal opioid with or without bupivacaine. J Pain Symptom Manage 1993; 8(8):539–48.

[25] Kanoff RB. Intraspinal delivery of opiates by an implantable, programmable pump in patients with chronic, intractable pain of nonmalignant origin. J Am Osteopath Assoc 1994;94(6):487–93.

[26] Hassenbusch SJ, Stanton-Hicks M, Covington EC, et al. Long-term intraspinal infusions of opiods in the treatment of neuropathic pain. J Pain Symptom Manage 1995;10(7): 527–43.

[27] Winkelmuller M, Winkelmuller W. Long-term effects of continuous intrathecal opioid treatment in chronic pain of nonmalignant etiology. J Neurosurg 1996;85(3):458–67.

[28] Paice JA, Penn RD, Shott S. Intraspinal morphine for chronic pain: a retrospective, multi-center study. J Pain Symptom Manage 1996;11(2):71–80.

[29] Yoshida GM, Nelson RW, Capen DA. Evaluation of contiuous intraspinal narcotic analgesia for chronic pain from benign causes. Am J Orthop 1996;25(10):693–4.

[30] Tutak U, Doleys DM. Intrathecal infusion systems for treatment of chronic low back and leg pain of noncancer origin. South Med J 1996;89(3):295–300.

[31] Angel IF, Gould HJ Jr, Carey ME. Intrathecal morphine pump as a treatment option in chronic pain of nonmalignant origin. Surg Neurol 1998;49(1):92–9.

[32] Anderson VC, Burchiel KJ. A prospective study of long-term intrathecal morphine in the management of chronic nonmalignant pain. Neurosurgery 1999;44(2):289–300.

[33] Willis KD, Doleys DM. The effects of long-term intraspinal infusion therapy with noncancer pain patients: evaluation of patient, significant-other, and clinic staff appraisals. Neuromodulation 1999;2(4):241–53.

[34] Kumar K, Kelly M, Pirlot T. Continuous intrathecal morphine treatment for chronic pain of nonmalignant etiology: long-term benefits and efficacy. Surg Neurol 2001;55:79–88.

[35] Roberts LJ, Finch PM, Goucke CR, et al. Outcome of intrathecal opioids in chronic non-cancer pain. Eur J Pain 2001;5(4):353–61.

[36] Anderson VC, Cooke B, Burchiel KJ. Intrathecal hydromorphone for chronic nonmalignant pain: a retrospective study. Pain Med 2001;2(4):287–97.

[37] Deer T, Chapple I, Classen A, et al. Intrathecal drug delivery for treatment of chronic low back pain: report from the National Outcomes Registry for low back pain. Pain Med 2004;5(1):6–13.

[38] Cherry DA, Gourlay GK, Eldredge KA. Management of chronic intractable angina: spinal opioids offer an alternative therapy. Pain 2003;102(1–2):163–6.

[39] Njee TB, Irthum B, Roussel P, et al. Intrathecal morphine infusion for chronic non-malignant pain: a multiple center retrospective study. Neuromodulation 2004;7(4):249–59.

[40] Du Pen S, Du Pen A, Hillyer J. Intrathecal hydromorphone for intractable nonmalignant pain: a retrospective study. Pain Med 2006;7(1):10–5.

[41] Yaksh TL, Hassenbusch S, Burchiel K, et al. Inflammatory masses associated with intrathecal drug infusion: a review of preclinical evidence and human data. Pain Med 2002;3(4):300–12.

[42] Paice JA, Penn RD, Ryan W. Altered sexual function and decreased testosterone in patients receiving intraspinal opioids. J Pain Symtom Manage 1994;9(2):126–31.

[43] Aldrete JA, Couto da Silva JM. Leg edema from intrathecal opiate infusions. Eur J Pain 2000;4(4):361–5.

[44] Sjoberg M, Nitescu P, Appelgren L, et al. Long-term intrathecal morphine and bupivacaine in patients with refractory cancer pain. Results from a morphine:bupivacaine dose regimen of 0.5:4.75 mg/ml. Anesthesiology 1994;80(2):284–97.

[45] Sjoberg M, Appelgren L, Einarsson S, et al. Long-term intrathecal morphine and bupivacaine in "refractory" cancer pain. I. Results from the first series of 52 patients. Acta Anaesthesiol Scand 1991;35(1):30–43.

[46] van Dongen RT, Crul BJ, De Bock M. Long-term intrathecal infusion of morphine and morphine/bupivacaine mixtures in the treatment of cancer pain: a retrospective analysis of 51 cases. Pain 1993;55(1):119–23.

[47] van Dongen RT, Crul BJ, van Egmond J. Intrathecal coadministration of bupivacaine diminishes morphine dose progression during long-term intrathecal infusion in cancer patients. Clin J Pain 1999;15(3):166–72.

[48] Deer TR, Caraway DL, Kim CK, et al. Clinical experience with intrathecal bupivacaine in combination with opioid for the treatment of chronic pain related to failed back surgery syndrome and metastatic cancer pain of the spine. Spine J 2002;2(4):274–8.

[49] Rainov NG, Heidecke V, Burkert W. Long-term intrathecal infusion of drug combinations for chronic back and leg pain. J Pain Symptom Manage 2001;22(4):862–71.

[50] Berde CB, Sethna NF, Conrad LS. Subarachnoid bupivacaine analgesia for seven months for a patient with a spinal cord tumor. Anesthesiology 1990;72(6):1094–6.

[51] Vanegas H, Schaible H. Effects of antagonists to high-threshold calcium channels upon spinal mechanisms of pain, hyperalgesia and allodynia. Pain 2000;85(1–2):9–18.

[52] McGivern JG. Targeting N-type and T-type calcium channels for the treatment of pain. Drug Discov Today 2006;11(5–6):245–53.

[53] Rauck RL, Wallace MS, Leong MS, et al. A randomized, double-blind, placebo-controlled study of intrathecal ziconotide in adults with severe chronic pain. J Pain Symptom Manage 2006;31(5):393–406.

[54] Thompson JC, Dunbar E, Laye RR. Treatment challenges and complications with ziconotide monotherapy in established pump patients. Pain Physician 2006;9(2):147–52.

[55] Hassenbusch SJ, Portenoy RK, Cousins M, et al. Polyanalgesic Consensus Conference 2003: an update on the management of pain by intraspinal drug delivery—report of an expert panel. J Pain Symptom Manage 2004;27(6):540–63.

[56] Kamibayashi T, Maze M. Clinical uses of alpha 2-adrenergic agonists. Anesthesiology 2000; 93(5):1345–9.

[57] Walker SM, Goudas LC, Cousins MJ, et al. Combination spinal analgesic chemotherapy: a systematic review. Anesth Analg 2002;95(3):674–715.

[58] Siddall PJ, Molloy AR, Walker S, et al. The efficacy of intrathecal morphine and clonidine in the treatment of pain after spinal cord injury. Anesth Analg 2000;91(6):1493–8.

[59] Uhle EI, Becker R, Gatscher S, et al. Continuous intrathecal clonidine administration for the treatment of neuropathic pain. Stereotact Funct Neurosurg 2000;75(4):167–75.

[60] Eisenach JC, De Kock M, Klimscha W. Alpha (2)-adrenergic agonists for regional anesthesia. A clinical review of clonidine (1984–1995). Anesthesiology 1996;85(3):655–74.

[61] Middleton JW, Siddall PJ, Walker S. Intrathecal clonidine and baclofen in the management of spasticity and neuropathic pain following spinal cord injury: a case study. Arch Phys Med Rehabil 1996;77(8):824–6.

[62] Raphael JH, Southall JL, Gnanadurai TV, et al. Long-term experience with implanted intrathecal drug administration systems for failed back syndrome and chronic mechanical low back pain. BMC Musculoskelet Disord 2002;3:17.

[63] Ackerman LL, Follett KA, Rosenquist RW. Long-term outcomes during treatment of chronic pain with intrathecal clonidine or clonidine/opioid combinations. J Pain Symptom Manage 2003;26(1):668–77.

[64] Cohen SP, Chang AS, Larkin T, et al. The IV ketamine test: a predictive response tool for an oral dextromethorphan treatment regimen in neuropathic pain. Anesth Analg 2004;99(6): 1753–9.

[65] Bion JF. Intrathecal ketamine for war surgery. A preliminary study under field conditions. Anaesthesia 1984;39(10):1023–8.

[66] Hawksworth C, Serpell M. Intrathecal anesthesia with ketamine. Reg Anesth Pain Med 1998;23(3):283–8.

[67] Kathirvel S, Sadhasivam S, Saxena A, et al. Effects of intrathecal ketamine added to bupivacaine for spinal anaesthesia. Anaesthesia 2000;55(9):899–904.

[68] Togal T, Demirbilek S, Koroglu A, et al. Effects of S(+) ketamine added to bupivacaine for spinal anaesthesa for prostate surgery in elderly patients. Eur J Anaesthesiol 2004;21(3): 193–7.

[69] Benrath J, Scharbert G, Gustorff B, et al. Long-term intrathecal S(+)-ketamine in a patient with cancer-related neuropathic pain. Br J Anaesth 2005;95(2):247–9.

[70] Muller A, Lemos D. Cancer pain: beneficial effect of ketamine addition to spinal administration of morphine-clonidine-lidocaine mixture. Ann Fr Anesth Reanim 1996;15(3): 271–6.

[71] Vranken JH, van der Vegt MH, Kal JE, et al. Treatment of neuropathic cancer pain with continuous intrathecal administration of S + -ketamine. Acta Anaesthesiol Scand 2004; 48(2):249–52.

[72] Yang CY, Wong CS, Chang JY, et al. Intrathecal ketamine reduces morphine requirements in patients with terminal cancer pain. Can J Anaesth 1996;43(4):379–83.

[73] Karpinski N, Dunn J, Hansen L, et al. Subpial vacuolar myelopathy after intrathecal ketamine: report of a case. Pain 1997;73(1):103–5.

[74] Stotz M, Oehen HP, Gerber H. Histological findings after long-term infusion of intrathecal ketamine for chronic pain: a case report. J Pain Symptom Manage 1999;18(3): 223–8.

[75] Vranken JH, Troost D, Wegener JT, et al. Neuropathological findings after continuous intrathecal administration of S(+)-ketamine for the management of neuropathic cancer pain. Pain 2005;117(1–2):231–5.

[76] Bowery NG. GABAB receptor pharmacology. Annu Rev Pharmacol Toxicol 1993;33: 109–47.

[77] Yaksh TL, Allen JW. The use of intrathecal midazolam in humans: A case study of process. Anesth Analg 2004;98(6):1536–45.

[78] Serrao JM, Marks RL, Morley SJ, et al. Intrathecal midazolam for the treatment of chronic mechanical low back pain; a controlled comparison with epidural steroid in a pilot study. Pain 1992;48(1):5–12.

[79] Borg PA, Krijnen JH. Long-term intrathecal administration of midazolam and clonidine. Clin J Pain 1996;12(1):63–8.

[80] Yanez A, Peleteiro R, Camba MA. [Intrathecal administration of morphine, midazolam, and their combination in 4 patients with chronic pain]. Rev Esp Anestesiol Reanim 1992; 39(1):40–2 [in Spanish].

[81] Ugur B, Basaloglu K, Yurtseven T, et al. Neurotoxicity with single dose intrathecal midazolam administration. Eur J Anaesthesiol 2005;22(12):907–12.

[82] Bahar M, Cohen ML, Grinshpon Y, et al. Spinal anaesthesia with midazolam in the rat. Can J Anaesth 1997;44(2):208–15.

[83] Johansen MJ, Gradert TL, Satterfield WC. Safety of continuous intrathecal midazolam infusion in the sheep model. Anesth Analg 2004;98(6):1528–35.

[84] Tucker AP, Lai C, Nadeson R, et al. Intrathecal midazolam. I. A cohort study investigating safety. Anesth Analg 2004;98(6):1512–20.

[85] Hwang JH, Yaksh TL. The effect of spinal GABA receptor agonists on tactile allodynia in a surgically-induced neuropathic pain model in the rat. Pain 1997;70(1):15–22.

[86] Slonimski M, Abram S, Zuniga R. Intrathecal baclofen in pain management. Reg Anesth Pain Med 2004;29(3):269–76.

[87] Taricco M, Adone R, Pagliacci C, et al. Pharmacological interventions for spasticity following spinal cord injury. Cochrane Database Syst Rev 2000;2:CD00131.

[88] Beard S, Hunn A, Wight J. Treatments for spasticity and pain in multiple sclerosis: a systematic review. Health Technol Assess 2003;7(40):1–111.

[89] van Hilten BJ, van de Beek WT, Hoff JI, et al. Intrathecal baclofen for the treatment of dystonia in patients with reflex sympathetic dystrophy. N Engl J Med 2000;343(9):625–30.

[90] Zuniga RE, Perera S, Abram SE. Intrathecal baclofen: a useful agent in the treatment of well-established complex regional pain syndrome. Reg Anesth Pain Med 2002;27(1):90–3.

[91] Herman RM, D'Luzansky JC, Ippolito R. Intrathecal baclofen suppresses central pain in patients with spinal lesions. Clin J Pain 1992;8(4):338–45.

[92] Taira T, Kawamura H, Tanikawa T, et al. A new approach to control central deafferentiation pain: spinal intrathecal baclofen. Stereotactic Funct Neurosurg 1995;65(1–4):101–5.

[93] Loubser PG, Akman NM. Effects of intrathecal baclofen on chronic spinal cord injury pain. J Pain Symptom Manage 1996;12(4):241–7.

[94] Zuniga RE, Schlicht CR, Abram SE. Intrathecal baclofen is analgesic in patients with chronic pain. Anesthesiology 2000;92(3):876–80.

[95] Lind G, Meyerson BA, Winter J, et al. Intrathecal baclofen as adjuvant therapy to enhance the effect of spinal cord stimulation in neuropathic pain: a pilot study. Eur J Pain 2004;8(4): 377–83.

[96] Denys P, Mane M, Azouvi P. Side effects of chronic intrathecal baclofen on erection and ejaculation in patients with spinal cord lesions. Arch Phys Med Rehabil 1998;79(5):494–6.

ELSEVIER
SAUNDERS

Anesthesiology Clin
25 (2007) 883–898

ANESTHESIOLOGY
CLINICS

Interventional Approaches to Pain Management

John D. Markman, MD[a,b,*], Annie Philip, MD[a]

[a]*Neuromedicine Pain Management Center, Departments of Neurosurgery and Neurology, University of Rochester School of Medicine and Dentistry, 601 Elmwood Avenue, Box 670 Rochester, New York 14642, USA*
[b]*The Pain Management Center at University of Rochester Medical Center, Rochester, NY 14642, USA*

Interventional approaches remain a mainstay of chronic pain treatment despite the many challenges to the study of their efficacy. When less invasive analgesic modalities provide inadequate relief, these techniques often play a complementary role. Interventional strategies typically target the neural structures that are presumed to mediate the experience of pain. The varied mechanisms of action range from reversible blockade with local anesthetics, to augmentation with spinal cord stimulation, and ablation with radiofrequency energy or neurolytic agents. Other techniques access intraspinal routes of medication delivery to improve an effective drug's therapeutic index. Many of the most common approaches are uniquely suited to offer rapid, potent, local control of pain with reduced systemic side effects.

Clinical indications for interventional pain management strategies encompass a broad range of conditions, from intractable neuropathic symptoms caused by advanced cancer to chronic, noncancer pain involving the spine. Each technique bears specific risks that pertain to its anatomic targets and therapeutic mechanism of action. Review of the evidence for the interventions considered raises practical issues common to virtually all procedures for chronic pain: (1) the validity of extending an indication for cancer pain to noncancer pain, (2) the timing and repeated use of a strategy with temporary benefit in the perioperative setting to a chronic pain condition, (3) the impact of neuroplasticity on the development of tolerance

A version of this article originally appeared in the 91:2 issue of Medical Clinics of North America.

* Corresponding author. Director, Neuromedicine Pain Management Center, Departments of Neurosurgery and Neurology, University of Rochester School of Medicine and Dentistry, 601 Elmwood Avenue, Box 670 Rochester, New York 14642.

E-mail address: john_markman@urmc.rochester.edu (J.D. Markman).

to analgesic effect, and (4) the clinical significance of a reduction in pain intensity in the absence of demonstrable function or benefit. This article traces the rationale and pivotal evidence for some representative, common interventional procedures, with the aim of helping nonspecialist physicians identify the patients most likely to benefit from these approaches.

Historical context and general considerations

The discovery of the local anesthetic properties of cocaine and the characterization of methods for subcutaneous and spinal injection in the late nineteenth century laid the groundwork for today's interventional pain management strategies [1]. These techniques were refined in the early twentieth century and were increasingly deployed beyond the operating room by the end of World War II. Anesthesiology-based "nerve block" clinics of that era have given way to an integrated treatment approach to chronic pain that incorporates psychologic and rehabilitative techniques [2].

A revolution in synthetic chemistry has paralleled refinements in neural blockade. The result has been a growing armamentarium of systemic analgesics, including acetaminophen, nonsteroidal anti-inflammatory drugs, semisynthetic and synthetic opioid analgesics, and the heterogenous group of medications known as adjuvants. Many of the medications in this latter group were developed for conditions such as epilepsy, and only later were found to have analgesic properties in conditions such as neuropathic pain [3]. In a similar way, interventional techniques shown to have temporary benefit in the perioperative setting have been extrapolated to chronic pain treatment. Despite the emergence of myriad pharmacologic and nonpharmacologic methods to treat chronic pain in an interdisciplinary environment, many of these are not well-tolerated or do not alleviate symptoms sufficiently [4]. The potential benefit of local and neuraxial approaches is often greatest when pain remains poorly controlled with pharmacologic and nonpharmacologic strategies.

Few placebo-controlled studies of invasive approaches for the treatment of chronic pain have been carried out. Factors complicating the study of procedures include the absence of consensus standards for block technique; the ethical questions and patient enrollment challenges posed by placebo-controlled research; limitations to treatment blinding; and the difficulty of quantifying psychosocial variables, such as litigation and family support, that influence treatment outcome [5]. As a consequence, the procedures developed for pain management have not been subject to placebo-controlled evaluation approaching the scale of newer pharmacologic agents. This limitation is balanced by the fact that most interventional techniques and associated drugs have been adapted from the perioperative context where their use is commonplace and the risks are well-characterized [6].

Symptom- and disease-based paradigms, rather than a mechanism-based understanding of pain, commonly inform treatment decisions. Drugs such as a gabapentin, for which there is strong evidence of analgesic benefit in a few neuropathic conditions, are used frequently to treat related symptom patterns [7]. Extrapolation of clinical trial data and individualized assessment of treatment response appears to be the norm in pharmacologic and procedural decision making alike [8]. For example, spinal cord stimulation is used to treat intractable lower extremity chronic pain characterized as "burning" following laminectomy and for a similar symptom characterization in complex regional pain syndrome [9,10]. Evidence does not show that these symptom patterns share a common underlying mechanism, despite the similar features. Patients undergo a defined trial of neuroaugmentation with different configurations of stimulation, just as they might engage in a titrated trial of a medication such as gabapentin. Treatment response, however defined, is not tantamount to a precise disclosure of the underlying pathophysiology of pain.

The diagnostic role of neural blockade is often overshadowed by its potential therapeutic benefit. The reversible interruption of neural conduction with local anesthetic may be used to disclose the localization and relative contribution of different structures along the nociceptive pathways that mediate the experience of pain. To some extent, this role has increased in importance because the widespread use of detailed imaging studies such as MRI and CT are sensitive and specific for anatomic changes but not for the presence of pain [11]. This problem is magnified when imaging correlation with patient report of symptoms is poor. Neural blockade may help determine a peripheral source of pain from a neuroma or entrapped nerve not amenable to visualization with advanced techniques. Blockade may assist in differentiating a local site of pain from a knee joint from that referred in a dermatomal distribution due to lumbar root injury. Alternatively, regional anesthetic techniques may distinguish somatic from visceral pain, as in certain pelvic pain syndromes. The diagnostic value of local anesthetic blockade for localization of chronic pain of spinal origin has limitations. For example, attempts to enrich study cohorts for the treatment of facet syndrome with diagnostic blocks have been hampered by low sensitivity and specificity [12]. Repetition of diagnostic blocks and the controversial use of sham blocks in the setting of clinical trials have been shown to improve sensitivity and specificity [13].

Intraspinal opioid delivery

Since the 1970s, when endogenous opioids and opioid receptors in the dorsal horn of the spinal cord were first identified, attempts have been made to optimize this form of therapy by delivering opioids centrally. In the small minority of cancer patients for whom oral and systemic opioid medication does not provide adequate pain control despite opioid rotation, changing the route of administration may enhance efficacy and minimize systemic side effects [14,15]. The principal benefit of intraspinal delivery appears to be the reduction in opioid side effects, rather than improved analgesia [16]. Adoption of these approaches has grown over the past 2 decades; as many as 20% of patients who had cancer were treated with spinal opioids in one series [17]. In patients who have cancer, the timing of intervention has proved to be among the most difficult clinical questions. Intolerance to systemic opioids, poorly controlled incident pain with movement, and intractable pain caused by neuroinvasive lesions, such as involvement of a plexus, are among the most common indications. The evidence for the use of these approaches in cancer pain is far more robust than for chronic noncancer pain where the risk-benefit balance may become less favorable with the course of time.

The delivery systems that introduce medication into the epidural and intrathecal spaces are varied. These include programmable, implanted pumps; implanted accessible reservoir systems; and tunneled, exteriorized catheters [18]. Epidural and external pump strategies have the greatest value when life expectancy is short (ie, <2 months). The type of trial that should precede implantation of a permanent device remains an unsettled issue and considerable variation in practice persists. In addition to morphine, which was until recently the only Food and Drug Administration–approved agent, dilute local anesthetic preparations and clonidine have been used effectively to augment analgesia [19]. The synergistic effects may confer greater relief in patients who have poorly controlled, incident pain and neuropathic pain [20]. Recently, intrathecal ziconotide, a selective N-type voltage-sensitive Ca^{2+} channel blocking agent, has demonstrated a significant reduction in pain in patients who have cancer or AIDS [21]. Intraspinal delivery systems enable logarithmic scale reductions in medication dosing, but require close monitoring of patients, especially early in the titration phases. The care of patients with tunneled subcutaneous catheters involves routine prophylactic measures (eg, bacterial filters, exit-site care) and monitoring for infection.

The preponderance of evidence supporting intraspinal opioid delivery is based on nonrandomized, uncontrolled series [22]. Two large studies have demonstrated improved analgesic efficacy and reduced toxic side effects in patients requiring a high dose of oral morphine [23,24]. The largest, randomized, prospective clinical trial compared an implantable drug delivery system with comprehensive medical management for refractory cancer pain (eg, Visual Analogue Scale [VAS] pain score ≥5 on a 0–10 scale). Clinical success was defined as a greater than or equal to 20% reduction in VAS scores, or equivalent analgesia with a greater than or equal to 20% reduction in opioid toxicity. Sixty of the seventy-one patients (84.5%) in the intraspinal treatment group achieved clinical success, compared with fifty-one of seventy-two comprehensive medical management patients. Patients receiving intrathecal therapy reported a significant reduction in fatigue and a depressed level of consciousness. Limitations of this study included the absence of controls for radiotherapy and chemotherapy, the younger age of the participants relative to the typical cancer population, and an inconsistent comparative benefit of the intrathecal route of delivery at different time points during the trial. Tight adherence to the algorithm for comprehensive medical management in the setting of a clinical trial produced a marked improvement in pain control. In a separate small, brief, double-blinded, crossover study of epidural and subcutaneous morphine, there was an advantage with regard to analgesia and a reduction in dose and side effects compared with oral morphine [25].

Lack of validated criteria for selection of patients and long-term data to evaluate the efficacy of intrathecal drug delivery systems in chronic, noncancer pain have limited adoption of this technology. Patients who have multiple types of intractable pain with nociceptive and neuropathic mechanisms inferred are described as the candidates most likely to benefit, but investigators who report treatment success in most cases concede patient selection remains difficult. A series by Kumar [26] reported significant opioid dose escalation with reduced analgesic benefit at 2 years. Favorable retrospective evidence from 12-month follow-up was seen in a small series of patients receiving intrathecal hydromorphone [27]. In one intriguing study, pump recipients demonstrated improvements in pain, mood, and function from baseline to 3 years following implant [28]. Despite this apparent benefit, these patients experienced a decline in function, an increase in self-rated pain, and more mood disturbances, compared with new patients referred to a pain specialist's practice. This finding suggests that pain severity remains high in these patients, despite the intervention. Uncontrolled studies with open follow-up have suggested benefit from long-term intrathecal treatment of spasticity and spasm-related pain with baclofen, a γ-aminobutyric acid agonist [29].

The risks and costs of intraspinal opioids exceed that of systemic opioids. The most common catheter-related problems, occurring in up to 25% of patients, include: kinking, obstruction, disconnection, and granuloma formation at the catheter tip with prolonged, high-rate infusion. Retrospective studies have shown the incidence of delayed respiratory depression with intrathecal narcotics to be 4% to 7% and with epidural infusion to be 0.25% to 0.5%. Pruritus occurs in up to 20% of patients, and urinary retention in as high as 15%. In one series of epidural delivery where nearly three quarters of patients achieved satisfactory relief, the investigators cautioned that the benefit was offset by the rate of deep infection, including epidural abscess, which reached 13% of patients [30].

Neurolytic blockade

Celiac plexus neurolysis in intra-abdominal cancer

Pancreatic adenocarcinoma and cancer of the upper abdominal viscera are commonly associated with severe, poorly controlled pain [31]. In pancreatic cancer, the pain is present early in the course of the disease and the prognosis is poor. Upper abdomen pain is mediated by the afferent nociceptive fibers that travel with the sympathetic fibers of the splanchnic nerves arising from T5-T12 and the parasympathetic efferent fibers that together form the celiac plexus. The ganglia are situated in the retroperitoneal space adjacent to the L1 vertebral body. Since the initial description almost a century ago, focal destruction of this nerve tissue has undergone numerous refinements that have improved both safety and efficacy [32]. The approach is reserved for pain associated with life-limiting illness largely because durable benefit in noncancer abdominal pain has not been demonstrated convincingly [33]. As with other interventional approaches in cancer pain management, some experts advocate the early use of these techniques because of superior pain relief, reduction in opioid side effects, and even improvement in quality-of-life measures [34]. The evidence is strongest for comparable relief with a reduction in opioid side effects.

Neurolytic celiac plexus blockade is the most extensively studied ablative procedure for the treatment of cancer pain. The most commonly used agent is alcohol, 50% to 100%, which provokes an extraction of lipids and a precipitation of proteins [35]. Phenol is also used for neurolysis and may carry a reduced risk of postinjection neuritis, but higher viscosity makes it more challenging to inject. With either agent, the variable duration of analgesia is typically on the order of months. The block has been performed using surface landmarks, fluoroscopy, CT, and ultrasound guidance. Numerous variations on the percutaneous, bilateral, retrocrural approach have been introduced over the past 2 decades, including transcrural, single-needle trans-aortic, and anterior, transabdominal approaches [36]. Most centers advocate a diagnostic block with a local anesthetic, such as bupivacaine 0.5%, before neurolytic blockade; a favorable diagnostic block strongly predicts analgesia from neurolysis [37]. More recently, endoscopic, ultrasound-guided approaches that may prove safer and more cost-effective are being pioneered by gastroenterologists [38].

Evidence for the analgesic efficacy of celiac plexus neurolysis in intra-abdominal cancer pain syndromes is compelling. A recent meta-analysis of multiple retrospective trials and a single prospective trial found a high rate of successful pain reduction, regardless of malignancy type [39]. The results of 21 retrospective studies of 1145 patients characterized "adequate" to "excellent" pain relief in 89% of the patients during the first 2 weeks after the block. Partial-to-complete pain relief continued in approximately 90% of the patients who were alive at the 3-month point, and in 70% to 90% until death. Wong [40] reported on a prospective, randomized, double-blinded, placebo-controlled trial of patients who had unresectable pancreatic cancer, which compared neurolytic celiac plexus block and opioid treatment with opioid treatment alone and sham injection. Pain intensity was reduced in patients undergoing celiac plexus neurolysis, but a reduction in opioid and improvement in quality of life were not demonstrated. Reduced need for analgesic drugs and fewer opioid-related side effects, have been demonstrated in additional double-blinded, prospective, randomized trials [41,42].

The most common adverse effects of blockade are transient local pain at the injection sites, diarrhea, and hypotension [39]. Neurologic complications, including lower extremity weakness and paresthesia, occurred at a rate of approximately 1%, although paraplegia and transient motor paralysis have occurred after celiac plexus block [43]. A meta-analysis by Eisenberg and colleagues [39] found nonneurologic complications such as pneumothorax, pleuritic chest pain, hiccoughing, or hematuria occurring at a rate of about 1%.

Intercostal nerve block

Intercostal neuralgia following thoracotomy

Chronic chest wall pain caused by postthoracotomy, intercostal neuralgia, as a cause of direct neural invasion of a tumor, is difficult to control. Poorly controlled perioperative pain appears to be a risk factor for this form of chronic neuropathic pain [44,45]. Temporary intercostal nerve blocks have been studied extensively in a randomized, controlled fashion in the perioperative setting, and analgesic benefit has been demonstrated convincingly [46,47]. Postthoracotomy pain, which requires a multidisciplinary approach, is a common motive for referral to pain management clinics. The intercostal nerves are the primary rami of the thoracic nerves T1-T11. Beyond the midaxillary line, the lateral cutaneous branch of the nerve arises; the optimal location for the intercostal nerve block is at the posterior angle of the rib, lateral to the paravertebral muscles [48]. Much like other regional blocks that are useful in the surgical setting, the technical challenge with intercostal blockade is achieving durable relief.

The use of intercostal nerve blockade in the context of chronic pain has undergone limited study, with mixed results. One retrospective series of 123 patients found intercostal nerve block in combination with trigger point injection compared favorably with chronic opioid use in patients who had advanced cancer and prolonged postthoracotomy pain [49]. High-concentration local anesthetic (eg, 5% tetracaine), 10% ammonium sulfate, and alcohol have been reported in small case series for the treatment of this neuropathic pain [50,51]. Reduction in pain in these cases has far exceeded a block with local anesthetic, but long-term efficacy is unknown.

The most commonly reported complications are the extended spread of the local anesthetic or neurolytic solution into the root cuff, epidural space, and cerebral spinal fluid. This last effect can cause weakness and sensory loss in the blocked dermatomes. Moore and Bridenbaugh [52] have reported the rate of pneumothorax by radiograph to be 0.42% in the perioperative setting.

Spinal cord stimulation

Neuropathic pain syndromes

The strategy of modulating neural transmission with an electrical stimulus dates to ancient Rome with Scribonius' observation that the pain of gout could be alleviated through accidental contact with a torpedo fish [53]. Acceptance of the gate theory of pain in the 1960s led to renewed interest in electrical stimulation [54]. Gate theory proposed that pain perception was influenced by the balance of firing between small and large neural fibers. Retrograde stimulation of large fibers would provoke nonpainful stimulation, thereby "closing" the gate through adjustment in the level of voltage.

Shealy [55] implanted the first spinal cord stimulator for the treatment of chronic pain in 1967. In spinal cord stimulation, an array of stimulating metal contacts is positioned in the dorsal epidural space. An electrical field is generated through connection of the contacts with a pulse generator, and subsequently programmed in combinations of anodes and cathodes. The resulting field stimulates the axons of the dorsal root and dorsal column fibers, leading to inhibition of activity in the lateral spinothalamic tract and increased activity in the descending antinociceptive pathways [56]. Optimal stimulation is achieved when paresthesias overlap with the anatomic distribution of pain reported by the patient [57]. Either cylindrical, catheter-like leads are introduced percutaneously through a needle, or flat, paddle-shaped leads are deployed by way of an open surgical approach (eg, laminotomy or laminectomy). The power source, similar in size to a cardiac pacemaker, is implanted in a subcutaneous pocket and connected to the leads by way of subcutaneous tunnel. Advances in consumer electronics have resulted in more precise targeting of neuronal stimulation, improved battery life, and smaller device sizes.

Neuropathic pain of peripheral origin and ischemic pain states are currently the most common indications for this therapy. As with other interventional techniques, patient selection is the key to sustained efficacy. Pain associated with a lesion of the nervous system, or dysfunction, or so-called neuropathic pain, in a fixed distribution amenable to stimulation coverage, comprise the most basic requirements. Among the most commonly treated syndromes in the United States are chronic radicular pain after lumbar surgery and complex regional pain syndrome [58]. Neuropathic pain arising from lesions of the central nervous system does not tend to respond to spinal cord stimulation [59]. A temporary trial of stimulation, most commonly performed with percutaneous lead placement, is used to identify patients who might benefit from this approach. Accepted end points for trial stimulation include a 50% reduction in pain intensity, patient tolerance of paresthesias, global satisfaction with therapy, and reduction in analgesic medications [60]. The inability to blind patients to the stimulus of spinal cord stimulation in clinical trials, for preimplant assessment or evaluation of the benefit of permanent placement, is cited as an important limitation to the study of this modality.

Two prospective studies of spinal cord stimulation in complex regional pain syndrome have demonstrated a statistically significant reduction in pain intensity [9,61]. A study of 29 patients by Harke [61] enrolled patients with a prior response to blockade of sympathetic efferents (presumably selecting for subjects with sympathetically maintained pain) and demonstrated a greater than 50% reduction in Pain Disability Index scoring. Nearly 60% of these patients discontinued oral analgesic medications. An important technical limitation of this study was the high rate of battery replacement (55%) and lead revision (41%). A randomized study by Kemler [9] compared spinal cord stimulation and physical therapy in combination, to physical therapy alone. At 6 months and 2 years, the mean reduction in pain intensity in the spinal cord stimulation group was greater than 50%. At 3 years, the benefit of stimulation was waning, and a statistically significant benefit was no longer observed [62]. Alterations in neuronal connectivity, or neural plasticity, may account for this "tolerance." Three prospective studies in complex regional pain syndrome demonstrated a statistically significant reduction in VAS and a marked reduction in analgesic requirements [63–65].

Spinal cord stimulation is used as a late-stage therapy in the treatment of chronic radicular pain after lumbar and cervical spine surgery when other nonpharmacologic, pharmacologic, and less invasive modalities have not provided adequate relief. A prospective, randomized, controlled trial demonstrated superior outcomes with spinal cord stimulation, compared with lumbar reoperation [66]. Patients randomized to stimulation were less likely to cross over to the surgical treatment arm (5 of 24 patients versus 14 of 26 patients, $P = .02$) and required reduced amounts of opioid analgesics. The long-term reduction in pain intensity was reported at 50% in a large cohort of patients [67]. A low rate of technical complication in this study was attributed to the development of multichannel devices that appeared to limit the need for revision because of electrode migration. Progress in the treatment of the axial distribution of low back pain with spinal cord stimulation has been reported more recently in two prospective trials [68,69]. In these studies, the analgesic benefit appeared to be more stable in the radicular component. The evidence in another indication, refractory angina pectoris is primarily retrospective, but a recent trial demonstrated no advantage over percutaneous myocardial laser revascularization with regard to angina-free exercise capacity, and complications were higher in the stimulation group [70].

The most common complication of spinal cord stimulation across 15 trials (N = 531) was lead migration, which occurred in 18% [71]. Infection occurred in 3.7% of cases and battery failure in 3.3%. No studies in the above series reported epidural hematoma or paralysis, but there are reports of these complications.

Radiofrequency neurotomy

Facet-mediated spinal syndromes

Pain of spinal origin is the most prevalent chronic noncancer pain syndrome [72]. Providers disagree as to the role of particular anatomic structures and the underlying pathophysiology of low back pain [73]. The poor understanding of low back pain, lack of accurate diagnostic methods, and difficulty of designing studies to assess treatment efficacy have impeded therapeutic progress for this common problem. Interventional treatments that target specific structures rarely provide complete relief, but have been shown to alleviate symptoms when first-line conservative therapies such as medication, rehabilitation, and pharmacologic strategies do not reduce pain intensity and activity limitation. This section considers the evidence for one such intervention, radiofrequency ablation, to highlight the complexity and possible benefit of interventional approaches for the complex problem of pain of spinal origin.

The facet joint (or zygapophyseal joint) was localized as the possible anatomic source low back pain by Ghormley [74] in 1933. The facet joints are paired synovial joints formed by the inferior articular process of one vertebra and the superior articular process of the vertebrae below. A tough fibrous capsule is present on the posterolateral aspect of the joint. These small joints are supplied by the medial branch from the posterior ramus of the spinal nerve root. For much of the past century, interest in pain syndromes attributed to the spine's posterior elements has been overshadowed by radicular localization attributed to intervertebral disc herniation. Large-scale radiologic studies confirm that arthritic changes in these joints were common in asymptomatic patients and, therefore, not strongly correlated with the symptom of low back pain [75]. In 1963, Hirsch [76] showed that pain in the back and upper thigh could be produced by injecting 11% hypertonic saline in the region of the facet joint. By the 1970s, reports of treatment success with radiofrequency denervation of the medial branches revived speculation in the facet joint as a target for the treatment of cervical and lumbar pain [77]. More recent animal models have offered a biochemical basis for the movement-evoked pains attributed to the facet joint [78].

The diagnostic criteria for facet syndrome remain a matter of controversy. Older age, relief of back pain with recumbency, exacerbation of pain with extension but not flexion, localized tenderness with palpation of the region overlying the facet joint, absence of leg pain, and radiologic characterization of hypertrophied joints have all been proposed as relevant features of "facet syndrome" [79–81]. The lack of sensitivity and specificity of these signs and symptoms has complicated attempts to define inclusion criteria for treatment trials. Attempts to define facet syndrome through prospective study of intra-articular facet joint injection have not produced consistent, validated criteria [82]. Intra-articular injections with local anesthetic and steroid have proved to be of little value diagnostically or therapeutically for the treatment of chronic low back pain [83,84].

Review of the clinical studies of radiofrequency ablation for facet syndrome attests to the difficulty of assessing treatment efficacy in the absence of well-validated, diagnostic criteria. Two prospective, double-blinded, randomized, controlled trials of percutaneous radiofrequency neurotomy demonstrated lasting relief [13,85]. In these trials, patients were enrolled based on response to local anesthetic blockade of the medial branches or the dorsal rami supplying the putatively symptomatic joints [86]. The study by Lord and colleagues [87] achieved a minimum of 50% reduction in pain intensity for 263 days in the active treatment group with cervical zygapophyseal-joint pain after motor vehicle accident, compared with 8 days in the placebo group. This study applied an uncharacteristically rigorous protocol of three blocks (ie, two active, with differing concentrations of local anesthetic, and one sham block) to identify patients who had zygapophyseal joint (ie, facet) syndrome. Van Kleef and colleagues [85] replicated this result in the lumbar spine with patients selected by response to diagnostic nerve block of the posterior primary ramus of the segmental nerves at L3, L4, and L5. The primary end point of a 50% reduction in pain, or a more than two-point reduction on numeric rating scale, was achieved, compared with placebo in those patients with at least 1 year of chronic low-back pain. The patients undergoing radiofrequency ablation reported a reduction in opioid use and improved Oswestry Disability Index scores. A third small prospective trial and a large retrospective series (outcome assessed by third party) demonstrated prolonged benefit in patients with a positive response to diagnostic block, compared with nonresponders [88,89].

Much as in recent large trials of analgesics for neuropathic pain, the positive trial results characterized above must be considered in the context of a well-designed trial with a negative result [90–92]. A relatively large (N = 70), placebo-controlled, double-blinded trial by Leclaire and colleagues [93] of patients who had low back pain for more than 3 months, selected by positive response to intra-articular facet injection, did not show a benefit over placebo. The high placebo-responder rates in interventional trials may reduce the likelihood of demonstrating statistical superiority versus placebo, as has been observed in oral analgesic trials [94]. Others have suggested that the use of intra-articular block by referring physicians may have resulted in greater heterogeneity of the study population (ie, patients whose pain was not truly of facet origin). Such a view highlights the importance of precision in diagnostic injection techniques and interpretation, and the broader challenge of matching treatment to patient in chronic pain of spinal origin.

Minor complications from fluoroscopically guided percutaneous radiofrequency ablation have occurred at the low rate of 1% per lesion site [95]. Localized pain at needle entry site lasting more than 2 weeks was rare (0.5%) and there were no cases of new motor or sensory deficits in this series of 116 procedures (616 sites). Intrathecal injection has been

reported in one case of chemical meningitis [96] and in a separate case of epidural abscess formation [97].

Summary

The patients who are candidates for interventional approaches are invari-
ably those with the most severe pain. Locally-targeted therapy offers the
possibility of improved pain control. These interventions do not supplant
pharmacologic and nonpharmacologic modalities to treat chronic pain;
their role is complementary. Intraspinal opioids, celiac neurolysis, spinal
cord stimulation, and radiofrequency neurotomy all have demonstrated analgesic efficacy and the potential to reduce exposure to the systemic side effects of other therapies. The most challenging aspect of implementing these
techniques is matching treatment to individual patient, and this is equally
true of the many techniques not covered here. Diagnostic neural blockade
with local anesthetics and temporary treatment trials of stimulation and intraspinal opioids enhance the likelihood of favorable outcomes. As the examination of intra-articular facet injection in low back pain reveals,
placebo effect, a favorable natural history, and regression to the mean all
may make it difficult to assess the actual benefit of interventions on
a case-by-case basis. Experience is not a substitute for larger, placebo-controlled, randomized, prospective trials. Further advances await a deeper understanding of the correlation between symptoms and pain pathophysiology
and a more precise understanding of the putative mechanisms of action of
interventional therapies.

References

[1] Katz N. Role of invasive procedures in chronic pain management. Sem Neurol 1994;14:
    225–35.
[2] Bonica JJ. Basic principles in managing chronic pain. Arch Surg 1977;112:783.
[3] Markman JD, Dworkin RH. Ion channel targets and treatment efficacy in neuropathic pain.
    J Pain 2006;7:S38–47.
[4] Rowbotham MC. Pain 2002—An updated review. Seattle (WA): IASP Press; 2002.
[5] North RB. Treatment of spinal syndromes. N Engl J Med 1996;335:1763–4.
[6] Block BM, Liu SS, Rowlingson AJ, et al. Efficacy of postoperative epidural analgesia:
    a meta-analysis. JAMA 2003;290:2455–63.
[7] Backonja M, Beydoun A, Edwards KR, et al. Gabapentin for the symptomatic treatment of
    painful neuropathy in patients with diabetes mellitus: a randomized controlled trial. JAMA
    1998;280:1831–6.
[8] Lenzer J. Pfizer pleads guilty, but drug sales continue to soar. BMJ 2004;328:1217.
[9] Kemler MA, Barendse GA, Van Kleef M, et al. Spinal cord stimulation in patients with
    chronic reflex sympathetic dystrophy. N Engl J Med 2000;343:618–24.
[10] Burchiel KJ, Anderson VC, Brown FD, et al. Prospective, multicenter study of spinal cord
     stimulation for relief of chronic back and extremity pain. Spine 1996;21:2786–94.

[11] Boden SD, Davis DO, Dina TS, et al. Abnormal magnetic-resonance scans of the lumbar spine in asymptomatic subjects. J Bone Joint Surg 1990;72:403–8.

[12] North RB, Han M, Zahurak M, et al. Specificity of diagnostic nerve blocks: a prospective randomized study of sciatica due to lumbosacral spine disease. Pain 1996;65:77–85.

[13] Lord SM, Barnsley L, Wallis BJ, et al. Percutaneous radio-frequency for chronic cervical zygapophyseal-joint pain. N Engl J Med 1996;335:1721–6.

[14] Davis MP, Walsh D, Lagman R, et al. Controversies in pharmacotherapy of pain management. Lancet Oncol 2005;6:696–704.

[15] Mercadente S. Controversies over spinal treatment in advanced cancer patients. Support Care Cancer 1998;6:495–02.

[16] Mercadente S. Problems with long-term spinal opioid treatment in advanced cancer patients. Pain 1999;79:1–13.

[17] Enting RH, Oldenmenger WH, van der Rijt CDC, et al. A prospective study evaluating the response of patients with unrelieved cancer pain to parenteral opioids. Cancer 2002;94: 3049–56.

[18] Waldman SD, Coombs DW. Selection of implantable narcotic delivery systems. Anesth Analg 1989;68:377–84.

[19] Sjoberg M, Nitescu P, et al. Long-term intrathecal morphine and bupivacaine in patients with refractory cancer pain. Anesthesiology 1994;80:284–97.

[20] Hanks GW, de Conno F, Cherry N, et al. Morphine and alternative opioids in cancer pain: the EAPC recommendations. Br J Cancer 2001;95:587–93.

[21] Staats PS, Yearwood T, Charapata SG, et al. Intrathecal ziconotide in the treatment of refractory pain in patients with cancer or AIDS. JAMA 2004;291:63–70.

[22] Ballantyne JC, Carwood CM. Comparative efficacy of epidural, subarachnoid, and intracerebroventricular opioids in patients with pain due to cancer. Cochrane Database Syst Rev 2004.

[23] Smith TJ, Staats PS, Lisa TD, et al. Randomized clinical trial of an implantable drug delivery system compared with comprehensive medical management for refractory cancer pain: impact on pain, drug related toxicity, and survival. J Clin Oncol 2003;20(19):4040–9.

[24] Rauck RL, Cherry D, Boyer MF, et al. Long-term intrathecal opioid therapy with a patient-activated, implanted delivery system for the treatment of refractory cancer pain. J Pain 2003; 4:441–7.

[25] Kalso E, Heiskanen T, Rantio M, et al. Epidural and subcutaneous morphine in the management of cancer pain: a double-blind cross over study. Pain 1996;67:443–9.

[26] Kumar K, Kelly M, Pirlot T. Continuous intrathecal morphine treatment for chronic pain of nonmalignant etiology: long term benefits and efficacy. Sugical Neurology 2001;55:79–86.

[27] Du Pen S, Du Pen A, Hillyer J. Intrathecal hydromorphone for intractable nonmalignant pain: a retrospective study. Pain Med 2006;7:10–5.

[28] Thimineur MA, Kravitz E, Vodapally MS. Intrathecal opioid treatment for chronic nonmalignant pain: a three year prospective study. Pain 2004;109:242–9.

[29] Emery E. Intrathecal baclofen: literature review of the results and complications. Neurochirurgie 2003;49:276–88.

[30] Smitt PS, Tsafka A, Zande FT, et al. Outcome and complications of epidural analgesia in patients with chronic cancer pain. Cancer 1998;83:2015–22.

[31] Grahm AL, Andren-Sandberg A. Prospective evaluation of pain in exocrine pancreatic cancer. Digestion 1997;58:542–9.

[32] Kappis M. Erfahrungen mit localanasthesie bie bauchoperationen. Verh Dtsch Gesellsch Chir 1914;43:87–9.

[33] Adolph MD, Benedetti C. Percutaneous-guided pain control: exploiting the neural basis of pain sensation. Gastr Clin North Am 2006;35:167–88.

[34] de Oliveira R, dos Reis MP, Prado WA. The effects of early or late neurolytic sympathetic plexus block on the management of abdominal or pelvic cancer pain. Pain 2004;110:400–8.

[35] Rumbsy MG, Finean JB. The action of organic solvents on the myelin sheath of peripheral nerve tissue-II (short-chain aliphatic alcohols). J Neurochem 1966;13:1513–5.

[36] De Cicco M, Matovic M, Bortolussi R, et al. Celiac plexus block: injectate spread and pain relief in patients with regional anatomic distortions. Anesthesiology 2001;94:561–5.

[37] Yuen TS, Ng KF, Tsui SL. Neurolytic celiac plexus block for visceral abdominal malignancy: is prior diagnostic block warranted? Anaes Intensive Care 2002;30:442–8.

[38] Abedi M, Zfass AM. Endoscopic ultrasound-guided (neurolytic) celiac plexus block. J Clin Gastr 2001;32:390–3.

[39] Eisenberg E, Carr DB, Chalmers TC. Neurolytic celiac plexus block for treatment of cancer pain: a meta-analysis. Anesth Analg 1995;80:290–5.

[40] Wong GY, Schroeder DR, Carns PE, et al. Effect of neurolytic celiac plexus block on pain relief, quality of life, survival in patients with unresectable pancreatic cancer: a randomized controlled trial. JAMA 2004;291(9):1092–9.

[41] Ischia S, Ischia A, Polati E, et al. Three posterior percutaneous celiac plexus block techniques; a prospective randomized study in 61 patients with pancreatic cancer pain. Anesthesiology 1992;76:534–40.

[42] Polati E, Finco G, Gottin L, et al. Prospective randomized double-blind trial of neurolytic celiac plexus block in patients with pancreatic cancer. Br J Surg 1998;85: 199–201.

[43] Van Dongen, Crul BJP. Paraplegia after celiac plexus block. Anesthesia 1991;46:862–3.

[44] Perkins FM, Kehlet H. Chronic pain as an outcome of surgery: a review of predictive factors. Anesthesiology 2000;93:1123–33.

[45] Katz J, Jackson M, Kavanagh BP, et al. Acute pain alter surgery predicts long term post-thoracotomy pain. Clin J Pain 1996;12:50–5.

[46] Richardson J, Sabanathan S, Eng J, et al. Continuous intercostal nerve block versus epidural morphine for postthoracotomy analgesia. Ann Thor Surg 1993;55:377–80.

[47] Concha M, Dagnino J, Cariaga M, et al. Analgesia after thoracotomy: epidural fentanyl/bupivacaine compared with intercostal nerve block plus intravenous morphine. J Cardiothor & Vasc Anes 2004;18:322–6.

[48] Moore DC. Intercostal nerve block: spread of India ink injected into the subcostal groove. Br J Anaesth 1981;53:325–9.

[49] Moriwaki K, Uesugi F, Kusunoki, et al. Pain management for patients with cancer. Masui 2000;49:680–5.

[50] Doi K, Nikai T, Sakura S, et al. Intercostal nerve block with 5% tetracaine for chronic pain syndromes. J Clin Anes 2002;14(1):39–41.

[51] Miller RD, Johnston RR, Hosobuchi Y. Treatment of intercostal neuralgia with 10 per cent ammonium sulfate. J Thor Cardiovascular Surg 1975;69(3):476–8.

[52] Moore DC, Bridenbaugh LD. Pneumothorax: its incidence following intercostal nerve block. JAMA 1962;182:1005–8.

[53] Stillings D. A survey of the history of electrical stimulation for pain to 1900. Med Instrum 1975;9:255–9.

[54] Melzack R, Wall PD. Pain mechanism: a new theory. Science 1965;150:971–9.

[55] Shealy CN, Mortimer JT, Resnick J. Electrical inhibition of pain by stimulation of the dorsal column: preliminary reports. J Int Anesth Res Soc 1967;46:489–91.

[56] Linderoth B, Foreman RD. Physiology of spinal cord stimulation: review and update. Neuromodulation 1999;2:150–64.

[57] North RB, Ewend MG, Lawton MT, et al. Spinal cord stimulation for chronic, intractable pain: superiority of "multi-channel" devices. Pain 1991;44:119–20.

[58] Alo KM, Holsheimer J. New trends in neuromodulation for the management of neuropathic pain. Neurosurgery 2002;50:690–703.

[59] Villavicencio AT, Burneikiene S. Elements of the pre-operative workup. Pain Med 2006;7: S35–46.

[60] Windsor RE, Falco FJ, Pinzon EG. Spinal cord stimulation in chronic pain. In: Lennard TE, editor. Pain procedures in clinical practice. 2nd edition. Philadelphia: Hanley and Belfus; 2003. p. 377–94.

[61] Harke H, Gretenkort P, Ladleif H, et al. Spinal cord stimulation in sympathetically maintainted complex pain syndrome type I with severe disability. A prospective study. Eur J Pain 2005;9:363–73.

[62] Kemler MA, de Vet CWH, Barendse GAM, et al. Spinal cord stimulation for chronic reflex sympathetic dystrophy-five year follow up. N Engl J Med 2006;354:2394–6.

[63] Calvillo O, Racz G, Didie J, et al. Neuroaugmentation in the treatment of complex regional pain syndrome of the upper extremity. Acta Orthop Belg 1998;64:57–62.

[64] Ebel H, Balogh A, Klug N. Augmentative treatment of chronic deafferent pain syndromes after peripheral nerve lesions. Minim Invas Neurosurg 2004;43:44–50.

[65] Oakley J, Weiner RL. Spinal cord stimulation for complex regional pain syndrome: a prospective study of 19 patients at 2 centers. Neuromodulation 1999;2:47–50.

[66] North R, Kidd D, Farrokhi F, et al. Spinal cord stimulation versus repeated lumbosacral spine surgery for chronic pain: a randomized controlled trial. Neurosurgery 2005;56(1): 98–106.

[67] North RB, Kidd DH, Zahurak M, et al. Spinal cord stimulation for chronic intractable pain: experience over two decades. Neurosurgery 1993;32:384–95.

[68] Barolat G, Oakley J, Law J, et al. Epidural spinal cord stimulation with multiple electrode paddle lead is effective in treating low back pain. Neuromodulation 2001;2:59–66.

[69] North RB, Kidd DH, Olin J, et al. Spinal cord stimulation for axial low back pain: a prospective controlled trial comparing dual with single percutaneous electrodes. Spine 2005;30: 1412–8.

[70] McNab D, Kahn SN, Sharples LD, et al. An open label, single-centre, randomized trial of spinal cord stimulation vs. percutaneous myocardial laser revascularization in patients with refractory angina pectoris: the SPiRiT trial. Eur Heart J 2006;27:1048–53.

[71] Bennett DS, Cameron T. Spinal cord stimulation for complex regional pain syndromes. In: Simpson B, editor. Electrical stimulation and relief of pain, in pain research and clinical management. Amsterdam: Elsevier Science B.V.; 2003. p. 111–29.

[72] Andersson GBJ. Epidemiologic features of chronic low-back pain. Lancet 1999;354:581–5.

[73] Deyo RA, Haselkorn J, Hoffman R, et al. Designing studies of diagnostic tests for low back pain or radiculopathy. Spine 1994;19:2057S–65S.

[74] Ghormely RK. Low back pain with special reference to the articular facets with presentation of an operative procedure. JAMA 1933;1773.

[75] Magora A, Schwartz A. Relation between the low back pain syndrome and X-ray findings. I. Degenerative osteoarthritis. Scand J Rehabil Med 1973;5:115.

[76] Hirsch D, Ingelmark B, Miller M. The anatomical basis for low back pain. Acta Orthop Scand 1963;33:1.

[77] Rees WS. Multiple bilateral subcutaneous rhizolysis of segmental nerves in the treatment of intervertebral disc syndrome. Ann Gen Prac 1974;26:126.

[78] Toshihiko Y, Cavanaugh JM, et al. Effect of substance P on mechanosensitive units of tissues around and in the lumbar facet joint. J Orthop Res 1992;11:205–14.

[79] Jackson RP. The facet syndrome. Myth or reality? Clin Orthop Relat Res 1992;279:110–21.

[80] Lewinnek GE, Warfield CA. Facet joint degeneration as a cause of low back pain. Clin Orthop Relat Res 1986;213:216–22.

[81] Schwarzer AC, Wang SC, O'Driscoll D, et al. The ability of computed tomography to identify a painful zygapophysial joint in patients with chronic low back pain. Spine 1995; 20:907–12.

[82] Schwarzer AC, Aprill CN, Derby R, et al. Clinical features of patients with pain stemming from the lumbar zygapophysial joints. Is the lumbar facet syndrome a clinical entity. Spine 1994;19:1132–7.

[83] Carette S, Marcoux S, Truchon R, et al. A controlled trial of corticosteroid injections into facet joints for chronic low back pain. N Engl J Med 1991;325:1002–7.

[84] Jackson RP, Jacobs RR, Montesano PX. Facet joint injection in low back pain. Spine 1988; 13:966–71.

[85] Van Kleef MV, Gerard AM, Barendse, et al. Randomized trial of radiofrequency lumbar facet denervation for chronic low back pain. Spine 1999;24:1937–42.

[86] Resnick DK, Choudhri TF, Dailey AT, et al. Guidelines for the performance of fusion procedures for degenerative disease of the lumbar spine. Part 13: injection therapies, low-back pain, and lumber fusion. J Neurosurg Spine 2005;2:707–15.

[87] Lord SM, Barnsley L, Bogduk. The utility of comparative local anaesthetic blocks in the diagnosis of cervical zygapophysial joint pain. Pain 1993;18:343–50.

[88] Gallagher J, Petriconne di Vadi P, Wedley J, et al. Radiofrequency facet joint denervation in the treatment of low back pain. A prospective controlled double-blind study to assess efficacy. Pain Clin 1994;7:193–8.

[89] North RB, Han M, Zahurak M, et al. Radiofrequency lumbar facet denervation: analysis of prognostic factors. Pain 1994;57:77–83.

[90] Backonja M, Glanzman RL. Gabapentin dosing for neuropathic pain: evidence from randomized, placebo-controlled clinical trials. Clin Ther 2003;25:81–104.

[91] Safirstein B, Tuchman M, Dogra S, et al. Efficacy of lamotrogine in painful diabetic neuropathy: results from two large double-blind trials [abstract]. J Pain 2005;6(suppl 3):S34.

[92] Thienel U, Neto W, Schwabe SK, et al. Topiramate in painful diabetic polyneuropathy: findings from three double-blind placebo controlled trials. Acta Neurol Scand 2004;110: 221–31.

[93] Leclaire R, Fortin L, Lambert R, et al. Radiofrequency facet joint denervation in the treatment of low back pain: a placebo controlled clinical trial to assess efficacy. Spine 2001;26:1411–7.

[94] Dworkin RH, Katz J, Gitlin M. Placebo response in clinical trials of depression and its implications for research on chronic neuropathic pain. Neurology 2005;65:S7–19.

[95] Kornick C, Kramarich S, Lamer TJ, et al. Complications of lumbar radiofrequency facet denervation. Spine 2004;29:1352–4.

[96] Thomson SJ, Lomax DM, Collet BJ. Chemical meningitis after lumbar facet joint block with local anesthetic and steroids. Anesthesia 1991;46:563–4.

[97] Alcock A, Regaard A, Browne J. Facet joint injection: a rare form cause of epidural abscess formation. Pain 2003;209–10.

ELSEVIER
SAUNDERS

Anesthesiology Clin
25 (2007) 899–911

ANESTHESIOLOGY
CLINICS

Invasive and Minimally Invasive Surgical Techniques for Back Pain Conditions

William Lavelle, MD[a,*], Allen Carl, MD[a], Elizabeth Demers Lavelle, MD[b]

[a]Department of Orthopaedic Surgery, Albany Medical Center, Albany Medical College,
1367 Washington Avenue, Albany, NY 12206, USA
[b]Department of Anesthesiology, Albany Medical Center, 43 New Scotland Avenue,
Albany, NY 12208, USA

Back pain is ubiquitous. More than 70% of people in developed countries experience low back pain at some time in their lives. Every year, one third to one half of adults suffer low back pain and 5% of people present to a nurse practitioner, physician's assistant, or physician with a new episode. Low back pain is most common in patients between the ages of 35 and 55 years [1,2]. In general, back pain can be attributed to a structural or neurologically mediated failure. Most cases of acute back pain are self-limited, with more than 90% of people recovering within 6 weeks. However, 2% to 7% go on to develop chronic and, at times, debilitating back pain. Back pain has a high recurrence rate with symptoms recurring in 50% to 80% of people within 1 year [3]. Looking at the epidemiology of back pain, female gender, older age, and lower socioeconomic status are associated with a higher risk for back pain. Lifestyle factors that predispose for back pain include lack of physical activity, obesity, and smoking [4].

Pain generators

There is a multitude of causes for low back pain. In a study evaluating the pathophysiology of back pain presenting to a primary care physician, 4% of patients had a compression fracture, 3% had spondylolisthesis, 0.7% had a tumor or metastasis of another tumor, 0.3% had ankylosing spondylitis,

---

A version of this article originally appeared in the 91:2 issue of Medical Clinics of North America.

* Corresponding author.
E-mail address: lavellwf@yahoo.com (W. Lavelle).

doi:10.1016/j.anclin.2007.08.003

and 0.01% had an infection [5,6]. The overwhelming cause of back pain remains nonspecific. It can be postulated that this nonspecific back pain is attributable, at least in some way, to the degenerative process of the spine.

Observing the natural history of spinal degeneration, one can witness a cascade of radiographic changes. Disc degeneration seems to occur first. The aging process causes progressive changes in intervertebral disc composition similar to the changes seen in other aging tissues in the body [7]. These changes to the biologic structure of the disc influence the mechanical properties of the disc. Aged discs have decreased stiffness and strength. Aging also causes an accumulation of degraded matrix material that can impair the normal metabolism of the remaining cells within the disc [7,8]. Some of these changes may be seen on MRI as "dark disc disease" [9]. Even though age-related changes are unavoidable and are found regularly in the discs and joints of patients who have back pain, a direct relationship between age-related changes and pain has not been proved [10]. Often, disc failure is the beginning of a domino effect in the spine. Loss of disc integrity often leads to lower anterior stability. This decreased stability from degenerative discs causes ligaments to buckle and hypertrophy from exposure to excessive forces, including new torsion forces. Finally, the facet joints often degenerate with hypertrophy [11–14]. Because degenerative joints may or may not be painful, back pain may result from this cascade of failure. Encroachment of bone spurs into the foramen of the exiting nerve roots may lead to sciatic pain involving the buttock and leg. The areas of the degenerating spine may fail at different rates. If the anterior disc and ligaments fail at the same rate as the posterior structures (eg, facet joints), anterior subluxation of one vertebra on another may occur and produce spondylolisthesis. This, in and of itself, may be painful, but it also may lead to compression of the lumbar nerves in the cauda equina and result in spinal stenosis [15].

Physicians attempt to explain back pain with radiographic findings. However, there is not always a relationship between radiographic findings and pain generators [10]. The overlap in terminology used to describe different symptoms exacerbates the diagnostic dilemma and leads to more confusion among referring physicians, consultants, and, ultimately, patients. The condition of neurologic leg pain or paresthesia carries the general term of sciatica. Sciatica can be attributed to several causes. In general, it is due to extrinsic compression of the fluid-filled thecal sac or to intrinsic nerve conduction dysfunction. Pressure on nerve roots may stem from a herniated disc, stenosis, or hypertrophy of the facet or ligament. Nerve conduction dysfunction may be caused by epidural fibrosis, arachnoiditis, neurologic tumors, or scar. However, disc herniation or degenerative stenosis from the failing and hypertrophied vertebral structures remains the most common cause of sciatic pain [16–19]. Sciatica cannot be explained entirely by a pressure phenomenon; inflammation of the nerve root also plays a role. The nucleus pulposus contains material that can cause inflammation and excite nerve roots [20,21]. Along with discs and joints, muscles and ligaments also can suffer the ails of degenerative disease and inflammation, which make muscles and ligaments potential sources of pain. Molecular biology and genetics have yet to yield conclusive information about the true etiology of spine-related pain.

Similar terms and definitions, based solely on radiographic findings, often confuse referring physicians as well as patients. Spondylosis is defined as the age-related changes seen on radiographs, with disc collapse and resultant spur formation as the hallmarks. Spondylolisthesis is the resultant vertebral translation that may accompany the degenerative processes. More advanced imaging, such as MRI, has increased the confusion. "Internal disc derangement" (IDD) is another ambiguous term used by spine physicians. Coined by Crock [22] in 1970, IDD was used to describe a large group of patients whose disabling back and leg pain worsened after operation for suspected disc prolapse [23]. IDD was intended to describe a condition marked by disc alterations—in the internal structure and metabolic functions—believed attributable to an injury or series of injuries that may even have been subclinical [23,24]. Annular tears are believed to be the major manifestation or cause of IDD [23,25]. The diagnostic criteria for discogenic pain attributable to IDD are based primarily on discography, which involves injection of contrast into the disc center and evaluating its morphology on CT and plain radiograph as well as monitoring the patient for a pain response. The criteria can be summarized as three steps:

1. CT discography reveals an IDD (eg, annular tear).
2. Pain is reproduced on provocative injection of the contrast.
3. As a control, stimulation of at least one other disc fails to reproduce pain.

Facet joint degenerative changes follow the degenerative process seen with the disc. When pain arises from this area, patients often complain of greater discomfort with spine extension or hyperextension. Once muscles weaken, any position can cause discomfort. As a minimally invasive diagnostic and therapeutic modality, facet injections may be offered. However, the diagnosis remains a clinical one. Studies with a high level of evidence that examined the true efficacy of facet injections are rare [26]. One study failed to find a statistically significant difference at 1 and 3 months between patients who were injected with corticosteroid and those who received saline injections. However, at 6 months, the patients treated with steroid had a significantly greater improvement in their pain compared with controls. Cointerventions were more frequent in the group that received steroids. Despite this, a small improvement in pain was noted [27,28].

Other similar-sounding terms for causes of low back pain are "spondylolysis" and "concomitant spondylolisthesis." The posterior elements of the vertebra may be disrupted by a stress fracture of an area of the spine called the pars interarticularis. This condition, called spondylolysis, also can lead to a slippage in the lateral plane (spondylolisthesis). Anatomically, the pars interarticularis is the lateral part of the posterior element that connects the superior and inferior facets. By definition, pars interarticularis means "part between the articulations." Repetitive flexion–extension and rotation lead to microtrauma at this junction and, thereby, fracture. In the athletic adolescent, spondylolysis is one of the most common causes of back pain. It should be investigated by spot radiographs in this population. In one series of 100 adolescent athletes who presented with low back pain, 47% had spondylolysis [29,30].

Even though scoliosis is described classically as a painless condition, up to 30% of patients who have adolescent idiopathic scoliosis complain of back pain [31]. It seems intuitive that spinal deformity would alter spine biomechanics and lead to increased stress, degeneration, and, therefore, pain. However, two recent studies found no difference in pain scores between a control group and patients who had scoliosis and were treated with a brace or surgery [32,33].

How discs fail

Each vertebral level of the spine must withstand numerous forces imparted from above and below. Put simply, repetitive mechanical loading is believed to cause, at least in part, intervertebral disc degeneration. This mechanical loading causes a disruption that affects the physical and biologic properties of the disc. The mechanical destruction is accompanied by a cascade of nonreversible cell-mediated responses that cause cell death. Cadaveric experiments and computer models show how various combinations of compression, bending, and torsion can cause the morphologic features of disc degeneration, such as endplate disruption, fissure formation in the annulus, radial bulging, disc prolapse, and internal collapse of the annulus [34]. As the repetitive trauma continues, nucleus pulposus material is pushed slowly into and sometimes through the annular ring of the disc. The added structural support and configuration of the posterior longitudinal ligament (which is diamond shaped) often deflects the protruded disc material to either side. However, central protrusions may be seen. This disc failure often develops as the result of additive microtraumas that patients experience in their daily lives.

As with most disease processes, one element of failure does not adequately explain all that we know about disc degeneration. Studies show that, as the disc ages, the number of blood vessels in the vertebral end plates decreases; most disappear by the third decade of life. The number of viable cells at the core of the disc also declines at this time [35]. The chemical structure and organization of the disc, including the collagen fibril organization, begin to change and eventually disappear [23]. Questions remain as to whether all of these changes are the predecessors to degeneration or if they truly are the result of the mechanical stresses described earlier.

Symptoms improve or resolve in about 50% of patients [36,37]. This improvement may be due to a decrease in the inflammatory response or reabsorption of the material causing compression. Those who fail conservative measures, such as oral analgesia, physical therapy, epidurals, or nerve-root injections for 6 to 12 weeks, may go on to surgical interventions. In 1983, Weber [38] prospectively studied 280 patients who were diagnosed with an L4–L5 or L5–S1 disc herniation. In the short term, the group that underwent surgery had better outcomes than did the group that did not undergo surgery. However, the difference was not significant after 4 years. Bowel, bladder, and sex-associated symptoms indicate that the central sacral neurologic structures are involved, and the patient should be considered for more urgent surgical intervention on the basis of cauda equina compression.

Surgical treatment for painful sciatica

Dandy [39] performed the first documented surgical decompression for a disc herniation. In the early 1930s, Mixter and Barr [40] popularized discectomy and laminectomy for the relief of sciatica-type pain. This surgical decompression involves removal of ligamentum and lamina. The surgeon then retracts the dural sac to access the disc material compressing the nerve root. Knowledge of the location of the exiting nerve roots in the surgical field and of the proper method of nerve retraction is necessary to perform this surgery safely. Because surgeon knowledge, skill, and experience vary, outcomes may vary as well. In the days of Dandy, Mixter, and Barr, patients underwent a much larger surgery, with a wide laminectomy and disc debridement. Over time, the size of the laminar resection has become smaller, and the soft tissue dissection has been minimized. A typical laminotomy is outlined in Fig. 1. It is hoped that minimally invasive techniques have decreased scar-tissue formation and the incidence of iatrogenic instability. However, such outcomes have not been proved in well-controlled, prospective, randomized studies. The use of a microscope or loops has

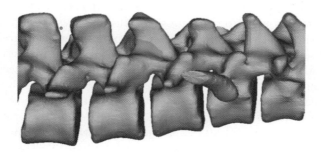

Fig. 1. A typical laminotomy for a modern discectomy.

assisted with minimally invasive surgery. More modern adaptations involve the use of tube-type tissue retraction devices. The tubular retractor system uses sequential, telescoping soft tissue dilators to establish a soft tissue corridor through the adjacent paraspinous musculature to the interspace of interest. Once this corridor is established, a tubular retractor of appropriate length is placed over the last dilator and is secured tightly using a table-mounted flexible arm [41].

Microdiscectomy by any method has become the operation of choice; it results in decreases in hospital cost, postoperative pain, and days missed from work [42–46]. The prevalence of recurrent disc herniation varies, and it may be related more to surgeon skill than to choice of operation [43]. Studies show no difference between the rate of recurrent disc herniation treated by open discectomy and that treated by microdiscectomy [47,48]. Patients who undergo decompression have a more rapid resolution of symptoms. However, long-term results are no different when compared with nonoperative management.

Percutaneous discectomy, microscopic discectomy, tube-assisted discectomy using METRx devices (Medtronic, Minneapolis, Minnesota), and energy-assisted discectomy using the Spine Wand (Arthrocare, Austin, Texas) are ways to minimize surgical exposure. However, minimal-access procedures require an even greater knowledge of spinal anatomy. Delineation of bone and nerve structures as they enter and exit an operative field is not possible with minimally invasive exposures. Better intraoperative imaging, such as computer-based image navigation devices (eg, products from BrainLAB AG, Munich, Germany) may help with this challenge in the future.

Surgery for painful motion segments

As with other joints in the body, painful spinal motion segments may be treated by arthroplasty or fusion. We are just embarking on the frontier of spinal arthroplasty and none of the current techniques is considered minimally invasive. Fusion has been and remains the standard of care for a painful motion segment that failed conservative treatment. From the standpoint of fusion procedures, the evolution of care started with using local and harvested autologous bone to facilitate spinal fusion. These fusion techniques have been supplemented with structural support systems (eg, rods, hooks, wires, and screws). The advent of pedicle screws allowed for shorter fusion masses. Pedicle screws may be performed by a percutaneous technique or used to augment other percutaneous procedures.

Percutaneous pedicle screw placement begins with accurate identification of the levels to be instrumented. In a manner similar to that for performing vertebroplasty or kyphoplasty, 22-gauge spinal needles are inserted under lateral fluoroscopy in a paramedian approach so that they bisect the superior and inferior pedicles. The medial to lateral position of the needles is confirmed on the anteroposterior (AP) fluoroscopic image. Depending on the vertical distance between the pedicles, a skin incision that connects the needle sites may be made or small, separate incisions may be made at each needle entry point.

The needle is passed through the skin under fluoroscopic guidance. Once the bone is reached, the needle is advanced down the pedicle. Biplanar fluoroscopic images are obtained throughout the procedure. When the needle tip reaches the posterior vertebral body line on the lateral image, the medial pedicle wall on the AP image should not be violated. If the medial wall is violated, the surgeon risks intrusion of the pedicle screw into the spinal canal. A Kirschner wire (K-wire) is placed through the cannulated needle, followed by needle removal. Sequential dilators are placed over the K-wire to develop a soft tissue corridor. The final dilator is left in place, and the pedicle is tapped under fluoroscopic guidance. Finally, a cannulated, polyaxial screw is placed over the K-wire, with the screw inserted under fluoroscopic guidance. Care is taken to avoid inadvertent advancement of the K-wire. This process is repeated for each screw.

After both screws are inserted, screw extenders are attached to the respective pedicle screws. The screw extenders are manipulated and mated. Rod templates are used to measure the correct rod length. A rod inserter is attached, and a separate incision is made at the site where a trocar will be placed to create the path of the rod through the soft tissues. The trocar is inserted until the most superior screw head is engaged. The trocar is removed, and the correct rod is inserted. The superior screw head is tightened, and compression or distraction is applied through the screw extenders. Finally, the rod inserter and screw extenders are removed [41].

Discs also may represent a painful motion segment. Posterior fusions alone may not alleviate pain at a particular vertebral level; anterior fusion may be necessary. Originally, this was performed through a second approach using an anterior or anterolateral exposure. This anterior exposure was popularized by surgeons from Hong Kong. The ability to accomplish similar stabilization procedures of the anterior column through a single posterior exposure would be a desirable next step. The posterior lumbar interbody fusion (PLIF) and, subsequently, the transforaminal lumbar interbody fusion (TLIF) approaches were soon popularized.

PLIF, performed first by Cloward [49] in 1943, was devised as a means to decompress nerve roots and perform a fusion procedure simultaneously. Because his technique was not reproduced easily, it was abandoned until new spinal instrumentation and devices made the technique more viable [41].

The biologic advantages of PLIF include the elimination of an anterior approach, which itself bears significant morbidity. From a mechanical standpoint, foraminal height is maintained, a well-vascularized fusion bed is created, and a shorter fusion distance is required [41,50]. Unfortunately, the preparation of the interbody region and placement of the device require significant nerve-root retraction.

The PLIF technique may be applied through two small paramedian skin incisions made at the level to be fused or in addition to a midline dissection that has been used for an open discectomy or decompression. The interlaminar space is accessed with any interposing soft tissue removed. Bilateral hemilaminotomies and medial facetectomies (Fig. 2) are performed, saving as much of the native bone as possible for the fusion. The traversing nerve roots are retracted medially, and a complete discectomy is performed. The endplates are prepared using decorticating instruments, such as rasps and curettes. The anterior disc space is packed with bone graft or a bone graft substitute (Fig. 3). Interbody devices, which may contain bone graft material, are placed. The fusion level is instrumented further with pedicle screws placed through the same midline or paramedian incision or percutaneously as described above (Fig. 4).

TLIF is similar to the PLIF procedure. However, TLIF was developed to address the concern of excessive nerve-root retraction [41,51–53]. The TLIF device is inserted through a unilateral approach and theoretically minimizes nerve-root retraction. Unfortunately, the approach sacrifices a facet joint [41,50]. The TLIF device also may be inserted in conjunction with another decompression procedure or through an isolated paramedian approach. The proper level is identified and the facet complex that is to be resected is approached surgically. As with a minimally invasive decompressive procedure, a tubular retractor system may be used to facilitate TLIF. A complete unilateral facetectomy is performed with the resected bone saved for the fusion procedure. Similar to PLIF, a complete discectomy is performed and the interbody region is prepared again with rasps and curettes. After the area is prepared, the interbody is packed with bone graft or bone graft substitute. As with PLIF, the levels to be fused by the interbody device are

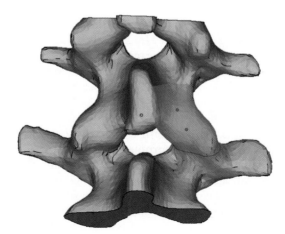

Fig. 2. The highlighted area illustrates the resection required for placement of an interbody device. The facet joint is removed, necessitating additional fixation (eg, pedicle screws).

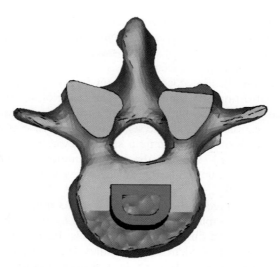

Fig. 3. Bone is placed within the anterior portion of the prepared interspace (*highlighted area*). An interbody device, which also may contain bone within its center, is placed.

instrumented with pedicle screws. The interbody device is placed diagonally across the interspace. The distraction across the interspace is released and compression is applied. With all interbody fusions, one must be cognizant of spinal alignment. Loss of balance in the sagittal plane can lead to a loss of normal contour and, subsequently, to flatback alignment complications (eg, fatigue and back pain after standing for extended periods of time).

Surgical treatment of spinal stenosis

Treatment of spinal stenosis is often surgical with the entirety of the offending areas of compression removed. This typically entails a posterior spine approach with excision of the lamina and a portion of the facet joints.

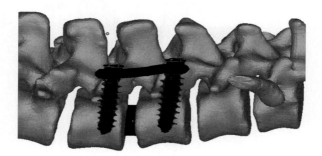

Fig. 4. Pedicle screws are placed to provide fixation across the interspace being fused.

Instability may result from the decompression, necessitating spinal fusion along with instrumentation. Dynamic spinal instability may also cause stenosis.

An alternative method to decompressive lumbar surgery involves the X Stop Interspinous Process Decompression System (St. Francis Medical Technologies, San Francisco, California). The mode of action of the device reflects the change in size of the spinal canal with normal flexion and extension. The cross-sectional area at one segment can increase as much as 50% from extension to flexion. By placing a spacer device between the spinous processes of the affected segment, the isolated motion segment is held in a relatively flexed position while the adjacent levels are allowed to freely flex and extend (Fig. 5).

The primary advantage of the device is that it accommodates a minimally invasive approach for implantation. The device is useful if the stenotic area of the spine encompassed one or two spinal levels. Early clinical trials have found good efficacy and excellent safety profiles. However, data is limited to 2 years. Patients who have undergone an X Stop procedure are still candidates for surgical decompression if their symptoms persist or recur.

Problems with current imaging

When an individual feels pain, he or she typically is upright and performing an activity. Yet, current imaging techniques are static images taken with patients in a recumbent position. Identifying areas for decompression may be difficult with this limited picture. Despite this, most spine surgeons

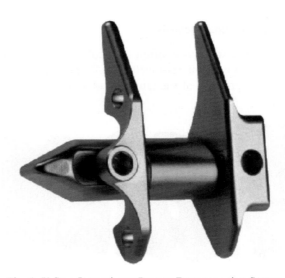

Fig. 5. X Stop Interspinous Process Decompression System.

believe that the current imaging studies are sensitive but not specific. Therefore, a careful history and physical examination that correlates with the radiographic abnormality are imperative. Active images, such as forward flexion and extension radiographs, are used to identify aberrant and painful motion. Upright MRI imaging is becoming more popular. However, despite the self-evident assumption that patients should be imaged in the position that provokes pain, no well-controlled studies have confirmed that such imaging is better for identifying sources of back pain.

The need for physical therapy

If pain relief ensues following any spinal procedure or injection, conditioning and strengthening of the surrounding structures are necessary to allow continued pain relief and function. It is of the utmost importance to improve the debilitated state of the patient once the pain is relieved. Physicians should have a low threshold for beginning physical therapy regimes for their patients. In addition, education about back pain is critical to its treatment. Studies show that the patient's understanding of his or her pain significantly predicted treatment success [54–56]. Because most back pain is self-limited, the most minimally invasive procedure is always no procedure.

Summary

The treatment of spine-related pain is an evolving area that requires a multidisciplinary focus. Our current fund of knowledge still relies on the decompression of compressed neurologic structures and the fusion of painful motion segments. Our approach for back pain management gives more attention to biologically favorable decompression and fusion techniques. The future may hold a better understanding of the genetics and molecular biology of disc degeneration and facet disease, with the possibility of even more direct and less invasive interventions.

References

[1] van Tulder M, Koes B. Low back pain (chronic). Clin Evid 2006;15:1634–53.
[2] Andersson GBJ. The epidemiology of spinal disorders. In: Frymoyer JW, editor. The adult spine: principles and practice. 2nd edition. New York: Raven Press; 1997. p. 93–141.
[3] Frymoyer JW. Back pain and sciatica. N Engl J Med 1988;318(5):291–300.
[4] Macfarlane GJ, Jones GT, Hannaford PC. Managing low back pain presenting to primary care: where do we go from here? Pain 2006;122(3):219–22.
[5] Koes BW, van Tulder MW, Thomas S. Diagnosis and treatment of low back pain. BMJ 2006;332(7555):1430–4.
[6] Deyo RA, Rainville J, Kent DL. What can the history and physical examination tell us about low back pain? JAMA 1992;268(6):760–5.
[7] Adams MA, Roughley PJ. What is intervertebral disc degeneration, and what causes it? Spine 2006;31(18):2151–61.

[8] Anderson DG, Li X, Tannoury T, et al. A fibronectin fragment stimulates intervertebral disc degeneration in vivo. Spine 2003;28(20):2338–45.

[9] Nissi MJ, Toyras J, Laasanen MS, et al. Proteoglycan and collagen sensitive MRI evaluation of normal and degenerated articular cartilage. J Orthop Res 2004;22(3):557–64.

[10] Battie MC, Videman T, Parent E. Lumbar disc degeneration: epidemiology and genetic influences. Spine 2004;29(23):2679–90.

[11] Garfin SR, Rydevik BL, Lipson SJ, et al. Spinal stenosis: pathophysiology. In: Herkowitz H, Garfin SR, Balderson RA, editors. The spine. 4th edition. Philadelphia: W.B. Saunders Co.; 1999. p. 791–826.

[12] Kirkaldy-Willis WH, Wedge JH, Yong-Hing K, et al. Pathology and pathogenesis of lumbar spondylosis and stenosis. Spine 1978;3(4):319–28.

[13] Garfin SR, Rydevik BL, Herkowitz H, et al. Spinal stenosis. Radiographic and electrodiagnostic evaluation. In: Herkowitz H, Garfin SR, Balderson RA, editors. The spine. 4th edition. Philadelphia: W.B. Saunders Co.; 1999. p. 791–875.

[14] Troup JD. Biomechanics of the lumbar spinal canal. Clin Biomech (Bristol, Avon) 1986;1: 31–43.

[15] Leong JC, Luk KD, Chow DH, et al. The biomechanical functions of the iliolumbar ligament in maintaining stability of the lumbosacral junction. Spine 1987;12(7):669–74.

[16] McLain RF, Kapural L, Mekhail NA. Epidural steroid therapy for back and leg pain: mechanisms of action and efficacy. Spine J 2005;5(2):191–201.

[17] Cornefjord M, Olmarker K, Farley DB, et al. Neuropeptide changes in compressed spinal nerve roots. Spine 1995;20(6):670–3.

[18] Howe JF, Loeser JD, Calvin WH. Mechanosensitivity of dorsal root ganglia and chronically injured axons: a physiological basis for the radicular pain of nerve root compression. Pain 1977;3(1):25–41.

[19] Rydevik B, Brown MD, Lundborg G. Pathoanatomy and pathophysiology of nerve root compression. Spine 1984;9(1):7–15.

[20] Cavanaugh JM. Neural mechanisms of lumbar pain. Spine 1995;20(16):1804–9.

[21] Takebayashi T, Cavanaugh JM, Cuneyt Ozaktay A, et al. Effect of nucleus pulposus on the neural activity of dorsal root ganglion. Spine 2001;26(8):940–5.

[22] Crock HV. A reappraisal of intervertebral disc lesions. Med J Aust 1970;1(20):983–9.

[23] Zhou Y, Abdi S. Diagnosis and minimally invasive treatment of lumbar discogenic pain—a review of the literature. Clin J Pain 2006;22(5):468–81.

[24] Crock HV. Internal disc disruption. A challenge to disc prolapse fifty years on. Spine 1986; 11(6):650–3.

[25] Merskey H, Bogduk N. Classification of chronic pain: descriptions of chronic pain syndromes and definitions of pain terms, 2nd edition. Seattle (WA): IASP Press; 1994. p. 180–1.

[26] Boswell MV, Shah RV, Everett CR, et al. Interventional techniques in the management of chronic spinal pain: evidence-based practice guidelines. Pain Physician 2005;8(1):1–47.

[27] van Tulder MW, Koes B, Seitsalo S, et al. Outcome of invasive treatment modalities on back pain and sciatica: an evidence-based review. Eur Spine J 2006;15(Suppl 1):S82–92.

[28] Carette S, Marcoux S, Truchon R, et al. A controlled trial of corticosteroid injections into facet joints for chronic low back pain. N Engl J Med 1991;325(14):1002–7.

[29] Lim MR, Yoon SC, Green DW. Symptomatic spondylolysis: diagnosis and treatment. Curr Opin Pediatr 2004;16(1):37–46.

[30] Micheli LJ, Wood R. Back pain in young athletes. Significant differences from adults in causes and patterns. Arch Pediatr Adolesc Med 1995;149(1):15–8.

[31] Sucato DJ. Spinal scoliotic deformities: adolescent idiopathic, adult degenerative, and neuromuscular in spine. In: Vaccaro AR, editor. Core knowledge in orthopaedics. Philadelphia: Elsevier Mosby; 2005. p. 137–56.

[32] Danielsson AJ, Nachemson AL. Back pain and function 22 years after brace treatment for adolescent idiopathic scoliosis: a case-control study—part I. Spine 2003;28(18): 2078–85.

[33] Danielsson AJ, Nachemson AL. Back pain and function 23 years after fusion for adolescent idiopathic scoliosis: a case-control study—part II. Spine 2003;28(18):E373–83.

[34] Adams MA, Bogduk N, Burton K, et al. The biomechanics of back pain. Edinburgh (UK): Churchill Livingstone; 2002.

[35] Trout JJ, Buckwalter JA, Moore KC. Ultrastructure of the human intervertebral disc. II. Cells of the nucleus pulposus. Anat Rec 1982;204(4):307–14.

[36] Weber H. Lumbar disc herniation. A prospective study of prognostic factors including a controlled trial. Part II. J Oslo City Hosp 1978;28(7–8):89–113.

[37] Weber H. Lumbar disc herniation. A prospective study of prognostic factors including a controlled trial. Part I. J Oslo City Hosp 1978;28(3–4):33–61.

[38] Weber H. The natural history of disc herniation and the influence of intervention. Spine 1994;19(19):2234–8.

[39] Dandy WE. Loose cartilage from intervertebral disk simulating tumor of the spinal cord. By Walter E. Dandy, 1929. Clin Orthop Relat Res 1989;238:4–8.

[40] Wisneski RJ, Garfin SR, Rothman RH, et al. Lumbar disc disease. In: Herkowitz H, Garfin SR, Balderson RA, editors. The spine. 4th edition. Philadelphia: W.B. Saunders Co.; 1999. p. 671–746.

[41] German JW, Foley KT. Minimal access surgical techniques in the management of the painful lumbar motion segment. Spine 2005;30(16 Suppl):S52–9.

[42] Gibson JN, Grant IC, Waddell G. The Cochrane review of surgery for lumbar disc prolapse and degenerative lumbar spondylosis. Spine 1999;24(17):1820–32.

[43] Awad JN, Moskovich R. Lumbar disc herniations: surgical versus nonsurgical treatment. Clin Orthop Relat Res 2006;443:183–97.

[44] Andrews DW, Lavyne MH. Retrospective analysis of microsurgical and standard lumbar discectomy. Spine 1990;15(4):329–35.

[45] Barrios C, Ahmed M, Arrotegui J, et al. Microsurgery versus standard removal of the herniated lumbar disc. A 3-year comparison in 150 cases. Acta Orthop Scand 1990;61(5):399–403.

[46] Bookwalter JW, Busch MD, Nicely D. Ambulatory surgery is safe and effective in radicular disc disease. Spine 1994;19(5):526–30.

[47] BenDebba M, Augustus van Alphen H, Long DM. Association between peridural scar and activity-related pain after lumbar discectomy. Neurol Res 1999;21(Suppl 1):S37–42.

[48] Toyone T, Tanaka T, Kato D, et al. Low-back pain following surgery for lumbar disc herniation. A prospective study. J Bone Joint Surg Am 2004;86(5):893–6.

[49] Cloward RB. The treatment of ruptured intervertebral discs by vertebral body fusion: indications, operative technique, after care. J Neurosurg 1953;10(2):154–68.

[50] Mummaneni PV, Haid RW, Rodts GE. Lumbar interbody fusion: state-of-the-art technical advances. J Neurosurg Spine 2004;1:24–30.

[51] Harms J, Rolinger H. [A one-stage procedure in operative treatment of spondylolistheses: dorsal traction-reposition and anterior fusion (author's translation)]. Z Orthop Ihre Grenzgeb 1982;120(3):343–7 [in German].

[52] Humphreys SC, Hodges SD, Patwardhan AG, et al. Comparison of posterior and transforaminal approaches to lumbar interbody fusion. Spine 2001;26(5):567–71.

[53] Lowe TG, Tahernia AD, O'Brien MF, et al. Unilateral transforaminal posterior lumbar interbody fusion (TLIF): indications, technique, and 2-year results. J Spinal Disord Tech 2002;15(1):31–8.

[54] Henrotin YE, Cedraschi C, Duplan B, et al. Information and low back pain management: a systematic review. Spine 2006;31(11):E326–34.

[55] Deyo RA, Diehl AK. Psychosocial predictors of disability in patients with low back pain. J Rheumatol 1988;15(10):1557–64.

[56] Fardon DF, Milette PC. Nomenclature and classification of lumbar discpathology. Spine 2001;26(5):461–2.

ELSEVIER
SAUNDERS

Anesthesiology Clin
25 (2007) 913–928

ANESTHESIOLOGY
CLINICS

Vertebroplasty and Kyphoplasty

William Lavelle, MD[a,*], Allen Carl, MD[a],
Elizabeth Demers Lavelle, MD[b],
Mohammed A. Khaleel, MS[a]

[a]Department of Orthopaedic Surgery, 1367 Washington Avenue, Albany Medical Center,
Albany, NY 12206, USA
[b]Department of Anesthesiology, Albany Medical Center, 43 New Scotland Avenue, Albany,
NY 12208, USA

The problem of osteoporosis

The aging population has brought new challenges to the medical community including osteoporosis, which is considered one of the most debilitating yet often ignored medical conditions. The National Osteoporosis Foundation estimates that more than 55% of Americans over the age of 50 suffer from either osteopenia or osteoporosis. Women bear the largest burden, making up approximately 80% of the affected population [1,2]. The hallmark of osteoporosis is fractures of fragility. A fragility fracture occurs as a result of a fall from standing height. The three sites that are typical of fragility fractures are the vertebra, hip, and wrist. Figs. 1–3 demonstrate a vertebral body fracture. With an annual incidence of 700,000, vertebral compression fractures occur more frequently than hip and ankle fractures combined [3]. Patients who have vertebral compression fractures often suffer such pain that it interferes with their daily living. Vertebral compression fractures account for 150,000 hospital admissions, 161,000 physician office visits, and more than 5 million restricted activity days annually [4]. In 1995, direct costs for osteoporotic fractures in the United States topped $13.8 billion, or $38 million daily [5,6].

Vertebral compression fractures frequently result in both acute and chronic pain, as well as leading to progressive vertebral collapse [5,7]. One thoracic vertebral compression fracture can cause enough overall sagittal kyphosis to cause a 9% loss of forced vital capacity [8–10]. Patients

A version of this article originally appeared in the 91:2 issue of Medical Clinics of North America.

* Corresponding author.
  E-mail address: lavellwf@yahoo.com (W. Lavelle).

doi:10.1016/j.anclin.2007.07.011 *anesthesiology.theclinics.com*

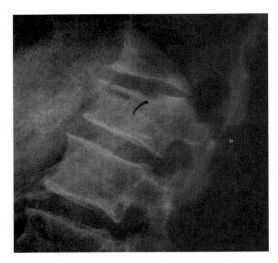

Fig. 1. A radiograph of a vertebral fracture is shown, demonstrating an osteoporotic compression fracture.

sustaining osteoporotic compression fractures also face increased risks for multiple comorbidities such as weight loss due to early satiety and poor psychologic well being [11–14]. Although these fractures are rarely a direct cause of death, they do frequently produce significant morbidities that

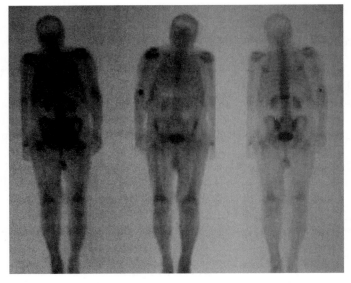

Fig. 2. Bone scan showing an acute vertebral fracture.

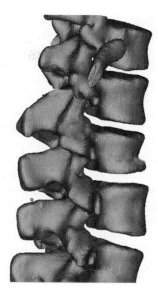

Fig. 3. Model showing a vertebral body fracture.

may eventually affect the mortality of the patient [12–19]. The 5-year survival of a patient who sustains a vertebral compression fracture is lower than that of a similar patient sustaining a hip fracture [12]. More commonly, elderly patients who were independent before their injury find themselves dependent on their adult children [20].

In the past, attempts at open surgical treatment of these injuries have been fraught with disaster. Poor bone quality would often lead to implant failure. Perioperative morbidity was often high because elderly patients bear other medical comorbidities. This has lead to patients being treated conservatively with oral, narcotic analgesia and an orthosis. Because this treatment offers little for those truly debilitated by their injury, physicians have become interested in new methods for pain relief and functional restoration to a degree that patients may return to their activities of daily living.

Use of cement in orthopaedics

Chemist Otto Röhm developed a new substance in the early twentieth century with novel structural properties and good biocompatibility. In the 1960s, Sir John Charnley began using Polymethyl methacrylate (PMMA) as bone cement on numerous patients for the fixation of both the femur and acetabulum for total hip replacement. Borrowing this idea from dentists of his era, bone cement acts as a grout, filling in the voids between the metal prosthesis and bone [21,22].

In the spine, PMMA was first used to treat a painful and aggressive variant of a vertebral haemangioma [21–26]. Bone cement was later used to treat painful vertebral lesions caused by metastatic disease to the spine [27–29]. Multiple explanations have been offered for the pain relief associated with introduction of PMMA into an osteoporotic compression fracture site. Thermal necrosis and chemotoxicity of the intraosseous pain receptors have been offered as explanations in addition to the obvious improvement in mechanical stability offered by the bone cement [30]. It has been proposed that the cement monomer itself may be neurotoxic [31–33] and possibly act on the interossious nerve endings in the vertebral body. To create less viscous cement with a longer working time for use in percutaneous vertebral augmentation, more monomer is typically added to the powder than is recommended by the manufacturer [4,34,35]. The polymerization reaction of PMMA cement is exothermic. During the polymerization, temperatures can reach up to 122°C [36,37]; however, cadaveric study of osteoporotic vertebrae found that temperatures generated during vertebroplasty may not be sufficient to result in widespread thermal necrosis of osteoblasts [38–40] or nerve endings [41]. Whatever its mechanism, injection of bone cement into painful vertebral compression fractures is a successful technique with well-published clinical efficacy.

Indications for percutaneous vertebral augmentation

As with any surgical procedure, the typical patient who is offered percutaneous vertebral augmentation is one who has already failed several weeks of conservative therapy consisting of oral nonsteroidal medications and mild opiate analgesia. Usually, patients have been offered a supportive orthosis as well. The prime issue is mobility. Osteoporotic patients are at risk of significant medical morbidity the longer they remain immobile. However, controversy exists as to what the exact number of weeks or months of conservative therapy is appropriate before offering percutaneous vertebral augmentation. Some physicians offer an early percutaneous vertebral augmentation to patients who have a documented inability to mobilize after their injury. Typically patients who are mobile but still have pain are given 4 to 6 weeks to improve [5].

There are particular fracture patterns that are less likely to improve with conservative treatment, such as fractures of the thoracolumbar junction (T11–L2), osteoporotic burst fractures, wedge anterior compression fractures with greater than 30° of sagittal angulation, and patients with continuing radiographic collapse upon subsequent follow-up radiographs [5].

Despite the feeling that percutaneous vertebral augmentation is effective, the technique does have limitations and relative contraindications. Patients who have cortical disruption that would preclude cement containment should not undergo a percutaneous vertebral augmentation. Patients who have preexisting radicular complaints are often disappointed and report a poor result. This is perhaps because patients are undereducated about the difference between the subaxial back pain that would be attributable to the compression fracture site and the more peripherial radicular pain that they are experiencing [5]. In the face of vertebra plana or complete verebral collapse, any technique of percutaneous vertebral augmentation is difficult [42]. Obtaining preoperative imaging such as sagittal CT or MRI images to assess trajectory and cortical integrity is often helpful [27,42,43]. Bone scan may also be useful in determining fracture acuity because these patients often have had previous fractures that may be obvious in a plain radiograph but inconsequential in the patient's current clinical state of back pain.

History of vertebroplasty

Galibert and Deramond [44] reported the first percutaneous vertebral augmentation, or vertebroplasty. This landmark procedure was performed in Amiens, France in 1984. These French physicians injected PMMA into a C2 vertebra that had been destroyed by an aggressive hemangioma. The authors reported that the procedure relieved the patient's long-standing pain. PMMA was then introduced by way of a similar percutaneous technique aided by fluoroscopic guidance into the vertebral bodies of veterbra that had sustained fractures caused by osteoporosis [45].

After the initial investigations in Europe, vertebroplasty was introduced in the United States by interventional neuroradiologists at the University of Virginia [46]. Veterbroplasty has gained increasing popularity with patients reporting rapid pain relief [21]. The technique used to perform vertebroplasty has been modified with time to include larger bore needles and additional barium in the cement to decrease the risk of extravasation.

Technique of vertebroplasty

Before attempting a procedure on the spine, it behooves the practitioner to have acceptable fluoroscopic imaging. It is the standard in the surgical community to confirm the spinal level for the procedure with the patient and the room staff. The procedure and level is again verified on the preoperative imaging and finally on the image intensifier before needle/cannula placement. Proper imaging is essential to performing the procedure with safety and precision. Proper cannula placement is observed on the fluoroscope before injection of the cement (Fig. 4). Fluoroscopic imaging also provides real-time images of the injection of the cement and the potential extravasation into surrounding tissues, which represents the most likely complication of the procedure [4,23,28,34,47].

As is done in many surgical procedures, prophylactic antibiotics are administered to the patient approximately 30 minutes before the actual procedure; however, the efficacy of this practice in preventing infection has never been affirmed by controlled study [4]. Some surgeons mix antibiotics such as tobramycin into the cement that will be injected into the vertebral

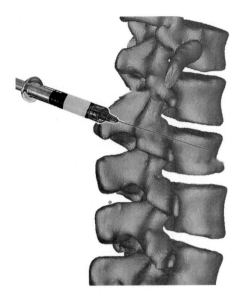

Fig. 4. For vertebroplasty, cement is injected directly into a fracture. The cement is injected under high pressure. The vertebral body is accessed through the pedicle.

body during the procedure; however, this practice is often reserved for the immunocompromised.

There are several anesthesia choices for percutaneous vertebral augmentation. Local anesthesia may be selected. The local anesthetic is injected in to the skin, subcutaneous tissues, and periosteum of the vertebra. Conscious sedation is often offered as an ajuant. General anesthesia is another possible choice. In cases that will involve CT guidance for needle localization, general anesthesia will best control for patient movement. General anesthesia is also the optimal choice for lengthy cases involving numerous levels of vertebral fractures.

After localization, a small incision is made and an 11-gauge cannulated trocar and bone biopsy needle is advanced to the posterior aspect of the vertebra. The cannula is passed through the pedicle into the vertebral body being treated. Both lateral and anteroposterior projections provide necessary visualization of the path of the needle. An alternative approach is a parapedicular. This is most often used to access the thoracic spine. The parapedicular approach involves inserting the cannula between the lateral margin of the pedicle of thoracic vertebrae and the rib head [23].

The most common approach involves accessing and injecting cement through both pedicles [23]. A unipedicular approach may also be employed. This approach does require a more oblique route because of the need to introduce the cement into the midline and anterior third of the vertebral body. The needle can be steered within the bone to allow injection into both sides of the injured body because of the beveled design [23]. Before injection of the cement, a vertebrogram may be performed to identify the basivertebral venous plexus and other large vessels that are susceptible for extravasation [48–50]. However this is often unnecessary, and in fractures that involve the endplate, the contrast material may leak into the disk and not drain. The remaining dye will mimic the contrast in the cement and preclude detection of cement leakage [48–50].

With single-plane fluoroscopic equipment, actual injection of the cement should be visualized with lateral fluoroscopy [23]. Anteroposterior images are checked regularly to monitor for lateral leaks. Deramond and colleagues [4] suggest that all the cements available currently do not contain enough barium sulfate for opacification on fluoroscopy; therefore approximately 30% wt/vol of pure barium sulfate may be added to the PMMA powder before mixing and injection. Biplane fluoroscopy will allow simultaneous visualization in two projections during injection. It allows the procedure to be performed more rapidly [51] and is often chosen when the procedure is performed in a radiology department because of equipment availability and familiarity. CT guidance has also been described [52], but often adds more to the cost of the procedure and has not become a popular adjuvant. It is useful in the anterolateral approach to the cervical spine where the carotid vessels must be avoided. It is also helpful down to the level of T4 where the shoulders will not allow for easy lateral fluoroscopy [52]. CT and MR imaging limit real-time monitoring, and many surgeons will use these modalities for placement of the needle and then use fluoroscopy during injection [4]. Typically the injection must be completed in 6 to 8 minutes and before the cement becomes too viscous to allow reinsertion of the stylus. Otherwise a "needle cast" or a "cement tail" may remain in the soft tissue as the needle is removed with the adherent cement [23].

The cement will set within 20 minutes and achieve 90% of its strength within an hour [4,23]. Patients can typically sit up and walk once they have recovered from anesthesia. On an outpatient basis, the patient should be observed for 1 to 3 hours postoperation. Pain relief is expected to be noticed in 4 to 24 hours. Clinical follow-up includes pain scale testing. Radiography is indicated if the patient fails to respond positively to the intervention because an incorrect level may have been treated or a new fracture may have occurred after the vertebroplasty procedure [3].

Results of vertebroplasty

Overall, vertebroplasty has been effective in relieving the back pain caused by vertebral compression fractures. Grados and colleagues [53] assessed pain relief with the use of the visual analog scale; they discovered a significant decrease in pain from 80 mm to 37 mm in just 1 month following the procedure. The improvement was stable with an average assessment of pain at 34 mm on the scale at a mean follow-up of 2 years. Zoarski and colleagues [54] at just 2 weeks follow-up also found significant improvement in pain and disability, physical function, and even mental function as reported by patients. Of the 23 patients treated, 22 reported satisfaction at 15 to 18 months following vertebroplasty. In a larger group of 75 patients, Kaufmann and colleagues [55] found positive effects of the procedure with regard to pain measurement, mobility, and the use of analgesics. However, they did find that the procedure was less effective in patients requiring narcotics for pain control before the operation and in those with longstanding fractures. Additionally, some reports have suggested a failure rate of up to 10%. Deramond and colleagues [56] suggest that failure rates much higher than this may indicate a flaw in patient selection; radiologists and clinicians should work as a team to select patients that stand to benefit the most from such procedures. These significant improvements result from a procedure that does not attempt to reduce the actual fracture, but only stabilizes it.

As would be expected with any surgical intervention, vertebroplasty is not without its risks. Complications may be medical, problems with anesthesia, and instrument misplacement or technical error. Unique complications to vertebroplasty and kyphoplasty include cement extravasation and fracture of vertebral bodies adjacent to the levels treated.

Grados and colleagues [53] suggest a rate of cement extravasation of 6% for vertebral level treated with vertebroplasty. Rates of neural compression from such leakage may range from 0% to 4% [5]. However, in cases of true vertebral compression fractures due to osteoporosis, the rate may be lower within the range. Treatment for angiomas and bone metastases tend to have a higher rate of this specific complication—as high as 10% in some reports [56]. Specific technical safeguards and the use of contrast within the cement mixture are ways to prevent the most frequent complication of percutaneous vertebral augmentation.

History of kyphoplasty

The possibility of injecting highly viscous cement into fractured trabecular bone was worrisome to spine surgeons. The fear that cement extravasation could have devastating neurologic consequences from intrusion was of particular concern. Spine surgeons were also concerned that the high pressures used to introduce the cement could potentially lead to the bolus embolization of cement through the venous channels in the vertebral bodies to the lungs. Additionally, vertebroplasty was felt to be an inadequate means of fracture reduction. As a solution to all these concerns, the kyphoplasty technique was devised and was first performed in 1998 [15,57]. The procedure seemed to result in the same type of pain relief.

Technique of kyphoplasty

All patients who undergo the procedure in our facility are anesthetized with general anesthesia. This form of anesthesia is chosen because the elderly patients in our population do not tolerate the prone position. The patients were prepared and draped in a normal sterile fashion. Fluoroscopic guidance is used to identify the fracture site to be treated.

A 1-cm incision is made just lateral to both pedicles of the vertebral body to be treated. A Jamshidi needle (Kyphon, Sunnyvale, California) is used to enter the superior lateral border of the pedicle under fluoroscopic guidance. Using a combination of manual pressure and light malleting, the Jamshidi needle is passed through the pedicle into the vertebral body. Frequent anteroposterior and lateral fluoroscopic images are used to confirm position. Once the Jamshidi needle enters the vertebral body, the needle is exchanged for an obturator (Kyphon, Sunnyvale, California) followed by a working cannula (Kyphon, Sunnyvale, California). A drill is then used to create a tract into the vertebral body. The balloon catheter is introduced into the fracture site and the process is repeated on the contralateral side. Both balloon tamps (Kyphon, Sunnyvale, California) are then inflated until either the fracture is reduced or it is felt unsafe to continue (PSIO300 or violation of one of the vertebral end plates). The balloons are then removed, and the cavities are filled with methyl methacrylate cement using a hand plunger system supplied by the manufacturer. Intraoperative radiographs are used to confirm containment of the cement in the vertebral body (Figs. 5–7) [3].

Results of kyphoplasty

Height restoration/fracture reduction

As one of the proposed device advances, fracture reduction results have been examined by several investigators. Within the confines of these studies, pre- and postprocedure images were reviewed to determine the degree of fracture reduction, particularly the restoration of vertebral height. Height restoration is determined by comparing the fractured vertebra to the adjacent vertebral segments.

Majd and colleagues [58] found in their series of 360 kyphoplasty procedures performed on 222 patients, a 30%-anterior fracture reduction or return of the relative anterior height was achieved. This study also looked at restoration of medial vertebral height; this restoration averaged 50%. Kyphotic angle was also examined, which is a relative measure that looks at how far forward a fracture causes a patient to bend as compared with the normal vertebral alignment. The average relative correction of the kyphotic angle was 7 degrees.

Boszczyk and colleagues [59] found a similar average correction of the kyphotic angle of 5 degrees with kyphoplasty. Within this study, a head-to-head comparison was made with vertebroplasty. No correction of the kyphotic angle was achieved through introduction of cement alone without use of a balloon tamp.

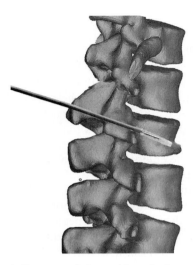

Fig. 5. For kyphoplasty, a balloon tamp is inserted into the fracture before cement injection.

Lieberman and colleagues [60] at the Cleveland Clinic reported on 30 patients who underwent 70 kyphoplasty procedures. Height restoration was again examined. When examining height restoration of the vertebral body as a whole, 35% of the relative height was restored in this series. With regard to correction of the kyphotic angle, a similar 6° of correction was achieved.

Crandall and colleagues [61] found the greatest degree of height correction at 86% in what were termed as "new" or acute fractures. Fractures

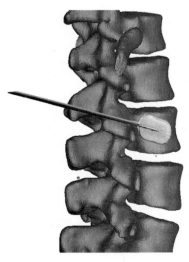

Fig. 6. An inflated balloon creates a void for the low-pressure injection of cement. Some feel the tamp acts as an aide for fracture reduction.

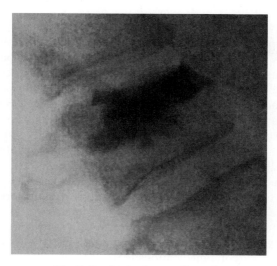

Fig. 7. Postkyphoplasty radiograph.

that were subacute (older than 4 months) a 79% correction was achieved. The kyphotic angle correction differed based on fracture age as well. Kyphoplasty of new fractures resulted in a 7° correction whereas subacute fractures were reduced by 5°.

The most recent study by Pradhan and colleagues [8] was a retrospective study of 65 patients who underwent one- to three-level kyphoplasty procedures. Measurements revealed that kyphoplasty reduced local kyphotic deformity at the fractured vertebra by an average of 7.3°. Overall angular correction decreased to 2.4° (20% of preoperative kyphosis at fractured level) when measured one level above and below. The angular correction further decreased to 1.5° and 1.0° (13% and 8% of preoperative kyphosis at fractured level), respectively, at spans of two and three levels above and below. With multilevel kyphoplasty procedures, the total gains seen over multiple vertebrae, such as 7.8° over two levels and 7.7° over three levels, compared with the 7.3° for a single level. In other words, the small correction in fracture height and angulation achieved through the use of kyphoplasty does not translate into a substantial improvement in the general sagital alignment of the spine as a whole.

All of these studies have examined fracture by way of pre- and postop imaging. Reduction of the fracture through positioning in hyperextension may achieve a degree of fracture reduction. This explanation has been proposed as the primary means of fracture reduction by some spine surgeons. However, if this were an effective means of osteoporotic fracture reduction, better fracture reduction results with vertebroplasty would have been noted in the literature.

Pain relief

The first report on the kyphoplasty procedure was published by Garfin and colleagues [15] in 2001. This group found that 95% of patients treated with kyphoplasty or vertebroplasty had significant improvement in pain. Lieberman and colleagues [60] published the results of a phase I study of the inflatable bone tamp used in the kyphoplasty procedure. Seventy kypho-plasty procedures were studied in 30 patients. Pain scores improved signifi-cantly as a result of the procedure from 11.6 to 58.7 ($P = .0001$). Physical function scores also demonstrated significant improvement. In 2003, Ledlie and Renfro [62] followed 133 kyphoplasty patients for 1 year. These patients realized a reduction in visual analog pain scores from an average of 8.6/10 preprocedure to 1.6/10 postprocedure. Thirty-five percent reported unas-sisted preprocedure ambulation, whereas 90% reported unassisted postpro-cedure ambulation. In a separate multicenter study, 90% of patients treated by kyphoplasty were able to return to their baseline activities with 90% also able to wean off narcotic medications [15].

Risk of another fracture after percutaneous vertebral augmentation

Much speculation and concern has been raised about recurrent vertebral compression fracture, particularly at adjacent levels [3,63–70]. Unfortu-nately, patients who experience one osteoporotic fracture have a high likeli-hood of sustaining a second fragility fracture [71,72]. There are few reports that are available in the literature describing the actual incidence of another fracture after a kyphoplasty procedure [58,68,70,72,73]. In one review by Fribourg and colleagues [68], 17 additional fractures occurred after 47 levels were treated by kyphoplasty. Another study by Majd and colleagues [58] found an overall recurrent fracture rate of 10% (36 additional fractures in 360 fractures treated). Finally, the recurrent fracture rate published by Lav-elle and Cheney [3] was 15% overall (16 of 109 treated levels) and 10% at 90 days. It seems from the literature that the incidence of a fracture after percutaneous vertebral augmentation falls within the realm of the incidence of a patient sustaining an additional veretebral fracture after a prior frac-ture. Although the incidence of a first-time vertebral fracture is 3.6%, the subsequent fracture rate may be as high as 19.2% within the first year [71].

Summary

Percutaneous veretebral augmentation offers a minimally invasive approach to a painful osteoporotic vertebral compression fracture. Both methods allow for the introduction of bone cement in to the fracture site with clinical results indicating substantial pain relief in approximately 90% of patients. Kyphoplasty offers the possibility of lower pressures for ce-ment introduction and the possibility of modest fracture reductions.

References

[1] Lemke DM. Vertebroplasty and kyphoplasty for treatment of painful osteoporotic compression fractures. J Am Acad Nurse Pract 2005;17(7):268–76.

[2] National Osteoporosis Foundation. 2005 Annual Report. Available at: http://www.nof.org/aboutnof/2005_Annual_Report_FINAL.pdf. Accessed December 20, 2006.

[3] Lavelle WF, Cheney R. Recurrent fracture after vertebral kyphoplasty. Spine J 2006;6(5):488–93.

[4] Mathis JM, Barr JD, Belkoff SM, et al. Percutaneous vertebroplasty: a developing standard of care for vertebral compression fractures. AJNR Am J Neuroradiol 2001;22(2):373–81.

[5] Truumees E, Hilibrand A, Vaccaro AR. Percutaneous vertebral augmentation. Spine J 2004;4(2):218–29.

[6] Michigan Department of Community Health. Michigan osteoporosis strategic plan. Available at: http://www.michigan.gov/documents/osteorpt_6772_7.pdf. Accessed December 20, 2006.

[7] Wasnich U. Vertebral fracture epidemiology. Bone 1996;18:1791–6.

[8] Pradhan BB, Bae HW, Kropf MA, et al. Kyphoplasty reduction of osteoporotic vertebral compression fractures: correction of local kyphosis versus overall sagittal alignment. Spine 2006;31(4):435–41.

[9] Schlaich C, Minne HW, Bruckner T, et al. Reduced pulmonary function in patients with spinal osteoporotic fractures. Osteoporos Int 1998;8(3):261–7.

[10] Leech JA, Dulberg C, Kellie S, et al. Relationship of lung function to severity of osteoporosis in women. Am Rev Respir Dis 1990;141(1):68–71.

[11] Leidig-Bruckner G, Minne HW, Schlaich C, et al. Clinical grading of spinal osteoporosis: quality of life components and spinal deformity in women with chronic low back pain and women with vertebral osteoporosis. J Bone Miner Res 1997;12(4):663–75.

[12] Kado DM, Duong T, Stone KL, et al. Incident vertebral fractures and mortality in older women: a prospective study. Osteoporos Int 2003;14(7):589–94.

[13] Jalava T, Sarna S, Pylkkanen L, et al. Association between vertebral fracture and increased mortality in osteoporotic patients. J Bone Miner Res 2003;18(7):1254–60.

[14] Silverman SL, Delmas PD, Kulkarni PM, et al. Comparison of fracture, cardiovascular event, and breast cancer rates at 3 years in postmenopausal women with osteoporosis. J Am Geriatr Soc 2004;52(9):1543–8.

[15] Garfin SR, Yuan HA, Reiley MA. New technologies in spine: kyphoplasty and vertebroplasty for the treatment of painful osteoporotic compression fractures. Spine 2001;26(14):1511–5.

[16] Cooper C, Atkinson EJ, Jacobsen SJ, et al. Population-based study of survival after osteoporotic fractures. Am J Epidemiol 1993;137:1001–5.

[17] Ismail AA, O'Neill TW, Cooper C, et al. Mortality associated with vertebral deformity in men and women: results from the European Prospective Osteoporosis Study (EPOS). Osteoporos Int 1998;8:291–7.

[18] Ensrud K, Thompson D, Cauley J, et al. Prevalent vertebral deformities predict mortality and hospitalization in older women with low bone mass. J Am Geriatr Soc 2000;48:241–9.

[19] Cauley JA, Thompson DE, Ensrud KC, et al. Risk of mortality following clinical fractures. Osteoporos Int 2000;11:556–61.

[20] Garfin SR, Reilley MA. Minimally invasive treatment of osteoporotic vertebral body compression fractures. Spine J 2002;2(1):76–80.

[21] Mathis JM, Maroney M, Fenton DC, et al. Evaluation of bone cements for use in percutaneous vertebroplasty [abstract]. In: Proceedings of the 13th Annual Meeting of the North American Spine Society (San Francisco, CA, October 28–31, 1998). Rosemont (IL): North American Spine Society; 1998:210–1.

[22] DiMaio FR. The science of bone cement: a historical review. Orthopedics 2002;25(12):1399–407.

926 LAVELLE et al

[23] Hide IG, Gangi A. Percutaneous vertebroplasty: history, technique and current perspectives. Clin Radiol 2004;59:461–7.

[24] Cortet B, Cotten A, Deprez X, et al. Value of vertebroplasty combined with surgical decompression in the treatment of aggressive spinal angioma. Apropos of 3 cases. Rev Rhum Ed Fr 1994;61(1):16–22.

[25] Ide C, Gangi A, Rimmelin A, et al. Vertebral haemangiomas with spinal cord compression: the place of preoperative percutaneous vertebroplasty with methyl methacrylate. Neuroradiology 1996;38(6):585–9.

[26] Feydy A, Cognard C, Miaux Y, et al. Acrylic vertebroplasty in symptomatic cervical vertebral haemangiomas: report of 2 cases. Neuroradiology 1996;38(4):389–91.

[27] Weill A, Chiras J, Simon JM, et al. Spinal metastases: indications for and results of percutaneous injection of acrylic surgical cement. Radiology 1996;199(1):241–7.

[28] Cotten A, Dewatre F, Cortet B, et al. Percutaneous vertebroplasty for osteolytic metastases and myeloma: effects of the percentage of lesion filling and the leakage of methyl methacrylate at clinical follow-up. Radiology 1996;200(2):525–30.

[29] Murphy KJ, Deramond H. Percutaneous vertebroplasty in benign and malignant disease. Neuroimaging Clin N Am 2000;10(3):535–45.

[30] Bostrom MP, Lane JM. Future directions. Augmentation of osteoporotic vertebral bodies. Spine 1997;22(24 Suppl):38S–42S.

[31] Dahl OE, Garvik LJ, Lyberg T. Toxic effects of methylmethacrylate monomer on leukocytes and endothelial cells in vitro. Acta Orthop Scand 1994;65(2):147–53.

[32] Danilewicz-Stysiak Z. Experimental investigations on the cytotoxic nature of methyl methacrylate. J Prosthet Dent 1980;44(1):13–6.

[33] Seppalainen AM, Rajaniemi R. Local neurotoxicity of methyl methacrylate among dental technicians. Am J Ind Med 1984;5(6):471–7.

[34] Deramond H, Depriester C, Toussaint P, et al. Percutaneous vertebroplasty. Semin Musculoskelet Radiol 1997;1(2):285–96.

[35] Jasper LE, Deramond H, Mathis JM, et al. The effect of monomer-to-powder ratio on the material properties of cranioplastic. Bone 1999;25(2 Suppl):27S–9S.

[36] San Millan Ruiz D, Burkhardt K, Jean B, et al. Pathology findings with acrylic implants. Bone 1999;25(2 Suppl):85S–90S.

[37] Jefferiss CD, Lee AJC, Ling RSM. Thermal aspects of self-curing polymethylmethacrylate. J Bone Joint Surg 1975;57B(4):511–8.

[38] Eriksson RA, Albrektsson T, Magnusson B. Assessment of bone viability after heat trauma: a histological, histochemical and vital microscopic study in the rabbit. Scand J Plast Reconstr Surg 1984;18:261–8.

[39] Eriksson RA, Albrektsson T. The effect of heat on bone regeneration: an experimental study in the rabbit using the bone growth chamber. J Oral Maxillofac Surg 1984;42(11):705–11.

[40] Rouiller C, Majno G. Morphological and chemical studies of bones after the application of heat. Beitr Pathol Anat 1953;113(1):100–20.

[41] De Vrind HH, Wondergem J, Haveman J. Hyperthermia-induced damage to rat sciatic nerve assessed in vivo with functional methods and with electrophysiology. J Neurosci Methods 1992;45(3):165–74.

[42] Cotten A, Boutry N, Cortet B, et al. Percutaneous vertebroplasty: state of the art. Radiographics 1998;18(2):311–20.

[43] Barr JD, Barr MS, Lemley TJ, et al. Percutaneous vertebroplasty for pain relief and spinal stabilization. Spine 2000;25(8):923–8.

[44] Galibert P, Deramond H, Rosat P, et al. Preliminary note on the treatment of vertebral angioma by percutaneous acrylic vertebroplasty. Neurochirurgie 1987;33:166–8.

[45] Bascoulergue Y, Duquesnel J, Leclercq R, et al. Percutaneous injection of methyl methacrylate in the vertebral body for the treatment of various diseases: percutaneous vertebroplasty [abstract]. Radiology 1988;169P:372.

[46] Jensen ME, Evans AJ, Mathis JM, et al. Percutaneous polymethylmethacrylate vertebroplasty in the treatment of osteoporotic vertebral body compression fractures: technical aspects. AJNR Am J Neuroradiol 1997;18(10):1897–904.

[47] Padovani B, Kasriel O, Brunner P, et al. Pulmonary embolism caused by acrylic cement: a rare complication of percutaneous vertebroplasty. AJNR Am J Neuroradiol 1999;20(3): 375–7.

[48] McGraw JK, Heatwole EV, Strnad BT, et al. Predictive value of intraosseous venography before percutaneous vertebroplasty. J Vasc Interv Radiol 2002;13(2 Pt 1):149–53.

[49] Gaughen JR Jr, Jensen ME, Schweickert PA, et al. Relevance of antecedent venography in percutaneous vertebroplasty for the treatment of osteoporotic compression fractures. AJNR Am J Neuroradiol 2002;23(4):594–600.

[50] Vasconcelos C, Gailloud P, Beauchamp NJ, et al. Is percutaneous vertebroplasty without pretreatment venography safe? Evaluation of 205 consecutives procedures. AJNR Am J Neuroradiol 2002;23(6):913–7.

[51] Wehrli FW, Ford JC, Haddad JG. Osteoporosis: clinical assessment with quantitative MR imaging in diagnosis. Radiology 1995;196(3):631–41.

[52] Gangi A, Kastler BA, Dietemann JL. Percutaneous vertebroplasty guided by a combination of CT and fluoroscopy. AJNR Am J Neuroradiol 1994;15(1):83–6.

[53] Grados F, Depriester C, Cayrolle G, et al. Long-term observations of vertebral osteoporotic fractures treated by percutaneous vertebroplasty. Rheumatology (Oxford) 2000;39:1410–4.

[54] Zoarski GH, Snow P, Olan WJ, et al. Percutaneous vertebroplasty for osteoporotic compression fractures: quantitative prospective evaluation of long-term outcomes. J Vasc Interv Radiol 2002;13:139–48.

[55] Kaufmann TJ, Jensen ME, Schweickert PA, et al. Age of fracture and clinical outcomes of percutaneous vertebroplasty. AJNR Am J Neuroradiol 2001;22:1860–3.

[56] Deramond H, Depriester C, Galibert P, et al. Percutaneous vertebroplasty with polymethylmethacrylate: technique, indications, and results. Radiol Clin North Am 1998;36:533–46.

[57] Armsen N, Boszczyk B. Vertebro-/kyphoplasty history, development, results. Eur J Trauma 2005;5:433–41.

[58] Majd ME, Farley S, Holt RT. Preliminary outcomes and efficacy of the first 360 consecutive kyphoplasties for the treatment of painful osteoporotic vertebral compression fractures. Spine J 2005;5(3):244–55.

[59] Boszczyk BM, Bierschneider M, Schmid K, et al. Microsurgical interlaminary vertebro- and kyphoplasty for severe osteoporotic fractures. J Neurosurg 2004;100(1 Suppl):32–7.

[60] Lieberman IH, Dudeney S, Reinhardt MK, et al. Initial outcome and efficacy of "kyphoplasty" in the treatment of painful osteoporotic vertebral compression fractures. Spine 2001;26(14):1631–8.

[61] Crandall D, Slaughter D, Hankins PJ, et al. Acute versus chronic vertebral compression fractures treated with kyphoplasty: early results. Spine J 2004;4(4):418–24.

[62] Ledlie JT, Renfro M. Balloon kyphoplasty: One-year outcomes in vertebral body height restoration, chronic pain, and activity levels. J Neurosurg 2003;98(Suppl. 1):36–42.

[63] Belkoff SM, Mathis JM, Fenton DC, et al. An ex vivo biomechanical evaluation of an inflatable bone tamp used in the treatment of compression fracture. Spine 2001;26:151–6.

[64] Villarraga ML, Bellezza AJ, Harrigan TP, et al. The biomechanical effects of kyphoplasty on treated and adjacent nontreated vertebral bodies. J Spinal Disord Tech 2005;18:84–91.

[65] Uppin AA, Hirsch JA, Centenera LV, et al. Occurrence of new vertebral body fracture after percutaneous vertebroplasty in patients with osteoporosis. Radiology 2003;226:119–24.

[66] Polikeit A, Nolte LP, Ferguson SJ. The effect of cement augmentation on the load transfer in an osteoporotic functional spinal unit: finite element analysis. Spine 2003;28:991–6.

[67] Spivak J, Johnson M. Percutaneous treatment of vertebral body pathology. J Am Acad Orthop Surg 2005;13:6–17.

[68] Fribourg D, Tang C, Sra P, et al. Incidence of subsequent vertebral fracture after kyphoplasty. Spine 2004;29:2270–6.

[69] Berlemann U, Ferguson SJ, Nolte LP, et al. Adjacent vertebral failure after vertebroplasty: a biomechanical investigation. J Bone Joint Surg Br 2002;84:748–52.

[70] Cohen D, Feinberg P. Secondary osteoporotic compression fractures after kyphoplasty. Am Acad Orthop Surg. Meeting; February 5–9, 2003; New Orleans (LA): Poster no. P31.

[71] Lindsay R, Silverman SL, Cooper C, et al. Risk of new vertebral fracture in the year following a fracture. JAMA 2001;285:320–3.

[72] Kanis J, Johnell O, Oden A, et al. The risk and burden of vertebral fractures in Sweden. Osteoporos Int 2004;15:20–6.

[73] Harrop J, Prpa B, Reinhardt M, et al. Primary and secondary osteoporosis incidence of subsequent vertebral compression fractures after kyphoplasty. Spine 2004;29:2120–5.

ELSEVIER
SAUNDERS

Anesthesiology Clin
25 (2007) 929–937

ANESTHESIOLOGY
CLINICS

Index

Note: Page numbers of article titles are in **boldface** type.

A

Acetaminophen, 815

Adenosine receptors, topical analgesia with, 829

Adjuvant analgesics, **775–786**
    algorithms for difficult-to-treat pain syndromes, 782
    alpha-2-adrenergic agonists, 777–778
    anticonvulsants, 776–777
    antidepressants, 775–776
    bisphosphonates and calcitonin, 780–781
    cannabinoids, 779–780
    corticosteroids, 778
    GABA agonists, 781
    local anesthetics, 778–779
    neuroimmunomodulatory agents, 781
    NMDA antagonists, 779
    topical agents, 779

Adverse reactions, of NSAID treatment, 812–814
        blood pressure, renal, and renovascular, 813–814
        cardiovascular, 813
        gastrointestinal, 812–813
        hypersensitivity, 814
        nephropathy, 814
        pharmacokinetics and pharmacodynamics, 814

Alpha-2 adrenoreceptor agonists, topical analgesia with, 832

Alpha-2-adrenergic agents, as adjuvant analgesics, 777–778
    intrathecal analgesia with, 872–873

Analgesics, *see also* Pain management.
    adjuvant, **775–786**
    nonopioid, **809–823**
    opioids, **787–807, 809–823**
    topical, **825–834**

Ancillary tests, in diagnostic workup of patients with neuropathic pain, 702–703

Anesthetics, local, as adjuvant analgesics, 778–779
        as topical analgesics, gels and creams, 827–828
        intra-articular injections of, for postoperative pain, 857
        intrathecal analgesia with, 867–871
        trigger point injections with, 848–849

Anti-inflammatory agents, as topical analgesics, 826–827
        nitrates, 826–827
        NSAIDs, 826

Anti-inflammatory uses, of nonopioid analgesics, 812

Anticonvulsants, as adjuvant analgesics, 776–777

Antidepressants, as adjuvant analgesics, 775–776
        tricyclic, topical analgesia with, 829–831
            adenosine receptors, 829
            animal evidence for antinociceptive effect of, 830–831
            sodium channels, 829–830

Antipyretics, NSAIDs use as, 812

Aquatic therapy, in physical therapy for pain conditions, 736

Assessment, of pain, in behavioral medicine, 711–712

Augmentation, vertebral. *See* Kyphoplasty *and* Vertebroplasty.

Autonomic function testing, in diagnostic workup of patients with neuropathic pain, 704–705

B

Back pain, invasive and minimally invasive surgical techniques for, **899–911**

doi:10.1016/S1932-2275(07)00096-1   *anesthesiology.theclinics.com*

United States Postal Service

Statement of Ownership, Management, and Circulation
(All Periodicals Publications Except Requestor Publications)

1. Publication Title	2. Publication Number									3. Filing Date
Anesthesiology Clinics	0	0	0	-	2	7	7	7		9/14/07

4. Issue Frequency	5. Number of Issues Published Annually	6. Annual Subscription Price
Mar, Jun, Sep, Dec	4	$202.00

7. Complete Mailing Address of Known Office of Publication (Not printer) (Street, city, county, state, and ZIP+4)

Elsevier Inc.
360 Park Avenue South
New York, NY 10010-1710

Contact Person
Stephen Bushing

Telephone (Include area code)
215-239-3688

8. Complete Mailing Address of Headquarters or General Business Office of Publisher (Not printer)

Elsevier Inc. 360 Park Avenue South, New York, NY 10010-1710

9. Full Names and Complete Mailing Addresses of Publisher, Editor, and Managing Editor (Do not leave blank)

Publisher (Name and complete mailing address)

John Schrefer, Elsevier, Inc., 1600 John F. Kennedy Blvd. Suite 1800, Philadelphia, PA 19103-2899

Editor (Name and complete mailing address)

Rachel Glover, Elsevier, Inc., 1600 John F. Kennedy Blvd. Suite 1800, Philadelphia, PA 19103-2899

Managing Editor (Name and complete mailing address)

Catherine Bewick, Elsevier, Inc., 1600 John F. Kennedy Blvd. Suite 1800, Philadelphia, PA 19103-2899

10. Owner (Do not leave blank. If the publication is owned by a corporation, give the name and address of the corporation immediately followed by the names and addresses of all stockholders owning or holding 1 percent or more of the total amount of stock. If not owned by a corporation, give the names and addresses of the individual owners. If owned by a partnership or other unincorporated firm, give its name and address as well as those of each individual owner. If the publication is published by a nonprofit organization, give its name and address.)

Full Name	Complete Mailing Address
Wholly owned subsidiary of	4520 East-West Highway
Reed/Elsevier, US holdings	Bethesda, MD 20814

11. Known Bondholders, Mortgagees, and Other Security Holders Owning or Holding 1 Percent or More of Total Amount of Bonds, Mortgages, or Other Securities. If none, check box ☑ None

Full Name	Complete Mailing Address
N/A	

12. Tax Status (For completion by nonprofit organizations authorized to mail at nonprofit rates) (Check one)
The purpose, function, and nonprofit status of this organization and the exempt status for federal income tax purposes:
☐ Has Not Changed During Preceding 12 Months
☐ Has Changed During Preceding 12 Months (Publisher must submit explanation of change with this statement)

13. Publication Title		14. Issue Date for Circulation Data Below	
Anesthesiology Clinics		June 2007	

15. Extent and Nature of Circulation		Average No. Copies Each Issue During Preceding 12 Months	No. Copies of Single Issue Published Nearest to Filing Date
a. Total Number of Copies (Net press run)		2200	2000
b. Paid Circulation (By Mail and Outside the Mail)	(1) Mailed Outside-County Paid Subscriptions Stated on PS Form 3541. (Include paid distribution above nominal rate, advertiser's proof copies, and exchange copies)	865	802
	(2) Mailed In-County Paid Subscriptions Stated on PS Form 3541 (Include paid distribution above nominal rate, advertiser's proof copies, and exchange copies)		
	(3) Paid Distribution Outside the Mails Including Sales Through Dealers and Carriers, Street Vendors, Counter Sales, and Other Paid Distribution Outside USPS®	593	592
	(4) Paid Distribution by Other Classes Mailed Through the USPS (e.g. First-Class Mail®)		
c. Total Paid Distribution (Sum of 15b (1), (2), (3), and (4))	▶	1458	1394
d. Free or Nominal Rate Distribution (By Mail and Outside the Mail)	(1) Free or Nominal Rate Outside-County Copies Included on PS Form 3541	108	111
	(2) Free or Nominal Rate In-County Copies Included on PS Form 3541		
	(3) Free or Nominal Rate Copies Mailed at Other Classes Mailed Through the USPS (e.g. First-Class Mail)		
	(4) Free or Nominal Rate Distribution Outside the Mail (Carriers or other means)		
e. Total Free or Nominal Rate Distribution (Sum of 15d (1), (2), (3) and (4))	▶	108	111
f. Total Distribution (Sum of 15c and 15e)	▶	1566	1505
g. Copies not Distributed (See instructions to publishers #4 (page #3))	▶	634	495
h. Total (Sum of 15f and g)	▶	2200	2000
i. Percent Paid (15c divided by 15f times 100)		93.10%	92.62%

16. Publication of Statement of Ownership

☑ If the publication is a general publication, publication of this statement is required. Will be printed in the December 2007 issue of this publication. ☐ Publication not required.

17. Signature and Title of Editor, Publisher, Business Manager, or Owner	Date
[signature] Jesse Fauver — Executive Director of Subscription Services	September 14, 2007

I certify that all information furnished on this form is true and complete. I understand that anyone who furnishes false or misleading information on this form or who omits material or information requested on the form may be subject to criminal sanctions (including fines and imprisonment) and/or civil sanctions (including civil penalties).

PS Form 3526, September 2006 (Page 1 of 3 (Instructions Page 3)) PSN 7530-01-000-9931 PRIVACY NOTICE: See our Privacy policy in www.usps.com

PS Form 3526, September 2006 (Page 2 of 3)

Moving?

Make sure your subscription moves with you!

To notify us of your new address, find your **Clinics Account Number** (located on your mailing label above your name), and contact customer service at:

E-mail: elspcs@elsevier.com

800-654-2452 (subscribers in the U.S. & Canada)
407-345-4000 (subscribers outside of the U.S. & Canada)

Fax number: 407-363-9661

Elsevier Periodicals Customer Service
6277 Sea Harbor Drive
Orlando, FL 32887-4800

*To ensure uninterrupted delivery of your subscription, please notify us at least 4 weeks in advance of move.

ELSEVIER